A Critical History of Psychotherapy, Volume 1

This unique book offers a comprehensive overview of the history of psychotherapy. The first of two volumes, it traces the roots of psychotherapy in ancient times, through the influence of Freud and Jung up to the events following World War II.

The book shows how the history of psychotherapy has evolved over time through different branches and examines the offshoots as they develop. Each part of the book represents a significant period of time or a decade of the 20th century and provides a detailed overview of all significant movements within the history of psychology. The book also shows connections with history and contextualizes each therapeutic paradigm so it can be better understood in a broader social context.

The book is the first of its kind to show the parallel evolution of different theories in psychotherapy. It will be essential reading for researchers and students in the fields of clinical psychology, psychotherapy, psychiatry, the history of medicine and psychology.

Renato Foschi is Professor of History of Psychology and History of Science at the Sapienza University of Rome, Italy.

Marco Innamorati is Professor of Dynamic and Developmental Psychology and History and Philosophy of Scientific Concepts at the University of Rome "Tor Vergata", Italy.

A Critical History of Psychotherapy, Volume I

From Ancient Origins to the Mid-20th Century

By Renato Foschi and Marco Innamorati

Routledge
Taylor & Francis Group

LONDON AND NEW YORK

First published in English 2023
by Routledge
4 Park Square, Milton Park, Abingdon, Oxon OX14 4RN

and by Routledge
605 Third Avenue, New York, NY 10158

Routledge is an imprint of the Taylor & Francis Group, an informa business

Published in Italian by Raffaello Cortina, Milano, 2020

British Library Cataloguing-in-Publication Data
A catalogue record for this book is available from the British Library

ISBN: 9781032169408 (hbk)
ISBN: 9781032172378 (pbk)
ISBN: 9781003252405 (ebk)

DOI: 10.4324/9781003252405

Typeset in Bembo
by Apex CoVantage, LLC

Contents

Editorial note for volume I

This is the first of two volumes that together make up a revised and edited translation of Foschi, R. and Innamorati, M. (2020). *Storia Critica della Psicoterapia*, Raffaello Cortina Editore, Milano.

This work intends to be above all a history of "Western psychotherapy" that critically discusses the way in which "traditionally" a movement composed of technicians and scholars who emphasized the treatment of mental pathologies developed, through means "à visée scientifique" that were not physical or chemical but behavioral and based on communication. Because of the monopoly on physical or chemical therapies, Western medicine became the first domain from which psychotherapy of psychopathologies emancipated itself. However, as we will see, discussing psychotherapy implies a broader disciplinary and even transdisciplinary horizon. Many of the scholars described were in fact not doctors, and others emancipated themselves from their medical identity to deal with psychotherapy. Therefore, we do not agree with a radical constructivism that considers psychotherapy a domain so full of aporias and ambiguities, a mythical construction of self-celebration of Western psychotherapists, that it is impossible to historicize. Although ours can be considered an attitude of old-fashioned historians, we believe it is more useful to use classical distinctions between a psychological and a neurological domain, but also between a magical and a sociological domain in order to "critically" illuminate the path that led Freud to what is now considered psychotherapy. Psychoanalysis is treated by us as a psychotherapy. Actually, most other psychotherapies either developed from psychoanalysis or used it as a point of reference, even if often a negative one. However, if we saw psychotherapy with the eyes of an orthodox psychoanalyst, but not of Freud himself, we could even exclude psychoanalysis from the history of psychotherapy! In fact, orthodox psychoanalysts consider psychoanalysis as a domain so different from psychotherapy that it should not be subjected to the laws regulating the professional practice of psychotherapy. In the same way, according to other categories we could reduce psychoanalysis to a myth with little value for the history of psychotherapy, but also for the history of psychology itself. Psychotherapy then would still be a patchwork full of different things from each other: Western, Eastern, esoteric, magical, initiatory notions, and so on. In all epistemological positions there is a grain of truth, but this grain of truth considered in an absolute way does not help to critically understand the history of Western psychotherapy because, willingly or unwillingly, psychoanalysis has had a central role in the history of psychological techniques for the treatment of psychopathologies. Psychoanalysis has also played a central role in the history of Western ideas and culture. Therefore, this work intends to present a brief excursus into the more distant past of psychopathology therapies, but then especially the history of psychotherapy from the late 18th century to the 2000s. The Italian edition published by Raffaello Cortina has been updated with some changes and additions. While the first volume ends with World War II, the second volume accompanies the reader from the 1950s to the third millennium. Well aware of being susceptible to criticism of various kinds, we have accepted the challenge of a history of psychotherapy that is neither merely an abstract critical exercise nor a mere celebration of specific professional techniques.

The authors discussed the contents of this volume in depth and appear on the cover in alphabetical order. Specifically, Renato Foschi dealt mainly with external history, the history of science, the 19th-century period, behavior therapies, early cognitivism, family and community therapy, hypnotherapy, Gestalt theory and therapy, phenomenological therapies, relationships between education and therapy, relationships between religion and psychotherapy, sex therapies, attachment and psychotherapy, the relationship between psychiatry and psychotherapy, and "crazy" therapies. Marco Innamorati dealt mainly with internal history, ancient philosophy and medicine, the relationship between science and philosophy, psychoanalysis, individual psychology, analytical psychology, psychodynamic psychotherapies, cognitive psychotherapies, Daseinsanalyse, psychodrama, group psychotherapy, research, and psychotherapy. Both have always tried to hybridize their point of view, each contributing to the work of the other. This is, therefore, a book in which responsibilities are fully shared.

Thanks are due to the colleagues and friends with whom the topics have been discussed over the years: Giuseppe Allegri, Mario Ambrogi, Mauro Antonelli, Saulo de Freitas Araujo, Antonello Armando, Bernd Bocian, Claudio Buccolini, James H. Capshew, Vincenzo Caretti, Jacqueline Carroy, Elisabetta Cicciola, Guido Cimino, Jean-Christophe Coffin, Daniele Cozzoli, Alejandro Dagfal, Nino Dazzi, Alessandra De Coro, Giancarlo Dimaggio, Paolo Fabozzi, Cristiana Facchinetti, Aude Fauvel, John Foot, Pier Francesco Galli, Nuccio Gennaro, Christopher D. Green, Patrizia Guarnieri, Horst Gundlach, Ben Harris, Suzanne Hollman, Costanza Jesurum, Ulrich Koch, Mauro La Forgia, Chiara Latini, Marco Lauriola, Martin Liebscher, Vittorio Lingiardi, Giovanni Pietro Lombardo, Sarah Marks, Pompeo Martelli, Jelena Martinovic, Luciano Mecacci, David Meghnagi, Paolo Migone, Alfonso Montuori, Annette Mülberger, Annick Ohayon, Francesca Ortu, Cecilia Panti, Lorenzo Perilli, Wade Pickren, Regine Plas, Tommaso Priviero, David K. Robinson, Rachel Rosner,

Giovanni Maria Ruggiero, Mariano Ruperthuz Honorato, Massimo Saccà, Diego Sarracino, Sonu Shamdasani, Chiara Simonelli, Maria Sinatra, Michael M. Sokal, Akihito Suzuki, Renata Tambelli, Ruggero Taradel, Marco Tarantino, Nadine Weidman, Robert H. Wozniak, and Phil Zimbardo. To all of them go our apologies, if we were not able to use all their suggestions correctly.

Mental health care from antiquity to modern times

The history and the histories of psychotherapy

The idea for this book arose primarily from the observation that, despite the importance of the topic, there are only a few books available specifically devoted to the history of psychotherapy. In contrast, many volumes have been devoted to the history of clinical psychology, psychiatry, and psychoanalysis. The latter are generally considered independent scientific disciplines, defined by their own methods and paradigms (in the sense of Kuhn, 1962), but psychotherapy seems to have a more problematic identity, the term sometimes being used as a synonym for the other three and sometimes for their applied field (Walker, 1957). Sometimes it is even used as an element of distinction between the other disciplines, in that, for example, many analysts have long contrasted their practice with "simple" psychotherapy.

In this book, psychotherapy will be defined as a cure for the psyche "by the psyche" or, even better, as a cure "through psychological interaction" (Trevi & Innamorati, 2000, pp. 126–127) or (mainly) psychological means, and so it can be understood that its overlap with the disciplines mentioned here is only partial. As such, it will also be possible to make only partial use of the historiographic categories of medicine and psychology, transcending the boundaries of both.

Our definition is necessarily provisional and may not be recognized as sound by all psychotherapists (and historians). However, it has, first, the advantage of excluding forms of psychological help that use nonpsychological means (e.g., assistive technology) and belong to the domain of clinical psychology but not to psychotherapy. Second, it includes forms of psychotherapy that are not defined as such by those who practice them: in particular, psychoanalysis. Many psychoanalysts have considered psychoanalysis and psychotherapy two completely distinct fields (where the latter is to be despised or at least considered inferior): still today this is valid at least for Lacanian psychoanalysts. Some behaviorist psychotherapists may not recognize epistemically sound either the term "psyche" or expressions such as "psychological interaction" or "psychological means": we recognize that in this case we apply an interpretation. All

DOI: 10.4324/9781003252405-1

this being said, we employ the proposed definition in the book because (1) we consider it necessary to define the field of research and (2) deflationary definitions may be even less precise. In fact, one cannot define psychotherapy simply as what psychotherapists have historically defined: for all that has been said, even psychoanalysis would risk being excluded.

It should also be added that the histories of disciplines related to psychotherapy have often been flattened by a collecting, celebratory, and often presentist vision, tending to describe only the events of the great personalities (the so-called founders) and the aspects of their scientific paths that, in the test of time, have met with success. These are often hagiographies filled with personal episodes. In the most useful cases, the history of psy-sciences refers to a periodization made up of ruptures, recompositions, changes, and innovations, like any other natural science. Many texts follow canons heavily conditioned by U.S. historiography, narratives that are often internal to the domains of psychiatry or, in a minority, clinical psychology (see, e.g., Alexander & Selesnick, 1966; Cushman, 1995; Ehrenwald, 1976; Freedheim et al., 1992; Harrington, 2019; Jackson, 1999; Millon, 2004; Norcross et al., 2011; Reisman, 1991; Zilboorg & Henry, 1941). The other stories, those of patients, failures, interdisciplinary contexts, cultures, associations, and institutions, are relatively neglected.

It is only in recent years that some historians have begun to describe the different scientific disciplines as a process of co-construction that includes all the cultural expressions that have conditioned them in different historical periods, taking into account the political and social context in which their actors were located. In the case of psychotherapy, the actors include psychologists, neurologists, and psychiatrists, but also patients, ideas, and institutions. A picture thus emerged that was characterized not only by linear periods of quiet, crises, and specific ruptures that led to paradigm shifts but also by more "subtle, twisted, and surprising" (Carroy, 1991, p. 30) vicissitudes. Such vicissitudes turn out to be tied to concepts that appear, disappear, and often reappear under other names. They are contextually constructed and de-constructed and they challenge domains that are not strictly concerned with psychology alone, but also the mores and balances on which contemporary society is founded. Examples of this complex history, which has been termed *croisée*, have been published primarily in France – the same nation in which modern psychotherapy emerged in the late 18th and 19th centuries (Carroy, 1991, 1993; Danziger, 1990; Hacking, 1995).

There have indeed been some attempts to reconstruct the history of the "psy" sciences, and especially of psychoanalysis, in complex terms, but most often, however, with the aim of pointing out the dark and collusive points of the conflicts and relationships between the founders (the therapists) and the patients (e.g., the emblematic cases of Sabina Spielrein and Marilyn Monroe; see Carotenuto, 1982; Mecacci, 2000). These attempts were certainly useful in inaugurating a history of psychotherapy that avoided pure celebration and restored humanity to an empirical domain that included, at the same time, art-craft, creation, and science.

Like all disciplines, psychotherapy has been conceived in multiple ways and in different cultures and has used different epistemological perspectives. Central and dominant cultures and peripheral and dominated cultures produced sciences that were integrated in diversity. Local knowledge was created in the various places of knowledge production, through a process of indigenization and hybridization, and also dynamically influenced the "center," or, conversely, generated no major changes (see Danziger, 2006; Pickren, 2009). The history of psychotherapy has thus also been the expression of central scientists and peripheral scientists. Patients, cultures, ideas, politics, institutions, exemplary histories, personal relationships, and major figures make up the fabric of our narrative. The task of the contemporary scholar is thus to move cautiously in a context that is, by nature, complex and interconnected.

Over the course of the last few years, international journals on the history of psychology and the human sciences have devoted articles and monographic issues to the history of psychotherapy (*History of Psychology, History of the Human Sciences, European Journal of Psychotherapy & Counseling*), and the category of the Cold War has become central to characterizing the impetuous development of psychotherapy in the 20th century (Herzog, 2017; Innamorati, 2017b). We see, on the one hand, the utilization of Foucauldian interpretations[1] and, on the other hand, a focus on micro-historical issues. Precisely because of its nature, however, even such a hermeneutic stance cannot take into account the different disciplinary levels (professional, medical, psychical, psychiatric, psychosomatic) that are interwoven into the history of psychotherapy. The historiographical point of view risks failing to meaningfully represent the major themes that characterize psychotherapy because it is actually located exclusively on a disciplinary history of psychiatry, medicine, and psychosomatics, rather than contextualized on the specificity of the psychological sciences (see Marks, 2017; Rosner, 2018). Such historiography has thus led to a fragmentation of the history of psychotherapy and has highlighted above all the potential negative aspects related to its diffusion, such as the idea that it was a technique at the service of political and cultural conflicts during the Cold War, a specific manipulative technique of consumerism, or, as identified in the most original psychotherapies (expressive, religious, meditative, oriental), a possible positive alternative to the contradictions of traditional psychotherapy enslaved to capitalism. The emphasis has recently been placed on the fact that psychotherapy is fundamentally a Western and Anglo-American phenomenon, while denying the importance of different cultures, such as those of Latin countries.[2] For example, the history of psychoanalysis in France has peculiarities (Ohayon, 1999; Roudinesco, 1982, 1986) that are very difficult to describe accurately in a general history of psychotherapy; and the history of psychoanalysis in Argentina has, in turn, peculiarities that could not be understood without taking French history into account (Dagfal, 2018). Instead, in the difficult enterprise of tracing a history of psychotherapy, it seems useful to understand how traditional and *à visée scientifique* theories and techniques have hybridized in different cultural contexts, and especially in industrialized countries (Pols, 2018; Shamdasani, 2018).

A complex reading of the history of psychotherapy brings this field closer to transdisciplinarity. In fact, we are faced with the solution of problems related to psychopathology through techniques that do not refer to a single discipline, but are meta-paradigmatic, and result from a hybridization not only of psychology and clinical psychiatry but which is constantly influenced by history, politics, and cultural anthropology – all those practices that investigate the production of meaning such as philosophy, linguistics, or art (Montuori, 2005).

From this point of view, it seems problematic to flatten the history of psychotherapy into the history of psychiatry and to describe it without taking into account the intertwining relationships, the dialectics, and the conflicts between psychiatry and psychology. The relationship between philosophy and psychotherapy is also significant: one can go so far as to define contemporary psychotherapies as ontologies aimed at changing the nature of patients (Shamdasani, 2017). Our books therefore aims to show how psychotherapy, especially in the 20th century, has been a field that developed more or less formalized techniques, almost always starting from a specific position with respect to psychoanalysis.[3] On the one hand, in fact, psychoanalysis has been a starting point from which to diverge (as in the case of Adler's individual psychology); or it has been a reference point with which to polemicize (as in the case of cognitive-behavioral psychotherapies).

History of psychotherapy is intertwined, on various levels, with that of philosophy and medicine, and then psychology, in the context of the encounters and clashes between these disciplines, without forgetting the subtle influences that other fields such as anthropology, classical studies, or the history of religions have had on the development of psychotherapy.

Our books wants, therefore, to contribute to the process of making psychotherapy autonomous from the domains of origin, by outlining a history that, while risking being interminable, attempts to provide new generations of "psy" with a knowledge base to start from.

A therapeutic patchwork

As is well known, Alexandre Koyré (1892–1964) introduced the fundamental historiographic categories of the *world of more-or-less* and the *universe of precision* in the history of the production of scientific knowledge. Science would pass through eras that led to a greater precision of concepts, measures, methodologies, and techniques (Koyré, 1948). This specific interpretation can be of great use in understanding the process of refinement, which led, from antiquity to the modern era, to the current psychotherapy techniques. The various notions were defined by a name, only to be re-contextualized, sometimes with different terms, sometimes in a strictly interconnected or completely disconnected way (consciousness, subconscious/unconscious, normality-pathology, mind-body, illness-healing, efficacy-inefficacy, etc.).[4] This nonlinear process has led to the coexistence of old and new, empirically verified and never verified, more and less homogeneous approaches.

The term "psychotherapy" has an as-yet unspecified genesis. In 1853, Walter Cooper Dendy (1794–1871) used the term "psychotherapeia" in his pamphlet on *Psyché; a Discourse on the Birth and Pilgrimage of Thought*, and Daniel Hack Tuke (1827–1895), the descendant of a generation of philanthropists who were very active in caring for the mentally ill), used the term "psycho-therapeutics" in his psychosomatic treatise *Illustrations of the Influence of the Mind upon the Body in Health and Disease Designed to Elucidate the Action of the Imagination* (1872); both physicians used the term in a highly medicalized, psychiatric context. In 1891, Hippolyte Bernheim (1840–1919), in his *Hypnotisme, Suggestion, Psychothérapie*, used the term with a meaning related to psychological intervention that became autonomous from the medical and hypnotic meaning, playing on the importance of the suggestive relationship for therapeutic purposes. Psychology probably entered the history of medical therapy with all its potential and its complexities (Carroy, 2000; Shamdasani, 2005, 2017).

The practices of the mind, on the other hand, are lost in the past, and finding a specific starting point for the history of psychotherapy is very unlikely. Human beings have always sought techniques to cope with disorders of the soul and reason, correlating them with the body, and these techniques were conditioned by the religious and cultural beliefs of the places in which they developed.

Greco-Roman mythology represented a narrative universe from which to draw prototypical models of normal and/or pathological behavior, as if the myth were *tout court* a projection outside the mind. Our history can therefore refer to ancient occidental medicine, and the history of catharsis and exorcism as the hypothetical beginning of "prescientific" psychotherapy.[5]

In order to fully understand the origins of what today is called psychotherapy, in fact, it may be necessary to go back to the moment in which human beings developed an awareness of the problem of psychological suffering and attempted in some way to understand its origin and to cure it, or at least to alleviate it.

The expression "psychological suffering" is imprecise, provisional, and only intended to offer an intuitive starting point since it is impossible, in many cases, to distinguish between, for example, physical and psychological suffering. The actual concept of the psyche (from which the adjective "psychological" derives) today involves very different definitions. Behaviorist psychology has basically considered it irrelevant, and "eliminative materialism" (e.g., Churchland, 1989) claims it is a false concept, a simple illusion, and a myth. The history of the meaning of psyche/psychological, moreover, is even more complex and articulated, as is that of the terms related to psyche, involving such things as the mind, spirit, and soul. It will be understood, however, that in order to define the field of psychological suffering, it is appropriate to refer to a broader concept than that of madness. In the common imagination madness defines a completely invalidating illness, for the purposes of an adequate personal and relational life. The history of the treatment of madness, moreover, coincides with the history of psychiatry rather than with the history of clinical psychology and psychotherapy: it is identified with the methods of treatment that today can be traced back to a medical or organicist approach, which, as we have said, only partially overlaps with psychotherapy. Madness, in any case, has not always been thought of as purely psychological suffering, as in several archaic cultures a mad person was considered endowed by the gods with special faculties, such as the ability to predict the future (Ellenberger, 1970).[6]

The field of psychotherapy, however, also takes into account milder modes of psychological distress and in some cases involves perfecting an already satisfactory experience that, however, it would like to improve. This attitude is related to the different possible meanings of *normality* at which psychotherapy can aim.[7] It should be also considered that there is no "absolute normality" because it is impossible to evaluate a condition as normal, regardless of the social and historical conditions in which a person can be evaluated. The evolution of attempts to cure or alleviate psychological suffering could therefore rightly be considered useful in understanding the very essence of psychotherapy.

Since psychological suffering has been perceived as a problem, there are several categories of actors who have also appeared in history, whose activities it is worth recalling: (1) technicians deputed to treat the suffering; (2) jurists devoted to protecting those who suffer, or rather to limit their actions; (3) artists aimed at depicting their conduct dramatically; and (4) philosophers interested in understanding the nature of suffering (Gourevitch, 1994). In the course of time, technicians have assumed different identities, according to the prevailing approach to psychological suffering: the magical-religious approach, the organic approach, or the psychological approach (Alexander & Selesnick, 1966). Originally, after all, the distinction between psychical and physical suffering must have been very vague, and the admixture of magic, religion, and medicine was even greater at the time (Alexander & Selesnick, 1966; Zilboorg & Henry, 1941).

The origin of some paradigmatic ideas, however, should also be considered among the historical roots of contemporary psychotherapy: we refer in particular to the ideas of ego, unconscious, continuity between the normal and pathological, and the clinical. We will try to give account of this origin, but it will be limited, for obvious reasons of space, to a systematic handling.[8] In this context, it would have been appropriate to clarify how the idea of "education" developed, since educational and psycho-educational interventions are part of the techniques applied by contemporary psychotherapy, but the task would have been either too broad or too superficial. The next paragraphs will therefore sketch the prehistory of psychotherapy, taking into account the premises described earlier.

Ancient medicine, suffering, and cure

According to a widely accepted classification, ancient interpretations of illness as such can be divided into three groups: (1) the loss of the soul or its escape from the body of the sufferer; (2) the magical penetration of an object into the body; and (3) the possession by evil spirits (Clements, 1932). The earliest modes of cure perhaps involved magical–religious rituals aimed at freeing the sufferer from the entity responsible for their condition, or at recovering the lost soul (Ellenberger, 1970). These rituals were not, however, the first step.

> Before humanity began to presume that the initiated, the priests or the saints, could cast out the devil, it was considered a matter of course that the mentally sick were in some way too sacred and good or too powerful for anyone to venture to reduce them to the unblessed state of normality. In other words, from the very outset it was taken for granted that medicine had no power, even had no right, over the mentally sick.
>
> (Zilboorg & Henry, 1941, p. 18)

There is evidence of the practice of rituals aimed at healing in the Meso-potamia of 2100 BC. The Babylonians sought to identify possessing demons through oracular and astrological methods and prayed to different deities to free the sick person, depending on which demon was believed to have been identi-fied (Ehrenwald, 1956). Drilled skulls have been found in prehistoric times, for example in South America, suggesting the practice of freeing the body of the possessed by creating an exit for the demon possessor (Mora, 1985). Originally, the distinction between psychical and physical suffering must have been very approximate: although the presence of the first lay physicians (*Azu*) is attested in Babylon, they used both primitive medicines and magical practices (Alexan-der & Selesnick, 1966).

Human suffering caused by supernatural entities was sometimes interpreted as blameless, sometimes as a possible violation of shared norms, especially if it involved taboos or cultic obligations. The use of amulets and talismans could then, according to common belief, prevent or pacify the intervention of spirits and demons (Brems et al., 1991).

Egyptian papyri dating back to 1550 BC testify to a certain distinction between diseases which were treatable by physical means and those which had a magical–spiritual origin. Spells were suggested as a remedy for the latter. On the other hand, the same sources describe the brain as the seat of mental functions for the first time (Castiglioni, 1927). Certainly, both Egyptian and Babylonian medicine influenced the Jewish culture, which testifies, from the beginning, to the development of a certain psychological wisdom. In addition to extensively describing different psychopathological pictures (Saul's psychotic depression, Nebuchadnezzar's lycanthropy – his belief to be a wolf – etc.), the Hebrews applied suggestion to enable the patient to speak freely about their discomforts and proposed distraction and a change of habits as a relief for psychological suffering (Gold, 1957). In general, health and illness, like wealth and poverty, were considered rewards or punishments given by God as a result of human conduct. According to the Bible, if psychological or even physical suffering (in the case of diseases such as asthma) was considered of demonic origin, then the presence of the demon was caused by a divine initiative. It was always up to God to free of the demon. The *Talmud* introduced a lesser belief in the supernatural origin of physical and psychological illnesses, however, and the presence of a para-hospital institution dedicated only to psychological sufferers is attested in Jerusalem in 490 BC (Whitwell, 1936).

Archaic and classical Greece

The basic grammar of ancient Greek thought and the history of what we today call psychotherapy are certainly deeply related. An obvious preliminary observation concerns the etymology of the word "psychotherapy" itself, which, although much later than the classical Greek, derives from *psychē* and *therapeía*, terms whose simplest translations (although not unique) are respectively "soul" and "care." *Therapeía*, however, was originally understood as "care of the body" (the alternative meaning is "service"), and the Greek *psychē* was initially described very differently from both the Christian tradition of the word "soul" and the more secular ways of describing the "psyche" or the "mind":

> The psyche of Homeric belief does not, as might have been supposed, represent what we are accustomed to call "spirit" as opposed to "body." All the faculties of the human "spirit" in the widest sense – for which the poet has a large and varied vocabulary – are indeed only active and only possible so long as a man is still alive. When death comes, the complete personality is no longer in existence. The body, that is the corpse, now becomes mere "senseless earth" and falls to pieces, while the psyche remains untouched. But the latter is by no means the refuge of the "spirit" and its faculties, any more than the corpse is.
>
> (Rohde, 1925/1897, p. 5)

The term *psychē* is onomatopoeic, designating the sound that human beings make when they breathe their last breath. In archaic Greece, "the only recorded function of the psyche in relation to the living man is to leave him" (Dodds, 1925, p. 16). In the Homeric poems, thinking is instead defined as a "speaking," whose seat is sometimes located in the heart, but more often in the *phrēn* (or *phrénes*), a term traditionally understood as *prechords* or *diaphragm*, while "deep reflection is the conversation of one's self with one's *thymós* or of one's *thymós* with one's self" (Onians, 1954, p. 13). On the other hand, it has been noted that even in Homer there are examples of the therapeutic use of speech, and not only in a magical sense: the power to help sick people with calming speeches is in some cases considered part of the therapeutic process used by Nestor and Patroclus with their "patients" (Laín Entralgo, 1958, pp. 28–31).

Only with the emergence of philosophy was human nature considered. If the origin of philosophy is certainly fundamental to understanding the beginnings of psychology (and consequently of psychotherapy), offering an objective picture is almost impossible: there are only scattered fragments and indirect testimonies of the first so-called philosophers, and they have led scholars to different and disparate interpretations. Perhaps a tradition of thought, which some identify with Orphism, began to identify the existence of a soul that was independent from the body and that could even detach itself from the body during life. Probably some of the earliest Greek philosophers, such as Empedocles (5th century BC) and Pythagoras (6th century BC), were carriers of the idea that the soul preexisted the body and survived it. However, it was Socrates (470 or 469–399 BC), or at least the character of Socrates that appears in Plato's (428 or 427–348 or 347 BC) more youthful *Dialogues*,[9] who clearly articulated this doctrine. Its consequences run through a very significant part of Western thought (all influenced by Christianity, which inherited the soul/body dualism from the Platonic tradition). Another line of thought, no less fundamental in the West, can be traced back to Aristotle (384 or 383–322 BC), a pupil but not a follower of Plato. In the Aristotelian conception, the human being is a *synol*, a compound-synthesis, of which the body constitutes the matter and the soul the form. It is therefore not possible for the soul to separate itself from the body and survive it. The archetype of the monist conceptions of the subsequent Western thought is therefore Aristotle. Socrates is thus a sort of singular fulcrum for the history of ancient Greek philosophy: his teaching was only oral, but all thinkers who lived before him are globally defined as Presocratics, while Plato and Aristotle, perhaps the two most important philosophers in the history of the West, are called Major Socratics, and other later schools of practical philosophy referred in some way to the Socratic teaching.

In a view of the psyche such as the Presocratic view, mental disorder consisted only of exceedingly strange behavior (Zilboorg & Henry, 1941, p. 30). With the passage of time, the possibility of altering human conduct became the specific task of a *daímon*, or an *alaster*, a demon. The demonic world became, in a paradoxical secularization, more and more distant from the divine one, until the poet Theognides (5th to 6th century BC) called fear and hope "dangerous demons." The *daímon* began to take on different features over time and was also identified with evil itself by other ancient peoples: "Evil spirits are often no more than the evil itself conceived as substantial and equipped with willpower" (Frankfort et al., 1947/1977, p. 17). The *daímon* could be identified with fate, as in the CXIV fragment of the pre-Socratic Heraclitus (6th to 5th century BC) *ēthos anthrōpō daimōn* (man's character is his fate; Kahn, 1979, pp. 80–81). It could also be identified with fortune (although *daímon* can form an endyad with fortune, as occurs in texts by 5th- to 4th-century orators such as Demosthenes and Lysias, who use expressions such as *daímon kaí týchē*; Dodds, 1925,

p. 41). He could become, finally, "a sort of lofty spirit-guide, or Freudian Super-ego" (Dodds, 1925, p. 42). Socrates spoke of his demon as an entity that urged him to work in the direction of goodness and justice. In the Platonic *Timaeus*, on the other hand, *daímon* is identified as the human element that represents pure rationality. Perhaps Empedocles even identified *daímon* and *psychē*: "The occult self which persisted through successive incarnations he called, not *psyche*, but *daemon*" (Dodds, 1925, p. 153). Such an articulated and polyphonic view of the human mind and its natural and supernatural influences also led philosophy to deal with mental health. Medicine dealt with it in parallel, as will be seen, especially thanks to another illustrious son of 5th-century Greece, Hippocrates (ca. 460–377 BC).

In this sense we can certainly say that Greek philosophical thought can be traced back to reflections concerning both the identification, classification, and prevention of psychological problems, and the treatment of the psyche. It has been argued, perhaps using a historical scheme a bit too univocal, that the Greek world between Homer and Plato saw a progressive transition in the use of words for therapeutic purposes from *prayer* to *incantation* and from the latter to *persuasion*, which is a real form of psychotherapy (Lain Entralgo, 1958). There is no doubt, however, that an important role in the history of the roots of psychology and psychotherapy can be attributed to Socrates and Plato, starting from the fact that it is the Socrates character of the *Charmides* (156e ff.) and of the *Lachetes* (185e) who identifies for the first time the need for a *therapeía psychēs* (therapy of the psyche), which has the same importance as a therapy of the physique. Indeed, it constitutes its foundation (the soul being instead unjustly neglected by doctors). It consists of "words of the right sort: by the use of such words is temperance engendered in our souls" (*Charmides*, 157a; Lamb, 1927, p. 21) and should be practiced by masters of the subject, who in turn have had excellent teachers (*Lachetes*, 156a-b). In all the *Dialogues* the human being was described as characterized by a condition of profound ignorance, of which they were not even aware: the oracle of Delphi had called Socrates the wisest of all the Greeks precisely because of his attitude toward reality, based on the principle "I know that I know nothing." In the *Apology of Socrates*, ignorance was explicitly defined as one of the two forms of madness (or – using the modern term – of psychopathology), the other being madness proper. Plato described Socrates as intent on revealing to his fellow Athenian citizens the need to change their existential beliefs by relying on two therapeutic tools: irony and maieutics (a term for the technique needed to help in childbirth). Thanks to irony it was possible to question prejudices. Maieutics, however, helped people to become aware of what they unconsciously already knew. To know, in fact, meant to remember. The myth of the cave in the *Republic* and the myths about *eros* in the *Symposium* illustrated how far human beings were from an ideal condition, and how much they had to correct themselves in order to aspire to a life worth living. Prevention, however, could only be ensured by a profound rethinking of the structure of society, which Plato described on several occasions in the *Republic*, the *Statesman*, and the *Laws*. For example, in order to prevent psychopathological conditions resulting from problematic family structures, Plato hoped in the *Republic* for a society in which no one would know the names of their parents, and all children would be brought up together on an equal footing.

As for proper madness, in the *Apology*, expounding (presumably) Socratic ideas, Plato distinguished between a divine madness, which is a gift and belongs to soothsayers and initiates, and a vulgar madness, the result of an illness. In the *Republic*, however, where Plato illustrated conceptions that were (Just as presumably) his own and not those of Socrates, the picture seemed to change. The conception of the soul was described in another well-known myth, that of the charioteer of the sun leading a chariot drawn by two winged horses, one of which tended to fly upward and the other downward. The first corresponded to the rational soul (which is immortal and survives the body); the second, to the irrational soul (mortal, bound to the body). Psychopathology could be traced back to the rational soul, if its action was too powerful for the body to which it was bound, or to the irrational soul, whose link with the body made it susceptible to an alteration of the humors of the body itself. Even clearer was the possibility of a negative influence of bodily humors (and the "vapors" from them) on mental health when Plato, in *Timaeus* (86b–89d), divided the soul into three parts (rational, irascible, and concupiscible), locating their presence in three parts of the body (brain, heart, and liver).

The theory of humors, however, was born long before Plato: perhaps even in ancient Egypt. Presumably developed on the basis of superficial observations made on bodily fluids, it was certainly reinforced by the pre-Socratic speculation on "opposites." Such a concept would later crystallize in the doctrine of the four elements of the universe: air, water, earth, fire. Alcmeon of Croton (6th century BC), traditionally considered the founder of Greek medicine, believed that health was the result of *isonomía* (i.e., the "democratic" balance) of opposites, and disease from the monarchy of one of them (Jones, 1923). However, the theory of humors assumed a long-lasting structure after Hippocrates, a contemporary of Plato (and cited by him in the *Dialogues*), or after the works that are attributed to Hippocrates.

Born in the island of Kos around 460 BC, Hippocrates was a pupil of Herodicus of Selimbria, the best-known doctor of the time, except for Alcmeon. But he was also a student, or at least a friend, of Democritus (between 470 and 457 BC – between 360 and 350 BC), who was the founder of atomic theory – that is, the idea that the whole cosmos was made up of indivisible material particles, called atoms. His materialistic vision influenced later Epicurus (341–270 BC).

The influence of Hippocrates on the history of medicine cannot be overestimated: "Except for the Bible, no document and no author from Antiquity commands the authority in the twenty-first century of Hippocrates of Cos and the Hippocratic Oath" (Nutton, 2004, p. 53). The prestige of Hippocrates induced his school to attribute to him even works that were certainly written after his death: consequently, the so-called *Corpus Hippocraticum* includes works written between the 5th and 3rd century BC, if not even later. Their content may even appear to have a unitary inspiration (Laín Entralgo, 1958), but identifying individual works that can be attributed with absolute certainty to Hippocrates seems to present insurmountable difficulties (Lloyd, 1991). The *Corpus Hippocraticum* is considered nothing less than the founding act of scientific medicine: its influence, direct or mediated by the work of the great Hippocratic Galen (ca. 130–200), is paramount. Hippocratic medicine was a technique, but also a general theory of man.

Therapy was no longer based on empirical attempts, or even on magical-religious rituals, it was related to a unitary conception. At the center of the Hippocratic vision of health and disease was the theory of humors. There were four humors in the human body: blood, phlegm, yellow bile, and black bile. Health derived from the right balance of the quantity of humors and the balance of the qualities that accompanied them (hot, cold, dry, wet). Each human being was distinguished, however, by the relative prevalence of one of the four humors in their body, the influence of which formed the temperament. The theory of the four temperaments, developed by the Hippocratic tradition, distinguished, respectively, the sanguine, the phlegmatic, the bilious, and the melancholic (*mélaina cholé* means precisely black bile), according to a terminology that has been used until recent times in scientific literature (e.g., in the construction of personality tests). The theory of humors, however, assumed that diseases were manifested mainly in their effects on individual parts of the body. The author of *De morbo sacro* believed that mental illnesses depended on the way the brain could be affected by humors. Since the brain is the only source of pleasures and joys, as well as sorrows and pains, the excess of heat or cold, dryness or moisture, in the same organ determined alterations in normal behavior such as insomnia, distraction, anxious states, and acts contrary to habits (*De morbo sacro*, XVII, 1–20). Psychopathology could be induced by excess bile or phlegm (*De morbo sacro*, XVIII, 1–2). A pseudo-Aristotelian work (*Problems*, XXX), which took its cue from Hippocratic notions, spread the idea that the intellectual's tendency to melancholy was related to the excessive accumulation of black bile due to a sedentary life. In the Hippocratic view, therefore, not only the diseases of the body but also psychological suffering had a physical origin. As such, they were treated with physical means, consisting of special dietary regimens and specific drugs. Melancholia, considered, as we have seen, the expression of an excess of black bile, had to be cured by the expulsion of this substance from the body.[10]

In spite of the fundamental value of the dialogue with the patient for anamnestic purposes, however, the verbal explanations of the doctor to the patient fulfilled, from the Hippocratic point of view, a more cognitive than therapeutic function (Laín Entralgo, 1958). The rejection of magical and purification rites led the Hippocratic school to the identification of human nature with the body. This attitude constituted both a great achievement and a great limitation, favoring the development of empirical medicine but conditioning, until very recent times, the development of modern psychotherapy (Laín Entralgo, 1958).

A fragment (Wellmann 92) of the Hippocratic physician Diocles of Charistos (375–295 BC) authorizes conjecture that he could believe in the curative effect of speech, even on a condition of physical pathology. This is insufficient to attribute to him a psychotherapeutic doctrine, however, and in any case it does not appear that such a doctrine would have subsequent influences. Instead, Diocles was considered by physicians of later generations, including Galen, to be a younger Hippocrates who specialized in theorizing about diet and exercise (Nutton, 2004).

Philosophy as existential practice: Cynicism, Stoicism, Epicureanism

Philosophers, starting from Socrates, tended to present themselves more and more not only as seekers of knowledge but also as masters of life and therapists of the soul. Plato, in the *Phaedon* (64a–70b), described philosophy as the only activity that could allow the best possible life, that is, the progressive liberation of the soul from the body. He also expressed on several occasions the thought that man should either philosophize or take leave of life (*Phaedon*, 64a; *Theetetus*, 176ab; *Gorgias*, 512a). Aristotle in turn devoted a specific work, the almost entirely lost *Protrecticus*, to illustrating how philosophy is necessary to a life worth living:

> The affirmation that among all men the philosopher is the one who pursues the highest happiness and noble joy is justified [by Aristotle] with the fact that only in the soul of the philosopher perfect harmony reigns. (. . .) He who devotes himself to philosophy, achieves the knowledge of the principles of nature, and discovers that order and regularity reign everywhere in nature. This knowledge also helps him to organize his personal existence.
>
> (Düring, 1966, p. 432)

The *Nicomachean Ethics* suggested, in turn, that the ideal life could only be pursued through the practice of knowledge and virtue, even though this was an extremely difficult path to follow:

> Well-being, we are told, must be activity in accordance with the virtue of the best part of us, which is reason. The activity which is well-being is theoretical. This is the best activity of which we are capable, since it is the exercise of the best in us on the best of all objects, those which are eternal and unchanging.
>
> (Ross, 1923/1995, p. 240)

It must be remembered that in Aristotle's works we find, in addition to philosophy, another area in which the power of speech can have therapeutic effects on human beings, namely theater, and in particular tragedy, "effecting, through pity and fear, the purification of such emotions" (*Poetics*, 1449b, 26–27: Kenny, 2013, p. 65).

The effect of purification or catharsis (*kátharsis*) on the spectator has been understood by several commentators literally, as purification from excessive humors in the Hippocratic sense (beginning even with Bernays, 1880). Whether it was a purification in the physical sense or rather in a more metaphorical sense (Laín Entralgo, 1958), this was the primary purpose of the tragic genre, and its value would have consisted for Aristotle "in its medicinal effect" (Ross, 1923, p. 242).

Three Greek philosophical schools can be considered as specifically addressed to the care of the existential human condition, through the adoption of a specific lifestyle, which could be accepted regardless of the social context (or individual economic possibilities). These are, in particular, Cynicism, Stoicism, and Epicureanism.

Cynicism was born, it seems, from the teachings of Antisthenes (ca. 445–365 BC), who in turn was a disciple of Socrates, and had a certain success in both classical and Hellenistic Greece, and in both republican and imperial Rome. It was also established as a popular philosophy, with followers even among the poorer classes. The best-known exponent of the movement was presumably Diogenes of Sinope (ca. 412–321 BC), who handed down (in addition to the habit of living in a barrel) provocations, such as walking around with a lantern in broad daylight shouting "I seek the man!" There are few, fragmentary, and late testimonies of ancient Cynicism. It seems certain, anyway, that the Cynics set human happiness as their goal, proposing bodily asceticism as a means to achieve it, practiced through the *pónoi*. These were exercises of abstinence and exposure to extreme privations, which had the purpose of letting people effortlessly endure poverty, in case of need. Happiness would then be achieved through the disregard of pleasure, which would make the individual able to overcome even the most adverse circumstances (Goulet-Cazé, 2000).[11]

It seems that the work of Antisthenes exerted a profound, though sometimes underestimated, influence on Stoicism (Caizzi, 2000). Stoicism had the exaltation of the ability to endure the adverse circumstances of life in common with Cynicism, precisely the attitude that ordinary language identifies as "stoic." It also seems likely that an underlying principle of all Stoicism originated from Cynicism: the idea that every human being, with the exception of the wise, is insane and should be treated as such (Ahonen, 2018). Paradoxically, however, the Cynics themselves behaved as fools, by common standards, and were often considered as such. Plato, asked what he thought of Diogenes, is said to have replied "a Socrates gone mad" (*Diog. Laert.*, 6.54).

Born in Athens, in the 4th century BC, Stoicism had a considerable following in Hellenistic Greece and Rome. Seneca (ca. 8–65), Epictetus (ca. 50–130), and Marcus Aurelius (121–180) belong, in fact, to the Roman imperial era. Stoicism has exerted a profound influence on Western thought through them, and this has come down to the contemporary world (Spanneut, 1973). Although

Stoicism did not disregard the traditional areas of Greek philosophical research, ethics was the main object of interest in Stoic philosophy, and its basic aim was the best possible life, which could be achieved by curing the psychical distress caused by wrong concerns. The underlying principles, as well as the conclusions, appear rather counterintuitive:

> The ancient Stoics (. . .) distinguished between "good," "bad," and "indifferent" things. The good ones are only moral, that is to say the virtues; the bad ones are, similarly, only the moral ones, that is to say the vices. This means that outside the moral sphere there is no good or evil, but only "indifferent" things, which are, precisely, "neither good nor evil." Such are life and death, health and illness, youth and old age, wealth and poverty, beauty and ugliness, etc.
>
> (Reale, 2009, p. 10)

Epictetus radicalized this subdivision, distinguishing two classes of things: those entirely dependent on our activity (e.g., desires, preferences, opinions) and those independent, or at least only partially dependent on it (e.g., health, wealth, reputation). He wrote in the *Handbook* that things per se do not lead human beings to worry, but judgments about them do: "Death, for instance, is nothing terrible, or else it would have seemed so to Socrates too; no, it is in the judgment that death is terrible that the terror lies" (*Handbook*, 5; Hard & Gill, 2014, p. 314). The goal to be pursued would thus have been the ability to make correct judgments about the world, seeking virtue that, in itself, is sufficient for happiness. Being happy is not so much a subjective feeling of satisfaction as an objective state of *achievement* (Brunschwig, 2000).[12] The virtuous attitude toward existence would have allowed one to accept one's own destiny anyway.

Epicurus also founded the philosophical school from which his teaching spread in Athens (in 306 BC), the Garden. It was not only an institution that provided for the learning of a doctrine: the members of the school of Epicurus lived together, philosophized together, and were united by bonds of friendship and solidarity. They also remained in touch by letter if they moved away from the Athenian seat, and sought proselytes. The Epicurean school thus bears similarities to religious or esoteric communities. It was, in fact, engaged in both the study of the founder's works and the worship of him (Laks, 2000).

The philosophy of Epicurus was entirely aimed at providing the conditions for people to live peacefully, to free them from worries, and to win them security. For a tradition as old as it was erroneous, the term "Epicureanism" has often been associated with the idea of debauchery, as a result of the slander by the opponents of his school and the misinterpretation of its principles. It is in fact Epicurus who states that "No pleasure in itself is a bad thing," but he adds that "the means which produce some pleasures bring with them disturbances many times greater than the pleasures" (*Ratae Sententiae*, 141, VIII; Bailey, 1926, p. 97).

The pillar of a happy life (sheltered from evils) was, according to Epicurus, the *tetraphármakon* (fourfold remedy), that is, knowledge about (1) the nature of the gods; (2) death; (3) pleasure; and (4) pain. The balance between pleasure and pain leaned in favor of the first if the human being learned to distinguish the nature of desires: "Among desires, some are natural and necessary, some natural but not necessary, and some neither natural nor necessary, but due to idle imagination" (*Ratae Sentientiae*, 149, XXIX; Bailey, 1926, pp. 101–103). The first were those whose satisfaction freed one from pain (e.g., the desire to drink to quench thirst); the second allowed people to vary their pleasure (e.g., eating refined foods, rather than those aimed simply at quenching hunger); the third were directed toward entirely futile goals (such as the desire for honors). A wise person was to orient themselves to natural and necessary desires, not despising but also not seeking too actively those that were natural and unnecessary, and shunning those that were unnatural and unnecessary altogether. The pursuit of natural desires was reflected in a conception of pleasure, for which the absence of pain is sufficient, and pain can be easily tolerated. Intense pain, in fact, is short-lived or, if it becomes chronic, will be endured out of habit as a sort of traveling companion, and if its intensity is considerable and persists, it will presumably lead to death, which will undo it.

The dream in the ancient world

If *The Interpretation of Dreams* by Sigmund Freud (1856–1939) was the iconic work that contributed most to the affirmation of psychoanalysis during the 20th century, following the beginnings of oniromancy in the prehistory of psychotherapy can be an interesting topic.

There were probably three basic modes of the ancient consideration of the dream world. A dream was considered (a) a somehow "objective" reality; (b) something that the soul saw as it detached itself from the body; (c) something endowed with symbolic content, subject to possible interpretation (Rose, 1925). Each of these concepts was developed before the advent of Greek civilization: the idea of possible symbolism (in this case of a prophetic nature) was also present in the Old Testament – for example, in the dream of the Pharaoh about the seven fat cows and seven thin cows, interpreted by Joseph as seven years of abundance followed by seven years of famine. The Egyptians had already developed an articulated oniromancy, testified in the Chester Beatty III papyrus. Individually, the basic interpretative principle was that the authentic meaning of the dream could be obtained by reversing its apparent content: a happy dream usually therefore had a nefarious meaning (Mancia, 1987).

A complex and varied conception was developed in Greece, which eventually led to a potential therapeutic use of dreams. It is possible to deduce from the Homeric poems, first, a distinction between different types of dream experience – dreams in which the dreamer received a visit from a character and passively assisted, dreams that expressed concerns (or actual nightmares), and dreams that expressed the realization of a desire – and, second, a dichotomy between dreams that can be interpreted because they have meaning (especially those sent by the gods) and dreams that cannot be interpreted (Dodds, 1925, p. 103ff). The *Iliad* and *Odyssey* testified to the existence of practitioners who specialized in interpreting the prophetic meaning of dreams. For example, Achilles, speaking to the Danaans in the first book of *Iliad*, wonders to whom it is necessary to turn in order to understand the origin of the current epidemic, whether to a priest, a soothsayer, or rather an interpreter of dreams.

Such a practice had to have continuity in time, since several sources allude to it, starting from the *Treatise of Dietetics* included in the *Corpus Hippocraticum*. Here the author claimed the role of interpreting dreams that could offer indications about the health of the dreamer for the medical arts, recognizing, however, the existence of dreams capable of predicting the future and the legitimacy of the role of their interpreters.

Both Plato and Aristotle dealt with the meaning of dreams. Plato wrote in *Timaeus*:

> For our makers remembered that their father had ordered them to make mortal creatures as perfect as possible, and so did their best even with this base part of us and gave it the power of prophecy so that it might have some apprehension of truth. And clear enough evidence that god gave this power to man's irrational part is to be found in our incapacity for inspired and true prophecy when in our right minds; we only achieve it when the power of our understanding is inhibited in sleep, or when we are in an abnormal condition owing to disease or divine inspiration.
>
> (*Timaeus*, 71d–e; Lee, 1977, p. 99)

However, he added immediately afterward, only a sensible man was able to interpret what had been seen in a dream (or in a vision), hence the legitimacy of the existence of professional interpreters (72a–b). There were allusions to the dream in previous dialogues, but they were very marginal. At the beginning of the ninth book of the *Republic*, dreams describing extreme behaviors, such as sex with one's mother (Freud's reader jumps up!), were attributed to a lack of moderation, especially in food and drink. In *Theetetus*, Socrates discusses the possibility that wakefulness coincides with sleep and vice versa with the aspect who gives his name to the dialogue, as part of an argument aimed at demolishing the idea that knowledge is sensation.

Aristotle composed two specific treatises on the topic: *On Dreams* and *On Divination in Sleep*. The Stagirite was careful to deny that the gods could send messages to humans through dreams (they could have chosen the system and recipients better), but he still called dreams, if not divine, at least demonic – a fact that was originally understood by Freud (1900/1958) as a kind of insight into their unconscious nature. Some dreams were also veridical, according to Aristotle. Sometimes they would provide information about the dreamer's state of health (presumably through the perception of symptoms that had escaped notice during waking), sometimes they would elaborate solutions to the dreamer's problems, and would thus have been a kind of self-fulfilling prophecy, and sometimes, finally, they might have turned out to be true by coincidence or through the perception of obscure stimuli in the air.

The first work preserved in Western antiquity, dedicated entirely to dreams, after the two Aristotelian treatises, is the *Oneirocritica* of Artemidorus of Daldis dating from the second half of the 2nd century. It is probable that more authors addressed the question of the nature of the dream in a systematic way after Aristotle and that Artemidorus took some elements of his own treatise from these authors (Dal Corno, 1975). It must thus be taken into account that the interpretation of dreams was, from the point of view of Artemidorus, a technique for predicting the future: one of the many known at his time (several of which, although not all, he himself branded as unreliable). However, the fact that Artemidorus was mentioned by his contemporary Galen, as well as in the *Suda*, a kind of late encyclopedia of the Greek world, is testament to the fact that the survival of this book rather than others was no accident.

Artemidorus distinguished the actual dream from the *enhypnion*, which was the hallucinatory realization of a wish (I, 1; Harris-McCoy, 2012, pp. 46–47), as stated by the Freudian *Interpretation of Dreams*. Among actual dreams, Artemidorus distinguished directly perceived dreams (whose prediction would be realized in the short term) from allegorical dreams (which would predict events of more distant realization) (I, 2; Harris-McCoy, 2012, pp. 48–49). The similarity between Artemidorus' theory of dream symbolism and Freud's is particularly significant: "if [one] should happen to love a woman, he will not observe his beloved but rather a horse or mirror or ship or the sea or a female beast or female apparel or some other thing that signifies a woman," Artemidorus writes, for example (IV, Praef.; Harris-McCoy, 2012, p. 303), or "A mortar signifies a woman, and a pestle a man" (II, 42; Harris-McCoy, 2012, p. 231).[13]

It is also surprising that "with regard to the dream of incest between son and mother, Artemidorus spoke of it as if he shared the ideas formulated by Freud on the oedipal complex" (Musatti, 1976, p. 17).[14] In short, in spite of the far from scientific nature of the treatise, there are enough analogies with psychoanalytic thought to lead the analyst Musatti to define Artemidorus as an "ancient colleague" (1976, p. 23).

Aelius Aristides (117–180) was a contemporary of Artemidorus, whose *Sacred Discourses* is a different and peculiar testimony to the use of dreams at the time, that of *incubation*. Aelius Aristides learned this practice at the Askelepeion in Pergamon, a large cultural-religious complex dedicated to the cult of Asclepius. Here the priests induced sick people to pass the night inside the temple in order to dream (this was the specific incubation). The dream resulting from such a night was considered direct inspiration from Asclepius, and its content was interpreted as the god's indication of the therapy necessary for the healing of the disease from which one was suffering. The cult of Asclepius was handed down and spread in the Mediterranean basin: the temple of Aesculapius (Roman name of the same divinity), near the Tiber island, became one of its main centers.

Interest in dreams and their interpretation did not wane during the Middle Ages. In a Christianized civilization, the basic question became the possible divine or diabolic origin of dreams, which naturally affected whether their meaning could be considered authentic or not (Le Goff, 1964). The dream was thus already an element of treatment for the fathers of the Church. Tertullian was convinced that a distinction between divine and diabolic dreams was possible according to their content, which appeared edifying in dreams sent by God and sinful in those sent by the devil (*De anima*). Clement Alexandrinus worked along similar lines (*Paedagogus*), although Augustine of Hippo seemed more optimistic, considering the dream as the manifestation of divine omnipotence, although the existence of erotic dreams instilled him with some doubts (Dulaey, 1973). The theme of the necessary distinction between divine and diabolic in the dream world seems to recur for centuries, so much so that the *Elucidarium*, a work influenced by Anselm of Canterbury and Scotus Eriugena, restates it in terms substantially similar to those proposed by Tertullian. The works of some authors, such as John of Salisbury (*Policraticus*) and Pascalis Romanus (*Liber thesauri occulti*), seem to identify a possible turning point toward a psychologization of the dream, around the 12th century (Mancia, 1987). In fact, however, this is nothing more than a recovery of the Greek tradition: Pascalis Romanus, in fact, draws all his interpretations of dreams directly from Artemidorus, or from other sources which in turn draw on Greek authors (Collin-Roset, 1963).

Medicine, philosophy, and mental health in Hellenistic and Roman times

After the Macedonian conquest of Greece, the city of Alexandria became the center of Hellenic culture, founded in 332 BC by Alexander the Great. The period from the founding of Alexandria to the Roman conquest of the entire Mediterranean area, in the first century of the Vulgar Era, is known in Greek culture as the Alexandrian or Hellenistic age. During this period, philosophy mainly saw the development of the skeptical school, the Stoic school, and the Epicurean school, while medicine was dominated by the influence of the Hippocratic culture. The birth of a *dogmatic school* in medicine, so called because his followers were convinced that, being already discovered everything essential in the medical field, further research was superfluous, is usually ascribed to the son of Hippocrates, Draco of Kos (4th century BC). The birth of an *empirical school* originated as a strong reaction to the attitude of the prevalent dogmatic school. The empiricists refused to submit themselves entirely to the authority of the preexisting medical culture and opposed the need for a doctor to have experienced every aspect of their practice firsthand. This, however, did not prevent them from an attitude of deep reverence toward Hippocrates (Nutton, 2004, p. 149).

In the Roman environment, the greatest success was initially achieved by the *methodical school*, whose founder is recognized as Asclepiades of Bithynia (born ca. 124 BC), who studied medicine, philosophy, and oratory in Alexandria and Athens but was mainly active in Rome, which gradually became not only the political but also the cultural center of the ancient West. The works of Asclepiades have been lost, but his ideas have come to us through the writings of Celius Aurelianus (5th century) and through the polemical references of Galen.[15] Asclepiades opposed the Hippocratic conception of the humors with a theory based on the solidity of the human body, which drew on the Epicurean atomistic theory (Vegetti, 1985). The dogmatic school, inspired by Hippocrates but also by Stoicism, had prescribed unpleasant therapies to patients, based on purification and restricted diet regimens, in order to recover the balance of the body's humors. Asclepiades, on the other hand, based his treatment on the idea of restoring atoms to their motility through mechanical means: massage, walking, and "all sorts of 'passive' exercises in which the body is content to let itself be agitated, such as walking in a chariot or traveling in a boat" (Gourevitch, 1994, p. 5). Particularly significant for the purposes of a prehistory of psychotherapy is the idea of the need for an improvement in the patient's morale, which was obtained through prescriptions that were very pleasant to follow, such as cycles of relaxing hot baths and wine tastings (Alexander & Selesnick, 1966). For Asclepiades, however, problems had to be solved quickly and without weighing on the sick person: "His saying 'cito, tute et iucunde' has come down to us to indicate that medical action must be expeditious, sure and serene" (Ottaviani et al., 2004, p. 19). This approach quickly met with favor among the Romans (Vegetti, 1984).

It seems appropriate to recall also that Asclepiades proposed a classification of diseases that were to be considered specifically mental, based on relatively subtle observations and considerations (e.g., Asclepiades correctly distinguished illusion and hallucination). His search for a pleasant condition for the sick person extended to mental illnesses: Asclepiades excluded, for example, the idea that the mentally ill should (or even could) be kept in darkness (Zilboorg & Henry, 1941), a practice that was widespread in his day and remained so for centuries – in fact, until Pinel's time.

Soranus of Ephesus (d. AD 98), who was known for his opposition to restrictive measures regarding psychopathological suffering, was also within the methodical school. He seems to have been the first to take into account cultural factors in the treatment of mental illness, proposing prescriptions regarding what should be said and possibly read to patients (who had to be involved in conversations that aroused their interest and were compatible with their previous activities). With Soranus we can speak of "the appearance of a new humanism in psychopathology (. . .) a keen interest in man and in the minutest aspects of his behavior, a flair for characteriological differentiations and a deeply seated and live therapeutic intent" (Zilboorg & Henry, 1941, p. 72). In fact, despite the belief that mental illnesses had an organic origin, Soranus prescribed treatment by psychological means, minimized the use of drugs, and emphasized the importance of the patient-therapist relationship (Alexander & Selesnick, 1966, p. 48). Soranus' ideas on mental health, like those of Asclepiades, are also known thanks to what survives of the work of Celius Aurelianus, the last major representative of the methodical school. From Celius Aurelianus himself it is worth remembering the tendency to distinguish between physical and psychological causes of mental illness (he even thought that philosophy itself could be a cause of alienation) and the idea that the diagnosis of all types of illness should be conducted *ex toto signorum consensu*, that is, taking into account all the symptoms and not isolating some of them from the context (Gourevitch, 1994).

The first historically ascertained representative of the so-called *eclectic school* was Cornelius Celsus, who lived at the time of the emperor Tiberius, in the first decades after Christ. In the proem of his work *De medicina* (Jones, 1948a), Celsus began with a summary of the history of medicine that can be described as "most fair and judicious" (Jones, 1948b, p. IX), making explicit his intention to find a middle way between dogmatists, empiricists, and methodists.

Celsus devoted a section of the *De medicina* (III, 18) to insanity – that is, madness – considering it a physical disease, referable to fevers (*febria*), during which, Celsus himself noted, transient delirious states were often observed. The opinions expressed on insanity in the *De medicina* can be considered a sort of summary of the medicine's debate on the subject at the time, with respect to which Celsus placed himself in a neutral position, proposing to apply the various techniques depending on the case. Celsus reported both the opinion of Asclepiades and the traditional opinion with regard to the illumination of rooms for the mentally ill, for example, arriving at the Solomonic conclusion that some patients could be made uncomfortable by light and others by darkness: it would therefore be necessary to empirically verify the appropriate solution. In the same way, Soranus' idea of awakening the interests of a sick person by reading a book seemed better to Celsus in some cases, in other cases, decoctions of various kinds and massages were prescribed, and for others, restrictive measures were proposed, even tying the mentally ill down if they were particularly agitated, so that they would not harm themselves or others, and that one should not believe immediately in their repentance, as this could be a trick to obtain release. In any case, in Celsus's view, if gentle treatment failed, it was necessary to use a stronger approach (*De medicina*, III, 18, 21). A sick person could be not only bound but also subjected to fasting or beatings. Celsus thus inaugurated a pseudoscientific practice in which anything that seemed to improve the condition of the individual patient could be useful.

Galen was also an exponent of the eclectic school, universally considered the most influential doctor of antiquity after Hippocrates, to the point of being the main authority in the field of medicine for almost a millennium and a half: for the doctors who came after him, Galen had said everything and everything was said by Galen (Boudon-Millot, 2012). This was certainly a singular fate for someone who, in a work entitled *De sectis* (i.e., "On the sects," referring to the medical schools), had proclaimed the need to recognize no one as an indisputable master. Before *De humani corporis fabrica* by Andreas Vesalius (1514–1564), it can be said that almost nobody questioned Galen's anatomy, and his therapeutic principles survived until the discovery of blood circulation by William Harvey (1578–1657), and in some ways even beyond. Equally enduring was, specifically, his influence on psychopathological thought, which for centuries was largely limited through Galen to the reworking of Hippocrates' doctrine of the four temperaments/humors. In fact, Galen was able to build a systematic medicine, synthesizing medical knowledge, starting mainly from the recovery of the Hippocratic tradition (questioned by methodists and empiricists), to which he attributed the root of any progress in the field. Like Celsus, Galen included medicine in a broader cultural project. Moreover, like Celsus, he belonged to an affluent family (although, in Galen's case, not a noble one) and never found himself in the position of practicing medical *téchnē* to earn a living (Menghi, 1984).

Born in Pergamum and having completed his education in Smyrna and Alexandria, Galen stayed for extended periods on multiple occasions in Rome, where he composed most of his works and where he achieved such resounding success that he almost abandoned his practical activity (really reduced to single episodes of *gratia*, i.e., generosity) to devote himself full time to the activity of a writer and lecturer.

Readers derived a total distrust of philosophy from the works of Galen, and in particular from the so-called moral works. In his opinion all philosophy, as it was taught at his time, was separate from both logic and facts. He exalted medicine against this philosophy, as able to offer a fundamental orientation to knowledge, even in a theological or teleological sense. The physician, however, in Galen's perspective, "remains a therapist of organs (above all [. . .], and only through them can he act on the faculties of the soul)" (Vegetti, 1984, p. 139). The idea of a mental illness independent of the physical remained completely absent from his perspective.

To Galen, however, can also be traced the matrix of a figure that is somehow similar to a psychotherapist. This figure is illustrated in *The Diagnosis and Treatment of the Affections and Errors Peculiar to Each Person's Soul*. Galen's starting point is that controlling the passions is an indispensable principle of individual health (not only psychological) and the best way to avoid existential errors: "Since errors arise from false belief, while affections arise from nonrational impulse, it seemed to me that one should first free oneself from the affections" (7K–7DB; Singer, 2013, p. 244). In order to control the passions, however, the first step was to diagnose them, and the diagnosis of oneself was impossible. It was therefore necessary to be helped by a neutral person, who led a moral life and was sincere. One could ask him "which (. . .) affections he sees in you, emphasizing the gratitude you will feel cowards him: he will be your saviour, even more so than the man who saves you when you have a bodily sickness" (9K; Singer, 2013, p. 246). Diagnosis was only the first step, the individual's effort then consisted of avoiding the most obvious manifestations of their passions, starting a path of improvement that could last a long time but that would still be of fundamental importance:

> It is a shameful thing that a man will make every effort for a period of many years to become a good doctor, orator, scholar or geometer, but that you should give up on ever becoming a good human being, because of the expenditure of time.
>
> (21K; Singer, 2013, pp. 255–256)

Medicine and philosophy in the late Roman Empire and in the Islamic East

Historians of medicine are used to identifying the death of Galen, in AD 200, with the beginning of a secular decline in medical culture. The decline of the philosophical culture of Greek inspiration had already begun, as had that of general Roman civilization. The Roman Empire had experienced its point of maximum expansion under Trajan and had maintained an almost total integrity until the time of Marcus Aurelius (i.e., in fact, the age of Galen). The following centuries saw the subdivision of the imperial territories between the Western Roman Empire (with its capital in Rome) and the Eastern Roman Empire (with its capital in Byzantium, or Constantinople). With the fall of the Western Empire and the deposition of its last emperor Romulus Augustulus in 476, the torch of Roman civilization remained feebly lit only thanks to the Eastern Empire.

The medical treatises written after the death of Galen were, as far as we know, essentially compilations of previous works. Among the authors who deserve a mention are Posidonius of Byzantium and Oribasius of Pergamon, both of the 4th century and both important sources for the last major medical compilations containing hints of the diagnosis and treatment of mental illness, by Aëtius of Amida (6th century), Paulus Nicaeus (6th century), and Paulus of Aegina (7th century). The expression "mental illnesses" must be used with particular caution here: none of these authors distinguished between diseases of the body and diseases of the mind, and indeed they discuss psychological disorders in the context of physical diseases of the head (Thumiger & Singer, 2018).

The rise of Christianity as the imperial religion led to a growing suspicion of pre-Christian culture in general, as dependent on "pagan" religious beliefs. Such suspicion eventually became a tendency to erase all traces of the previous civilization. After the closure of the philosophical schools, there was a sort of exodus to the Near East of the remaining intellectuals, who began the translation of the Greek classics into local languages (in addition to founding medical schools, which flourished in the following centuries). Only when Europe began to have cultural exchanges with the Islamic world, after 1100, was the Western environment able to recover a significant part of Greek culture, enriched in the meantime by the contribution of Persian and Arab scholars. The Muslims built very early hospitals, in order to allow the dignified care of sick people, even the poor. Hospitals appear to date from the 8th century, and several contained specific wards for the mentally ill. Some were even exclusively for them. It is significant that most of the mentally ill (those who were not considered dangerous to themselves or others) enjoyed a certain freedom of movement within the hospitals (Dols, 1992).

The relationship between medicine and philosophy was very close in the history of Islamic culture, and the two most important Arab philosophers, Avicenna (980–1037) and Averroes (1126–1198), as well as many others, were also physicians. Perhaps for this reason, the conscious use of speech for therapeutic purposes (through suggestion) is attested by some of the most illustrious representatives of the medical tradition. Among them must be counted al-Rāzī (865–925), "without doubt the greatest clinical and observational physician of Islam, and along with Avicenna, the most influential, both East and West" (Nasr, 1968, p. 196). He wrote – among dozens of volumes dedicated to religion, philosophy, and astronomy as well – what in the West is known by the Latin name *Liber Continens*, a *summa* of all the medical knowledge accumulated up to that time. Al-Rāzī reported that he had cured a powerful emir, who was refractory to all physical treatment, through a complex process of psychological shock. After leading the emir, who had long been unable to stand, to the baths and subjecting him to a certain ritual, al-Rāzī suddenly began to threaten him with a dagger. The emir, in an attempt to defend himself, stood up and from that moment he became able to walk again (Nasr, 1968, pp. 196–197). Ishaq ibn Imran (died ca. 903–909), however, clearly expressed the idea that if, as per the Hippocratic-Galenic tradition, the soul follows the temperament of the body, then in turn the temperament can be influenced by the soul, perhaps even before al-Rāzī (Omrani et al., 2012).

Avicenna, the author of the *Canon*, the most respected medical work in the history of Islam, once had to deal with a prince who was convinced that he was a cow, and consequently asked to be slaughtered and cooked. Faced with the futile efforts of the court physicians to convince him of his human identity, the young man had also lost his appetite and become very weak. Avicenna initially indulged the prince's delirium, explaining, however, that he was too thin to be slaughtered and that he would have to feed himself to offer meat of the best quality. When the prince had recovered his strength thanks to the nourishment, it was also possible to convince him of his humanity (Dols, 1987).

Keikavus (Kay Kā'ūs ibn Iskandar, b. 1021, d. after 1082), Persian prince, in the *Qabus Nama* (which was written after 1000 and was influenced by Avicenna) apparently stated that suggestion could be fundamental in any medical therapy, when he noted that "encouragements from the doctor produce, among other things, beneficial effects on natural heat" (Zipoli, 1981, p. 199).

Some believe that the most famous book handed down by the Arab-Persian tradition, *The Thousand and One Nights*, can be interpreted as the story of a real psychotherapy which lasted three years. The story develops from the madness of Sultan Shariyar, who, betrayed by a wife, decides to take revenge by killing every new bride after their wedding night. The sequence of killings stops when Sharhazad, one of the predestined, implements a talking cure, every night telling the sultan a story that is concluded the next night, until the sultan falls in love with her and comes to his senses (Clinton, 1985).

Soul suffering between the Middle Ages and the Renaissance

Between the Middle Ages and the Renaissance, the filter of Christianity affected the general culture and the development of ideas about mental suffering:

> The culture of medieval Latin Christendom absorbed and made use of both of the Greek alternatives (madness as moral trauma, madness as disease). But it also fitted them with a cosmic Christian scheme – madness as divine Providence – which could impart a higher significance to either. Christian theology could also, of course, treat madness in quite distinctive ways, ones essentially alien to Greek man-centred philosophy: this lay in seeing mental disorder as a mark of the war for the possession of the soul (the "psychomachy" waged between God and Satan). Medieval and Renaissance minds could regard madness as religious, as moral or as medical, as divine or diabolical, as good or bad.
>
> (Porter, 1987, p. 25)

De anima of Tertullian (160–220), written in 205, was already a significant step in this direction, because it examined

> the theories of physicians and classical philosophers, the Church Fathers, the texts of the Old and New Testament, the physiological theories of Hippocrates, Diocles of Charistus, Erophilus, Erasistratus and Soranus of Ephesus, both in order to criticize them but also to justify a synthesis between the old culture and the new Christian vision of man.
>
> (Roccatagliata, 1973, p. 319)

The synthesis of the Greek-Roman world and Christianity found its highest expression in the figure of Augustine of Hippo (354–430), who must be remembered above all for the extraordinary finesse of his psychological analyses, which recall the depth of the phenomenological method, especially in the sort of spiritual autobiography constituted by the famous Confessions. For example, Augustine wrote: "The weakness then of infant limbs, not its will, is its innocence. Myself have seen and known even a baby envious; it could not speak, yet it turned pale and looked bitterly on its foster brother" (Confessions, 1, 7, 11; Parker, 2005, p. 8).

The attraction that the *Confessions* exerted on psychoanalysts, after all, is widely understandable. At the very instance when he depicted sexuality as temptation and sin, Augustine emphasized its importance in human life in accents that had rarely been touched upon before (Flasch, 1971). In describing the love of his own mother, intent on drawing him closer to the Christian life, Augustine revealed an Oedipal triangle in his own youthful history.[16]

Diabolic possession was a recurring theme in medieval narratives concerning psychopathology. The great power that Satan, the "prince of this world," could exert over humans (Luke 13:11) began to be used as an explanation of both mental and physical illnesses. Since Satan was supposed to brand his acolytes, the search for diabolical *stigmata* (signs) became part of the diagnostic procedure. After all, the idea of demonic possession as the cause of psychopathology, as well as that of the influence of spirits on illnesses, had antecedents dating back to the dawn of civilization (Zilboorg & Henry, 1941). In any case, exorcism practices became part of the necessary treatment of both mental and physical illnesses as early as the time of St. Cyprian (ca. 210–258; Innamorati et al., 2019). Some Church Fathers, such as Gregory of Tours (ca. 538–594), gradually tended to consider spiritual medicine as the only legitimate one. The recitation of prayers and formulas always accompanied the administration of any other forms of treatment.

On the one hand, Christianity monopolized the care of souls in the West, inserting the Greek tradition into a thought pattern that focused on eternal life rather than earthly life. On the other hand, the care of bodies also became a specifically religious domain. Medicine tended to be practiced for a long time, especially in monasteries. The first secular medical centers began to acquire particular importance when the Council of Clermont and the Second Lateran Council (in the 12th century) imposed a number of restrictions on the practice of medicine by monks, including a prohibition on leaving the monastery to treat patients (Alexander & Selesnick, 1966).

The first centers to develop important schools of medicine were Montpellier and especially Salerno, a port city known for its cosmopolitanism: it was said to have been founded in the 9th century by a Jew, an Arab, a Greek, and a native. The fundamental impulse for establishing the medical school of Salerno was in any case offered by Constantine the African (1020–1087), a Jew converted to Catholicism, who brought the Greek tradition back to Italy, translating into Latin the Arabic medical works, which had absorbed the lessons of Hippocrates and Galen.

The influence of Hippocratic-Galenic medicine fostered a long tradition of treatises that tiredly renewed the principle of the influence of temperaments and moods on mental health (Just think of the renewed idea of the influence of black bile on the origin of melancholy, which culminated in the monumental work of Robert Burton, *Anatomy of Melancholy* [1621]). Finally, taking the historical scheme inaugurated by Foucault with his *History of Madness* very cautiously, we can see that the attitudes of the rulers toward the mentally ill oscillated between a substantial indifference and the conviction that it was necessary to imprison them rather than to find a cure. This attitude became prevalent over time (Porter, 1987). There is no lack of examples of the hospitalization of mental illness: in 1203, in a hospital near the cathedral of Le Mans, frenzied lunatics were admitted, "and later, in the West, certain hospitals specialized in mental cases, as did the Royal Bethlehem or Bedlam in London at the end of the 13th century" (Crombie, 1952, p. 211).

During the Middle Ages, however, philosophers tended to attribute mental suffering to neither the body nor the presence of demons (or at least not only to it). Thomas Aquinas (1225–1274), author of a profound reinterpretation of Aristotelian thought in the light of Christian theology, was a fundamental expression of this tendency. According to Thomas, human beings became *amentes*, that is, inaccessible to human relationships (*Summa Theologica*, Ia IIae, 10.3), or *furiosi* (furious; III, 68.11) because of the loss of reason, which could not be caused by an organic lesion. Another form of loss of reason was insanity, the result of the abandonment of the human being to the basest and most material appetites (*Summa Theologica*, Ia IIae, q. 77, a. 2). If the loss of reason was the cause of the pathological condition, its recovery was the possible cure:

> Everything that is suitable for stimulating reason must be used: teaching, well-regulated asceticism, through which man recovers his perfection, despite the obstacles. In case of failure, the community surrounding the insensate person will have to make up for the paralysis of his reason, taking strict account of the dignity of this spirit, even though paralyzed in its manifestation.
>
> (Simonnet, 1994, p. 54)

The lack of specialization that characterized culture for a long time contributed to preventing the treatment of mental suffering from becoming the task of a specific professional figure. Often the same person could be a doctor, a theologian, and a philosopher, even in the period in which – between the 12th and the 13th century – the training and professionalization of doctors were "regulated and normalized: in a word, institutionalized" (Agrimi & Crisciani, 1988, p. 11). In fact, if philosophy was called *ancilla theologiae* (servant of theology) in ancient Christian thought, medicine was defined, with a saying attributed (apocryphally) to Tertullian, *soror philosophiae* (sister of philosophy) (Rialdi, 1968). The fact that philosophy and medicine were sisters is also confirmed in the *Conciliator differentiarum* of Peter of Abano (1257–1313), which also insisted on the indissoluble link between medicine and astrology: the latter offered the possibility to mediate between universal knowledge (astronomical) and the application of knowledge to individuals (Alessio, 1976).

Clinical method and psychopathology

Between the end of the Middle Ages and the beginning of the Renaissance, medicine was still strongly conditioned by the Galenic paradigm, but some characters introduced a series of innovations, especially in the field of anatomical and clinical studies, which laid the foundations of modern medicine. Anatomy in particular, thanks to the work of pioneers (Vesalius, Harvey, Borrelli, Morgagni), gradually detached itself from the theory of humors, hybridizing medicine with studies of mechanics, chemistry, physics. The causes of diseases were then sought in natural facts other than the dyscrasia of the humors.[17] The observation and classification of symptoms then led, in the 18th century, to the formulation of major medical systems. Together with anatomy, clinical medicine acquired an increasing importance, leading to an anatomical and clinical synthesis according to a method of diagnosis and treatment that, from the observation of symptoms of the body, assumed the presence of physical impediments or injuries, confirmed or disconfirmed by postmortem anatomical dissection. Nosographies were thus created, which led to a rationalization of different pathologies and places of care (Grmek, 1996).

The clinical study of diseases became essential, and the term "clinical," from the Greek word *klíne*, which indicated the bed that in ancient times was used for banquets and meetings, but also for the sick, began to define medical schools that taught their lessons in front of the sickbeds. In the 16th century, Giovanni Battista da Monte (1498–1551), in Padua, taught medical practice by basing it on clinical observation. The word "clinical" began to refer both to the perceptible signs of a disease and to the inscription of these signs in a nosography, a set of symptoms of a particular disorder. Between the 17th and 18th centuries, first Thomas Sydenham (1624–1689) and then Hermann Boerhaave (1668–1738) were the true systemizers of the clinical approach. Sydenham started a research program in order to identify the specific symptoms of diseases and thus distinguish and classify them into categories. Boerhaave, at the University of Leiden, instead, established a clinic with twelve beds, six for men and six for women, where he conducted a careful observation of cases for research and treatment purposes. The Age of Enlightenment brought innovations in medicine that opened the door to modernity. Leopold Auenbrugger (1722–1809) and Jean-Nicolas Corvisart (1755–1821) introduced auscultation, later, René Laennec (1781–1826) created the stethoscope (1816). Thus was opened a pioneering period in which scientific medicine increased its space and its power in society. Anatomy and clinical method became the pillars on which modern medicine was founded (Lombardo & Foschi, 1999).[18]

Psychiatric clinics ran on parallel tracks to those of medical clinics, with peculiarities deriving from the complexity of the psychopathological phenomenon, which could be justified by resorting to beliefs that were not only medical but also religious, sociological, and philosophical. The psychiatric patient, bereft of reason, did not correspond to the ideal of "the Renaissance man," author of his own destiny, which led to the emergence of the bourgeoisie, especially during the 17th and 18th centuries. According to Foucault (1961/2006), in 17th-century Europe there was even a sort of great internment of diversity that did not conform to the ideal of the bourgeois. Dörner (1969/1981) has shown that all European countries, each with its own peculiarities, saw the creation of places of confinement for those who suffered from alterations in reason. It was a varied humanity, and just as varied were the homes for the insane and the theories behind the different internments.[19] Madhouses, hospices, sanatoriums, and prisons were the first institutions to contain the insane, along with a whole series of undesirables (the poor, vagrants, heretics, political suspects, unemployed people, rebels, and criminals). The Enlightenment then led to a rationalization of clinical psychiatry, and the asylum. The Madhouses Act of 1774, enacted in England, was one of the first regulations aimed at preventing the various abuses committed in the management of these places of confinement, which were then set under the control of official medicine, authorized and inspected by the Royal College of Physicians.

In France, Philippe Pinel (1745–1826) initiated a psychiatric nosography on new rational bases and the organization of new asylums. The asylum thus became the site in which a patient could be studied through the clinical observation of their daily behavior, which became possible only through their liberation from previous systems of internment (i.e., liberation from chains). Philippe Pinel and his principal pupil Jean Esquirol (1772–1840) thus formulated the first systematic categorizations of mental illnesses (Pinel, 1801, 1809; Esquirol, 1805). The trend toward an increasingly meticulous classification of psychopathology deepened during the 19th century and saw its greatest expression in German psychiatrist Emil Kraepelin (1855–1925), who initiated contemporary clinical and descriptive psychiatry (Pietikäinen, 2015; Porter, 2002). The purpose of diagnostic classifications in psychiatry was in every way similar to those of any other medical classification. It was necessary to formulate general descriptive categories of disease with the aim of recognizing the symptoms accurately and then arriving at the causes and formulating a specific therapy and prognosis.

Toward a clarification of the therapy: the moral treatment

In this cultural context, there were at least two initial therapeutic approaches in the field of medical treatment for various forms of psychopathology: one that used physical and chemical factors of treatment (e.g., cold baths – a sort of thermal shock that anticipated the chemical and electrical ones of later psychiatry – light baths, psychosurgery, psychotropic drugs) and one that instead used behavioral or communicative techniques. At the same time, there were reforms of treatment spaces. Over time, within the psy-sciences, these two approaches met and clashed, dividing and characterizing different disciplinary domains.

A particular expression of the second method was promoted by the Tuke Quaker family of philanthropists, active in the field of mental health.[20] The Tukes were the creators in York, England, of a "retired habitation" of unprecedented conception for the time, aimed at a more humane treatment of the mentally ill. William Tuke (1732–1822) was the founder of the York Retreat in 1796. Conceived and financed by the local Quaker community and then opened to other citizens, it was a pioneering organization and an alternative to public psychiatric hospitals. The idea for a new place for the treatment of mental disorders came to William, who was not a physician, as a result of his outrage over the death of Hannah Mills, a woman from his religious community, which was caused by the mistreatment she suffered in the city's asylum. He obtained funding from the Quakers – or Society of Friends – to create an institution in which the patient was treated with dignity, in order to recover their reason by therapeutic means that made use of work, prayer, and order in a comfortable environment. The Quakers were a religious community confident in the potential of human reason – the inner light – which came directly from God: they were also influenced by a communitarian and egalitarian conception that drew on the cenacles of the early Christians. The York Retreat became a place of experimentation for new therapeutic approaches to mental illness, in a context in which religion inspired by a radical Protestantism found a foothold in the Enlightenment. The Enlightenment reformers opposed the classic means of psychiatry of the time, which had become inhumane and dangerous (purges, coercion, isolation, bloodletting, punishment, chains, etc.), advancing a new moral approach to treatment. It was necessary to intervene with patients using a human and supportive attitude, trying to bring reason where behavior was chaotic and excessively passionate. They tried to achieve the moralization of patients through a set of new practices, which reformed places of care by making them more spacious and attentive to the needs of the patient. Samuel Tuke (1784–1857), William's grandson, described the therapeutic setting at the York Retreat in 1813 as a moral treatment, likening York's practices to those of Pinel in France (Tuke, 1813; see also Pietikäinen, 2015; Porter, 2002).

Moral treatment was then taken up as the main therapeutic practice of psychiatry, especially in revolutionary France, and spread to other European nations as an alternative psychiatric treatment context to the coercive or violent treatments that degraded sick people and yet were still commonly practiced.

Disciplining passions

Between the end of the 18th century and the beginning of the 20th century, the pathology of the passions was the territory in which medical, psychiatric, and psychological approaches that constituted the French psychiatry – especially Parisian – clustered around the *Annales médico-psychologiques*. The treatment of dyscrasias of the passions, which were a kind of psychological metaphor for the moods, was the goal of *traitement moral* (Esquirol, 1805; Descuret, 1841; see also Foucault, 1961/2006, 2003; Goldstein, 1987).

Compared to the Tukes, the French were revolutionary doctors with a decidedly secular outlook. As masterfully analyzed by Gauchet and Swain (1980/2012), a new organization of medical institutions began in Parisian public and university hospitals, in particular, beginning with the revolution of 1789, which went hand in hand with the search for an empirical and experimental unification of physiology and clinical method on the part of the Medical School of Paris, achieved later in the mid-19th century (Grmek, 1996). Gauchet and Swain (1980/2012) have, moreover, shown that the early French asylums were fundamentally an attempt to rationalize and humanize psychiatric care. The new psychiatric hospitals were conceived as ideal cities created to control deranged behavior by restoring, through physical and moral techniques, to patients their lost reasoning. Pinel described moral treatment as a therapeutic reform elaborated from the observation of the nursing work carried out by the married couple Jean-Baptiste (1746–1811) and Marguerite Pussin who, as non-doctors, were in charge of organizing mental health in Bicêtre. Pinel, who became a leading figure in Parisian psychiatry and director of the clinics of Bicêtre and Salpêtrière, was assisted in his duties by Jean-Baptiste, who was a prototype for the particular professional figure who would become the nurse in psychiatry (Pinel, 1801, 1809). Pinel was thus portrayed as a savior who advocated a humanistic organization of the hospital. We have paintings of him with an order freeing the sick from their chains, and indeed this first generation of alienists or enlightened psychiatrists devoted themselves with extraordinary commitment to the diagnosis and treatment of mental illness and to the establishment of their own new psychiatric profession (see also Castel, 1976; Pietikäinen, 2015; Porter, 2002; Shorter, 1997).[21]

Moral treatment was essentially characterized by a pedagogical attitude whereby the patient would be able to regain their reason by following an appropriate dietary regimen, resting, and enhancing their resources, and supported in this by the hospital organization, paramedics, and physicians. *La médecine des passions* and moral treatment were also characterized by a paternalistic dimension that consoled, classified, and guarded in order to correct the behavior of the mentally ill, which was deemed deviant. Goldstein (1987) pointed out that moral treatment was also based on a sort of kindness therapy toward the mentally ill, which had its roots in both folk medicine and the religious treatment of the sick.[22] For his part, Foucault (2003) argued that the treatment of patients was entirely arranged according to a familial model of relationships and had the goal of disciplining the inner world of the sick person. From this point of view, the doctor-patient relationship would have been conditioned by a power which advantaged the doctor, who thus performed a disciplining function, recognized and accredited by postrevolutionary society itself.[23]

Moral treatment then also took root – especially in the United States – as a work cure in psychiatry (which was counterbalanced by a rest cure), especially useful to patients with high functioning and able to be productive. In some ways, the term "psychotherapy" in psychiatric hospitals became synonymous with moral treatment or work therapy. Asylums became veritable citadels or self-sufficient farms that functioned through the work of the inmates. This idea of work as a cure even led to the exploitation of the inmates' labor. It was only with the dismantling of psychiatric hospitals, due to the late twentieth-century anti-institutional movement, the entrenchment of a new psychiatry, and the influences of psychotherapy, but also due to real lawsuits brought against the labor exploitation of the patients, that "therapeutic work" disappeared, only very recently, from the horizon of therapies of the mental (Harris, 2016; see Goffman, 1961).

Children and moral treatment

Among the postrevolutionary alienists and, later, also among the positivists, there even spread an idea of children as individuals in a lower state of evolution than adults and who, for this reason, needed an *orthophrenic* education, that is, able to straighten out and amend their nature, favoring the normality of a growth that, if left to itself, would have deviated toward an irremediable perversion of the personality (see Guarnieri, 2006). A moral therapy for children similar to that for adults was thus developed, and the first departments dedicated to them were founded (Foucault, 2003). It is necessary to point out the presence of some revolutionary doctors in this field, however, who expressed an optimistic view of the child's capacity for development. These doctors developed the principle of "educability," which later had considerable success.

As is well known, Jean-Jacques Rousseau (1712–1778) spread the fortunate enlightenment principle, according to which children, theoretically, would have virtues disposed to goodness and directed toward evil and the loss of innocence only because of an inadequate society. Education was considered useful, in this sense, to foster and accompany the development of the true and positive nature of the child. This positive idea of educability was destined during the 19th and 20th centuries to attain a certain fortune among some pioneers of psy-sciences, inspired by a version of evolutionism for which the characters could be modified and transmitted from one generation to another, from an optimistic and Lamarckian perspective (transformism).[24] Two French doctors in particular, Jean Marc Gaspard Itard (1775–1838) and his pupil Édouard Séguin (1812–1880), in the midst of an optimistic attitude toward childhood, did not limit themselves to elaborate tools and techniques for observing children, but were concerned with modifying their personalities, and greatly influenced subsequent history. For them, infantile idiocy was not a disease but the sign of a developmental arrest that could be recovered by appropriate education.

The treatment of Victor, the wild child who grew up in the Aveyron countryside at the beginning of the 19th century and was diagnosed as incurable by Pinel and the inner circle of alienists, but was partially recovered by Itard,[25] was prototypical of both the history of clinical developmental psychology and education. Itard thus elaborated a series of behavioral techniques that should have moralized the behavior of the wild child and also enriched his linguistic and symbolic baggage in order to potentially rehabilitate him in society. Victor's case started a long and inexhaustible debate on the specific weight of nature or nurture in individual development. The idea emerged with the case of the wild child, that there were sensitive periods of education, and that, given certain conditions of learning, individuals would have a natural aptitude to learn. Victor was subjected to a therapeutic practice that was supposed to help him recover the cognitive, linguistic, and moral skills he had never developed. Itard helped Victor to name things, to control his passions, to speak. Itard and Séguin were thus among the first to deem children with mental retardation educable (Douthwaite, 2002).[26] This psycho-pedagogical tradition later had various outcomes, leading to the founding of child neuropsychiatry, modern teaching methods, and clinical developmental psychology.[27]

Notes

1 We refer here to the thought of Michel Foucault (1926–1984), a French intellectual who trained in the school of pathological psychology (see infra, Ch. 2) and later became a historian of science and a philosopher. In the history of "psy" sciences, the Foucauldian concept of governmentality has been particularly successful, that is, the critique, also historical, of all those disciplinary devices that have been used to manage people for practical and political purposes in institutions (factories, schools, hospitals, prisons).

2 The final 2018 issue of the journal *History of the Human Sciences* (Vol. 31, issue 4) and the first 2018 issue of the *European Journal of Psychotherapy & Counselling* (Vol. 20, issue 1) partially remedied this lack of cross-cultural history of psychotherapy at least for different European nations (see Marks, 2018; Martin, 2018; Shamdasani, 2018).

3 A possible exception is the origin of family therapy. See Vol. 2, Ch. 6, pp. 43–49.

4 As highlighted by Robert M. Young (1990), a historian of science and Kleinian psychoanalyst, dichotomies and categorizations seem to be a characteristic means of the production of scientific knowledge, even though, on the other hand, they move us away from a unified understanding of phenomena.

5 The problem of epistemological ruptures in the description of the psy-sciences is currently at the center of a particularly lively historiographical debate between authors of different sets in search of continuity between the history of philosophical and pre-19th-century psychology, and that of contemporary psychology (Robinson, 2013; Araujo, 2017), and historians who value discontinuities in order to have a more complex and multifactorial view of contemporary psychology (Danziger, 2013; Brock, 2017). The history of psychotherapy, in our opinion, defies historians of discontinuity in that psychotherapeutic theories have more or less overtly always referred to pre-19th-century traditions in a way that today can be called transdisciplinary (Montuori, 2005). Jackson (1999) wrote a volume assuming that there is continuity among those who treat the psyche over a historical period thousands of years long, through the use of similar modalities in different periods. A long history of psychotherapy has thus been described from practices of various kinds. The expression of feelings through catharsis and abreaction, confession and confiding, consoling and comforting, the use of the passions and imagination, suggestion and persuasion, reward and punishment, explanation and interpretation, introspection and cognitive approaches would thus all be metatheoretical techniques shared by therapists far apart in space and time. A disciplinary history of psychotherapy would therefore give way to a long history related to the treatment of the mind via communication in a period that runs from antiquity to the present day, using a diachronic approach.

6 It should be considered, after all, that in the classical Greek language the words *manía* (madness) and *mantikḗ* (divination) have a common etymological root (Liddell & Scott, 1925).

7   The word "normality," in fact, has a juridical term (norm) as its root, and already for this reason refers to convention rather than to presumed objective data. Normality can in fact be understood as (a) the condition that characterizes the majority of a population; (b) a certain level (average or statistical norm) on a scale of measurement, which represents the average of the population itself (this is the case of the level 100 of the Intelligence Quotient); (c) a previous condition experienced on the subjective level as adequate (which could be better or worse than the average norm); (d) conversely, a condition-objective that one sets oneself (again, higher or lower than the average norm); (e) a state of complete absence of psychological problems (being perfectly normal) that is as distant from common experience as the full and perfect functionality of all tissues, organs, and systems of the physical human body (Scharfetter, 1980).

8   For example, see, on the history of the unconscious: Whyte, 1960; Ellenberger, 1970; Tallis, 2002; on the history of the concept of self: Taylor, 1989; on the history of the idea of the clinical: Foucault, 1963/2012; on normal and pathological: Canguilhem, 1966/2012; Lombardo & Pedone, 1995.

9   Socrates taught philosophy to the young Athenian aristocrats but wrote nothing, while his most important pupil, Plato, left an abundant harvest of philosophical works, written in the form of dialogues between different characters. Socrates is the main character in several of these dialogues. It has been much discussed over time whether what is said by Socrates in the Platonic works is attributable to himself or rather to the thought of his illustrious and original pupil. Generally, however, there is a tendency to believe that at least the Socrates of the early Platonic *Dialogues* is a faithful mirror of true Socratic thought (see, e.g., Capizzi, 1990).

10   Doctors were convinced that administering hellebore (a very toxic plant) would accomplish this. The black stool that a person evacuated after taking hellebore seemed to prove, in their eyes, that the body had rid itself of black bile (Onians, 1954). In fact, the ingestion of hellebore causes bleeding in the digestive tract, and the black stools were naturally the result of the presence of blood from the stomach, partially digested afterwards in the intestine. This circumstance is an archaic, but far from historically unique, example of how empirical observation, conditioned by erroneous assumptions, can lead to egregious errors and not without consequences (in this case, the risk of poisoning).

11   Indifference is what the ancient and the modern meanings of "cynicism" have in common, but they are so different that the German language uses two different terms to distinguish them. In this sense, Sloterdijk (1983) opposes modern *Zynismus* and proposes, as a solution to get away from it, the use of ancient *Kynismus*.

12   Epictetus argued that we can become ill with misjudgments, just as contemporary cognitivist therapists such as Ellis and Beck claim (Sellars, 2019).

13   See infra, Section 3: 88–91.

14   See infra, Section 3: 88–89; 141–147.

15   See pp. 21–23.

16   Augustine recounts that, having gone to the baths with his father when he was 16, his father had the opportunity to observe that Augustine had an erection. Back home, the father was happy to tell his wife about the episode, wishing for a future descendant. The mother, on the other hand, was only concerned about the possible sinful consequences, foreshadowing the possibility of a life consecrated to God for Augustine, that is, the possibility of not sharing him with another woman (*Confessions*, 2, 3, 6–7).

17   Galen's influence on psychiatry and psychology, on the other hand, was exceptionally long-lasting and generated an articulated system of beliefs. The personality and the body were believed to be conditioned by the mixture of the four humors. Health and personality depended on the balance and imbalance of the humors, which also corresponded to the four elements, four temperaments, four colors, and four planets, which therefore influenced individual destiny. Being born under the influence of a planet would lead to

a personality influenced by the planet: the connection between Saturn and the melancholic temperament is particularly well known, mediated, as we have seen, by black bile (see Klibansky et al., 1964). Such a pseudo-rational system survived for a long time. Terms such as rebalancing or stabilizing (e.g., by means of psychotropic drugs), dyscrasia, and fusion/defusion all distantly reference the theory of the harmonic/disharmonic functioning of the elements/humors of nature. Even today, however, people still speak of a sanguine or bilious temperament to describe a person's character (see Lombardo & Foschi, 2002a, 2002b).

18 Along these lines, Claude Bernard (1813–1878) was the scholar who implemented a research program fundamental to the birth of modern scientific medicine, integrating anatomy, clinical method, and experimentation (Bernard, 1865).

19 The idea that this was indeed a large European internment in quantitative terms has been questioned by Porter (2002) and recently analyzed by Pietikäinen (2015). Porter (2002) lumped Foucault (1961/2006) and Dörner (1969) together by labeling the story as "conspiratorial" (p. 98). In reality, Dörner's volume (1969) highlighted the different European cultures of internment in the pre-psychiatric era, which then favored the establishment of true clinical psychiatry, containing various historiographic innovations and discontinuities with respect to Foucault's history that were later underestimated by Anglo-Saxon historiography. Similarly, in Italy there was a prehistory of psychiatry, intimately connected to the particular culture of our country, which led to the internment of diversity in hospices, which were also precursors of the asylum (Giacanelli, 1975; Babini, 2009).

20 Quakers are the followers of a reformed Christian movement that arose during the English Revolution of the 17th century led by George Fox (1624–1691), founder of the Society of Friends. It is a religion that spreads a spirituality in which the possibility of a direct experience of divinity through meditative, disciplined, and silent prayer, promoting a social and peaceful cooperation among human beings, is emphasized.

21 While there is a tendency to mythologize Pinel as the first liberator of patients from chains, others before him embodied similar ideals. William Battie (1703–1776) at the Bedlam Hospital around 1750 in England, Abraham Joly (1748–1812) in 1787 in Geneva, Vincenzo Chiarugi (1759–1820) in 1789 in Pisa all implemented reforms with similar intentions to Pinel's.

22 Moral treatment can also be considered a primordial form of cognitive-behavioral psychotherapy, aimed at restoring to individuals both appropriate behaviors and better interpretative categories with which to adapt to the environment. It was not an antecedent of psychodynamic therapies, which, on the contrary, were born with the idea of re-evaluating the passions and their influences on consciousness.

23 More recently, other researchers have remarked on the hereditary nature of this psychiatry, which tended, however, to consider mental illness as the expression of a biological degeneration, manageable only with an asylum device with custodial functions, rather than transformative of the personality (see Coffin, 2003; Dowbiggin, 1991; Pick, 1993). See infra, Ch. 2, note 44, p.?.

24 Transformism is an approach derived from the evolutionary ideas of Jean-Baptist Lamarck (1744–1829), spread mainly in France and Europe, that education and environment could genetically modify individuals, leading to the improvement of generations and populations. It was therefore particularly useful to psy-scientists as a theory, to affirm the goodness of their practices. The theory was empirically disconfirmed by August Weismann (1834–1914) and fell into disfavor during the 20th century. However, Lamarckism survived for a long time and is now taking a sort of revenge in studies of epigenetics, which actually demonstrate the importance of the environment in the regulation, from generation to generation, of DNA expression.

25 As is well known, François Truffaut dedicated a famous film to Victor's case: *The Wild Child* (1970).

26 Séguin's volume entitled *Traitement moral, hygiène et éducation des idiots* (1846), for example, became the main source of inspiration for Maria Montessori (1870–1952), as well as
for many other 20th-century psy-scientists (Foschi, 2012).
27 Clinical psychology, at least nominally, was founded at the University of Pennsylvania by
Lightner Witmer (1867–1956), an American psychologist who, inspired by this psycho-
pedagogical tradition begun by Itard, inaugurated a psychological clinic in 1896 and the
journal *The Psychological Clinic* in 1907, dealing exclusively with children with learning
disorders (McReynolds, 1997; Reisman, 1991; Routh & Barrio, 1996).

References

Agrimi, J., & Crisciani, C. (1988). *Edocere medicos. Medicina scolastica nei secoli xiii-xv* [Teach the
physicians: Scholastic medicine in the centuries XIII-XV]. Guerini.
Ahonen, M. (2018). Making the distinction: The stoic view of mental illness. In C. Thu-
miger & P. N. Singer (Eds.), *Mental illness in ancient medicine* (pp. 341–364). Brill.
Alessio, F. (1976). Filosofia e scienza. Pietro da Abano [Philosophy and science: Peter of
Abano]. In *Storia della cultura veneta* [History of Venetian culture] (Vol. II). Neri Pozza.
Alexander, F. G., & Selesnick, S. T. (1966). *The history of psychiatry: An evaluation of psychiatric
thought and practice from prehistoric times to the present.* Harper & Row.
Araujo, S. D. F. (2017). Toward a philosophical history of psychology: An alternative path for
the future. *Theory & Psychology, 27*(1), 87–107.
Babini, V. P. (2009). *Liberi tutti. Manicomi e psichiatri in Italia: Una storia del Novecento* [Free all.
Asylums and psychiatrists in Italy: A history of the twentieth century]. Il Mulino.
Bailey, C. (Ed.). (1926). *Epicurus. The extant remains.* Clarendon Press.
Bernard, C. (1865). *Introduction à l'étude de la médicine expérimentale* [Introduction to the study
of experimental medicine]. Baillière.
Bernays, J. (1880). *Zwei Abhändlungen über die Aristotelische Theorie des Dramas* [Two essays on
the Aristotelian theory of drama]. Hertz.
Boudon-Millot, V. (2012). *Galien de Pergame* [Galen]. Les Belles Lettres.
Brems, C., Thevenin, D. M., & Routh, D. K. (1991). The history of clinical psychology. In
C. E. Walker (Ed.), *Applied clinical psychology* (pp. 3–35). Springer.
Brock, A. C. (2017). Alternative path for the future or a return to the past? Araujo's "philo-
sophical" history of psychology. *Theory & Psychology, 27*(1), 108–116.
Brunschwig, J. (2000). Stoicism. In J. Brunschwig & E. R. Lloyd (Eds.), *Greek thought*
(pp. 977–996). Belknap Press.
Caizzi, F. D. (2000). Antisthenes. In J. Brunschwig & E. R. Lloyd (Eds.), *Greek thought*
(pp. 536–543). Belknap Press.
Canguilhem, G. (2012). *On the normal and the pathological.* Springer. (Original edition 1966)
Capizzi, A. (1990). *The cosmic republic.* Brill.
Carotenuto, A. (1982). *A secret symmetry: Sabina Spielrein between Jung and Freud.* Pantheon.
Carroy, J. (1991). *Hypnose, suggestion et psychologie* [Hypnosis, suggestion and psychology]. PUF.
Carroy, J. (1993). *Les personnalités doubles et multiples* [Double and multiple personalities]. PUF.
Carroy, J. (2000). L'invention du mot psychothérapie et ses enjeux [The invention of the
word psychotherapy and its issues]. *Psychologie Clinique, 9*, 11–30.
Castel, R. (1976). *L'ordre psychiatrique. L'âge d'or de l'aliénisme* [The psychiatric order. The
golden age of alienism]. Minuit.
Castiglioni, A. (1927). *Storia della medicina* [History of medicine]. Unitas.

Churchland, P. M. (1989). *A neurocomputational perspective: The nature of mind and the structure of science.* MIT press.

Clements, F. E. (1932). *Primitive concepts of disease.* University of California Press.

Clinton, J. W. (1985). Madness and cure in the 1001 nights. *Studia Islamica,* 61, 107–125.

Coffin, J.-C. (2003). *La transmission de la folie: 1850–1914* [The transmission of madness: 1850–1914]. Harmattan.

Collin-Roset, S. (1963). Le "Liber Thesauri Occulti" de Pascalis Romanus: Un traité d'interpretation des songes du XIIe Siècle [The "Liber Thesauri Occulti" by Pascalis Romanus: A treatise on the interpretation of dreams of the XII century]. *Archives d'histoire doctrinale e littéraire du Moyen Age, 30,* 111–198.

Crombie, A. C. (1952). *The history of science from Augustine to Galileo.* Heinemann.

Cushman, P. (1991). Ideology obscured: Political uses of the self in Daniel Stern's infant Relational psychoanalysis as political resistance. *American Psychologist, 46,* 206–219.

Cushman, P. (1995). *Constructing the Self, constructing America: A cultural history of psychotherapy.* Addison-Wesley.

Dagfal, A. A. (2018). Psychology and psychoanalysis in Argentina: Politics, French thought, and the university connection, 1955–1976. *History of Psychology, 21*(3), 254–272.

Dal Corno, D. (1975). *Introduzione* [Introduction]. In Artemidoro (Ed.), *Il libro dei sogni* [The book of dreams] (pp. IX–LVIII). Adelphi.

Danziger, K. (1990). *Constructing the subject: Historical origins of psychological research.* Cambridge University Press.

Danziger, K. (2006). Universalism and indigenization in the history of modern psychology. In A. C. Brock (Ed.), *Internationalizing the history of psychology* (pp. 208–225). New York University Press.

Danziger, K. (2013). Psychology and its history. *Theory & Psychology, 23*(6), 829–839.

Descuret, J. B. F. (1841). *La médecine des passions ou Les passions considérées dans leurs rapports avec les maladies, les lois et la religion* [The medicine of passions or The passions considered in their relations with the diseases, the laws and the religion]. Labé.

Dodds, E. R. (1925). *The Greeks and the irrational.* University of California Press.

Dols, M. W. (1987). Insanity and its treatment in Islamic society. *Medical History, 31*(1), 1–14.

Dols, M. W. (1992). *Majnum: The madman in medieval Islamic society.* Clarendon Press.

Dörner, K. (1981). *Madmen and the bourgeoisie: A social history of insanity and psychiatry.* Blackwell. (Original edition published 1969)

Douthwaite, J. V. (2002). *The wild girl, natural man, and the monster.* University of Chicago Press.

Dowbiggin, I. (1991). *Inheriting madness: Professionalization and psychiatric knowledge in nineteenth-century France.* University of California Press.

Dulaey, M. (1973). *Le rêve dans la vie et la pensée de saint Augustin* [The dream in the life and thought of St, Augustin]. Études Augustiniennes.

Düring, I. (1966). *Aristoteles* [Aristotle]. Carl Winter.

Ehrenwald, J. (1956). *From medicine man to Freud.* Dell.

Ehrenwald, J. (Ed.). (1976). *The history of psychotherapy: From healing magic to encounter.* Jason Aronson.

Ellenberger, H. F. (1970). *The discovery of the unconscious: The history and evolution of dynamic psychiatry.* Basic Books.

Esquirol, J. É. D. (1805). *Des passions considérées comme causes, symptômes, et moyens curatifs de l'aliénation mentale* [Passions considered as causes, symptoms, and curative means of insanity]. Didot Jeune.

Flasch, K. (1971). *Augustin: Einführung in sein Denken* [Augustine: Introduction to his thought]. Reclam.

Foschi, R. (2012). *Maria Montessori*. Ediesse.

Foucault, M. (2003). *Le pouvoir psychiatrique. Cours au Collège de France 1973–1974* [Psychiatric power. Course at the Collège de France 1973–1974]. Gallimard.

Foucault, M. (2006). *History of madness*. Routledge. (Original edition published 1961)

Foucault, M. (2012). *The birth of the clinic*. Routledge. (Original edition published 1963)

Frankfort, H., Frankfort, H. A., Wilson, J. A., Jacobsen, T., & Irwin, W. A. (1977). *The intellectual adventure of ancient man*. University of Chicago Press. (Original edition published 1947)

Freedheim, D. K., Freudenberger, H. J., Kessler, J. W., Messer, S. B., Peterson, D. R., Strupp, H. H., & Wachtel, P. L. (1992). *History of psychotherapy: A century of change*. American Psychological Association.

Freud, S. (1958). The interpretation of dreams. First part. In *The standard edition of the complete psychological works of Sigmund Freud. Vol. 5*. Hogarth. (Original work published 1900).

Gauchet, M., & Swain, G. (2012). *Madness and democracy*. Princeton University Press. (Original work published 1980)

Giacanelli, F. (1975). Appunti per una storia della psichiatria in Italia [Notes for a history of psychiatry in Italy]. In K. Dörner (Ed.), *Il borghese e il folle* [Madmen and the bourgeoisie] (pp. V–XXXII). Laterza.

Goffman, E. (1961). *Asylums: Essays on the social situation of mental patients and other inmates*. Aldine Transaction.

Gold, H. R. (1957). *Psychiatry and the Talmud* (Vol. 1/1). Jewish Heritage.

Goldstein, J. E. (1987). *Console and classify: The French psychiatric profession in the nineteenth century*. University of Chicago Press.

Goulet-Cazé, M.-O. (2000). Cynicism. In J. Brunschwig & E. R. Lloyd (Eds.), *Greek thought* (pp. 843–857). Belknap Press.

Gourevitch, D. (1994). La psychiatrie de l'antiquité gréco-romaine [Psychiatry in the Greek-Roman age]. In J. Postel & C. Quétel (Eds.), *Nouvelle histoire de la psychiatrie* [New history of psychiatry] (pp. 3–23). Dunod.

Grmek, M. D. (1996). Il concetto di malattia [The concept of disease]. In *Storia del pensiero medico occidentale. Dal Rinascimento all'inizio dell'Ottocento, Vol. 2* [History of western medical thought. From the renaissance to the beginning of the nineteenth century] (pp. 259–289). Laterza.

Guarnieri, P. (2006). Un piccolo essere perverso. Il bambino nella cultura scientifica italiana tra Otto e Novecento [A perverse little being. The child in the Italian scientific culture between the nineteenth and twentieth centuries]. *Contemporanea, 9*(2), 253–284.

Hacking, I. (1995). *Rewriting the soul: Multiple personality and the sciences of memory*. Princeton University Press.

Hard, R., & Gill, C. (Eds.). (2014). *Epictetus. Discourses, fragments, handbook*. Oxford University Press.

Harrington, A. (2019). *Mind fixers: Psychiatry's troubled search for the biology of mental illness*. W. W. Norton.

Harris, B. (2016). Therapeutic work and mental illness in America, c. 1830–1970. In W. Ernst (Ed.), *Work, psychiatry and society, 1800–1950* (pp. 55–76). Manchester University Press.

Harris-McCoy, D. E. (Ed.). (2012). *Artemidorus' oneirocitica*. Oxford University Press.

Herzog, D. (2017). *Cold war Freud*. Cambridge University Press.

Innamorati, M. (2017b). Review of Cold War Freud, Psychiatry in communist Europe, and psiquiatría, psicoánalisis y cultura comunista: Batallas ideológicas en La Guerra

Fria [Psychiatry, psychoanalysis and communist culture: Ideological battles in the Cold War]. *History of Psychology, 20*(3), 330–335.

Innamorati, M., Taradel, R., & Foschi, R. (2019). Between sacred and profane: Possession, psychopathology, and the Catholic church. *History of Psychology, 22*(1), 1–16.

Jackson, S. W. (1999). *Care of the psyche: A history of psychological healing.* Yale University Press.

Jones, W. H. S. (1923). General introduction. In *Hippocrates (Works) I.* William Heinemann.

Jones, W. H. S. (Ed.). (1948a) *Cornelius Celsus. De Medicina.* Harvard University Press.

Jones, W. H. S. (1948b). Introduction. In *Cornelius Celsus. De Medicina* (pp. vii–xiv). Harvard University Press.

Kahn, C. (Ed.). (1979). *The art and thought of Heraclitus: An edition of the fragments with translation and commentary.* Cambridge University Press.

Kenny, A. (Ed.). (2013). *Aristotle. Poetics.* Oxford University Press.

Klibansky, R., Panofsky, E., & Saxl, F. (1964). *Saturn and melancholy.* Basic Books.

Koyré, A. (1948). Du monde de l'à peu près à l'univers de la précision [From the world of more-or-less to the universe of precision]. *Critique, 28*, 806–823.

Kuhn, T. S. (1962). *The structure of scientific revolutions.* University of Chicago Press.

Laín Entralgo, P. (1958). *The therapy of the word in classical antiquity.* Yale University Press.

Laks, A. (2000). Epicurus. In J. Brunschwig & E. R. Lloyd (Eds.), *Greek thought* (pp. 586–605). Belknap Press.

Lamb, W. R. M. (Ed.). (1927). *Plato with an English Translation. Vol. VIII.* William Heinemann.

Le Goff, J. (1964). *La civilisation de l'Occident medieval* [The civilization of the West during the Middle Ages]. Arthaud.

Lee, D. (Ed.). (1977). *Plato. Timaeus and Critias.* Penguin.

Liddell, R., & Scott, H. (1925). *A Greek-English Lexicon.* Oxford University Press. (Original work published 1819)

Lloyd, G. E. R. (1991). *Methods and problems in Greek Science.* Cambridge University Press.

Lombardo, G. P., & Foschi, R. (1999). Storia e categorie storiografiche della psicologia clinica [History and historiographic categories of clinical psychology]. In J. M. Reisman (Ed.), *Storia della psicologia clinica* [History of clinical psychology] (pp. IX–XL). Raffaello Cortina.

Lombardo, G. P., & Foschi, R. (2002a). The European origins of "personality psychology". *European Psychologist, 7*(2), 134–145.

Lombardo, G. P., & Foschi, R. (2002b). *La costruzione scientifica della personalità* [The scientific construction of personality]. Bollati Boringhieri.

Lombardo, G. P., & Pedone, G. (1995). *Normale e patologico nelle teorie della personalità* [Normal and pathological in the theories of personality]. Laterza.

Mancia, M. (1987). *Il sogno come religione della mente* [The dream as religion of mind]. Laterza.

Marks, S. (2017). Psychotherapy in historical perspective. *History of the Human Sciences, 30*(2), 3–16.

Marks, S. (2018). Suggestion, persuasion and work: Psychotherapies in communist Europe. *European Journal of Psychotherapy & Counselling, 20*(1), 10–24.

Martin, K. (2018). Transcultural histories of psychotherapy. *European Journal of Psychotherapy & Counselling, 20*(1), 104–119.

McReynolds, P. (1997). *Lightner Witmer: His life and times.* American Psychological Association.

Mecacci, L. (2000). *Il caso Marilyn M. e altri disastri della psicoanalisi* [The case Marilyn M. and other disasters of psychoanalysis]. Laterza.

Menghi, M. (1984). Introduzione [Introduction]. In Galeno (Galen) (Ed.), *Le passioni e gli errori dell'anima. Opere morali* [Passions and mistakes of the soul: Moral works] (pp. 7–20). Marsilio.

Millon, T. (2004). *Masters of the mind: Exploring the story of mental illness from ancient times to the new millennium.* Wiley.

Montuori, A. (2005). Gregory Bateson and the promise of transdisciplinarity. *Cybernetics & Human Knowing, 12*(1–2), 147–158.

Mora, G. (1985). History of psychiatry. In H. Kaplan & B. J. Sadock (Eds.), *Comprehensive textbook of psychiatry* (Vol. 4, pp. 1034–1054). Williams & Wilkins.

Musatti, C. (1976). Introduzione [Introduction]. In Artemidoro (Ed.), *Dell'interpretazione de' sogni* [On the interpretation of dreams]. Rizzoli.

Nasr, S. H. (1968). *Science and civilization in Islam.* Harvard University Press.

Norcross, J. C., VandenBos, G. R., & Freedheim, D. K. (2011). *History of psychotherapy: Continuity and change* (2nd ed.). American Psychological Association.

Nutton, V. (2004). *Ancient medicine.* Routledge.

Ohayon, A. (1999). *L'impossible rencontre. Psychologie et Psychanalyse en France 1919–1969* [The impossible encounter: Psychology and psychoanalysis in France 1919–1969]. La Découverte.

Omrani, A., Holtzman, N. S., Akiskal, H. S., & Ghaemi, S. N. (2012). Ibn Imran's 10th century treatise on melancholy. *Journal of Affective Disorders, 141*(2–3), 116–119.

Onians, R. B. (1954). *The origins of European thought.* Cambridge University Press.

Ottaviani, R., Vanni, D., & Vanni, P. (2004). *Trenta lezioni di storia della medicina* [Thirty lessons in history of medicine]. FrancoAngeli.

Parker, P. M. (Ed.). (2005). *The confessions of St. Augustine.* Icon.

Pick, D. (1993). *Faces of degeneration: A European disorder, c. 1848–1918.* Cambridge University Press.

Pickren, W. E. (2009). Indigenization and the history of psychology. *Psychological Studies, 54,* 87–95.

Pietikäinen, P. (2015). *Madness: A history.* Routledge.

Pinel, P. (1801). *Traité médico-philosophique sur l'aliénation mentale* [Medical-philosophical treatise on mental alienation]. Richard, Caille et Ravier.

Pinel, P. (1809). *Traité médico-philosophique sur l'aliénation mentale. Seconde édition, entièrement refondue et très-augmentée* [Medical-philosophical treatise on mental alienation. Second edition, entirely recast and much enlarged]. Brosson.

Pols, H. (2018). Towards trans-cultural histories of psychotherapies. *European Journal of Psychotherapy & Counselling, 20*(1), 88–103.

Porter, R. (1987). *A social history of madness.* Weidenfield & Nicolson.

Porter, R. (2002). *Madness: A brief history.* Oxford University Press.

Reale, G. (2009). Introduzione [Introduction]. In Epitteto (Ed.), *Opere* [Works]. Rusconi.

Reisman, J. M. (1991). *A history of clinical psychology.* Taylor & Francis.

Rialdi, G. (1968). *Introduzione allo studio della medicina nei Padri della Chiesa* [Introduction to the study of medicine of Church fathers]. Giardini.

Robinson, D. N. (2013). Historiography in psychology: A note on ignorance. *Theory & Psychology, 23*(6), 819–828.

Roccatagliata, G. (1973). *Storia della psichiatria antica* [History of ancient psychiatry]. Hoepli.

Rohde, E. (1925). *Psyche: The cult of souls and belief in immortality among the Greeks.* Kegan Paul, Trench, Trubenr & Co. (Original edition 1897)

Rose, H. J. (1925). *Primitive culture in Greece.* Methuen.

Rosner, R. I. (2018). History and the topsy-turvy world of psychotherapy. *History of Psychology, 21*(3), 177.

Ross, D. (1995). *Aristotle.* Routledge. (Original edition published 1923)

Roudinesco, E. (1982). *Histoire de la psychanalyse en France* [History of psychoanalysis in France] (Vol. 1). Seuil.

Roudinesco, E. (1986). *Histoire de la psychanalyse en France* [History of psychoanalysis in France] (Vol. 2). Seuil.

Routh, D. K., & Barrio, V. D. (1996). European roots of the first psychology clinic in North America. *European Psychologist, 1*(1), 44–50.

Scharfetter, C. (1980). *General psychopathology: An introduction.* CUP Archive.

Sellars, J. (2019). *Lessons in stoicism.* Penguin.

Shamdasani, S. (2005). 'Psychotherapy': The invention of a word. *History of the Human Sciences, 18*(1), 1–22.

Shamdasani, S. (2017). Psychotherapy in society: Historical reflections. In G. Eghigian (Ed.), *The Routledge history of madness and mental health* (pp. 363–378). Routledge.

Shamdasani, S. (2018). Towards transcultural histories of psychotherapies. *European Journal of Psychotherapy & Counselling, 20*(1), 4–9.

Shorter, E. (1997). *A history of psychiatry. From the era of the asylum to the age of Prozac.* Wiley.

Simonnet, J. (1994). Folie et notations psychopathologiques dans l'oeuvre de Thomas d'Aquin [Madness and psychopathological notes in the work of THomas Aquinas]. In J. Postel & C. Quétel (Eds.), *Nouvelle histoire de la psychiatrie* [New history of psychiatry] (pp. 48–56). Dunod.

Singer, P. N. (Ed.). (2013). *Galen. Psychological works.* Cambridge University Press.

Sloterdijk, P. (1983). *Critique of cynical reason.* Verso.

Spanneut, M. (1973). *Permanemce du Stoicisme: De Zénon à Malraux* [Permanence of stoicism: From zeno to malraux]. Gembloux.

Tallis, F. (2002). *Hidden minds: A history of the unconscious.* Arcade Publishing.

Taylor, C. (1989). *Sources of the self: The making of the modern identity.* Harvard University Press.

Thumiger, C., & Singer, P. N. (2018). Introduction. In C. Thumiger & P. N. Singer (Eds.), *Mental illness in ancient medicine* (pp. 1–32). Brill.

Trevi, M., & Innamorati, M. (2000). *Riprendere Jung* [The heritage of Jung]. Bollati Boringhieri.

Tuke, S. (1813). *Description of the retreat, an institution near York, for insane persons of the Society of Friends.* Peirce.

Vegetti, M. (1984). La terapia dell'anima. Patologia e disciplina del soggetto in Galeno [The therapy of the soul: Pathology and discipline of the soul]. In Galeno (Galen) (Ed.), *Le passioni e gli errori dell'anima. Opere morali* [Passions and mistakes of the soul: Moral works] (pp. 131–155). Marsilio.

Vegetti, M. (1985). *Tra Edipo e Euclide* [Between Oedipus and Euclides]. il Saggiatore.

Walker, N. (1957). *A short history of psychotherapy: In theory and practice.* Routledge & Kegan Paul.

Whitwell, J. R. (1936). *Historical notes on psychiatry.* Lewis.

Whyte, L. L. (1960). *The unconscious before Freud.* Basic Books.

Young, R. M. (1990). *Mind, brain, and adaptation in the nineteenth century: Cerebral localization and its biological context from Gall to Ferrier.* Oxford University Press.

Zilboorg, G., & Henry, G. W. (1941). *A history of medical psychology.* W. W. Norton.

Zipoli, R. (Ed.). (1981). *Kay Kā'ūs ibn Iskandar, Il libro dei consigli* [The book of suggestions]. Adelphi.

2

From hypnotism to psychotherapy

Exorcism, Enlightenment, and Magnetism

Many ancient practices of mind healing can be considered exemplary for later history. They developed in very ancient times and were not classically related to medicine: ritual dances, mystical-religious beliefs, shamanism, practices against the evil eye, quacks, magicians, and so on. They were based on a liberating function that was culturally legitimized and, like moral theories, aimed at socializing and regulating individual emotions and passions.[1] These practices shared with psychotherapy the general idea of warding off the evil that lurked in people's souls. They were magical forms of intervention that ran parallel to other attempts to heal people physically and psychically.[2]

Pastoral guidance and confession, on the other hand, have represented a mystical-religious approach to caring for the soul, which seems to have more points of contact with the origins of psychotherapy. Christianity has always taken care of the souls of the faithful, working with techniques of conviction and persuasion to direct them on the right path and, where necessary, to make them understand the truth.

It seemed necessary to control, with institutions such as the Inquisition, heterodox individuals, finally eliminating the irreducible (see Ginzburg, 1980). In the pastoral setting, exorcism deserves special attention. As is well illustrated by Ellenberger (1970), exorcism was conventionally schematized into phases, paradoxically similar to those of diagnosis and treatment in psychotherapy. First of all, the exorcist had to verify the real presence of the evil (the pathology). Then, through prayer, he had to drive away the entity that he presumed possessed the sick person. In this context, it is clear that the line between reality and fiction, sacred and profane, mental pathology and religious belief, was very blurred.

Exorcist priest Johann Joseph Gassner (1727–1779) played a pivotal role in the transition from religious to secular cures, which emerged based on Enlightenment demands. Gassner was a Catholic who attempted to cure the most varied diseases as if they were all the work of the devil. He operated with complex exorcistic practices in 18th-century central Europe, both among Catholics

DOI: 10.4324/9781003252405-2

and Protestants. Somehow his work was a problem for both theology and the Enlightenment. His idea of finding a common ground for diseases was followed by Franz Anton Mesmer (1734–1815), who, however, achieved the same results as Gassner through nonreligious practices. He showed that phenomena that Gassner attributed to the supernatural could be brought back into the natural sciences (see Crabtree, 2008; Ellenberger, 1970; Midelfort, 2005).[3] Mesmer, drawing heavily from the science of the day, used the ideas of electricity, gravity, and terrestrial magnetism as the foundation of his belief that a system of forces conditioned not only nature and the Earth but also body and mind. In the case of human beings, health and disease were linked to the so-called *magnetism* (Traetta, 2007). If, for Gassner, the disease depended on the action of the Evil, according to Mesmer, it was due to an imbalance of a *magnetic fluid* (especially to a deficiency of it), which, through the practices of magnetization, could be harmonized (see Mesmer, 1779).

Magnetism was also used in what one can consider the first form of "group therapy,"[4] consisting of meetings held around a *baquet*, a large wooden container with iron *cannulae*, that were held by the hands of the participants, placed around the *baquet* and also tied together by ropes. By means of this procedure it would be possible to rebalance the hidden force that conditioned the nervous system. The therapeutic process also took place through *magnetic crises*, conveyed by the magnetizer, in individual therapy, and by the *baquet*, in group therapy.

In Vienna, Mesmer had made his home a meeting place to circulate his ideas on animal magnetism. In addition to his suggestive practices, the use of magnets and the *baquet*, Mesmer used music. In particular, he used the *glass harmonica*. This instrument had been developed by Benjamin Franklin (1706–1790) and could spread melodies that seemed particularly suggestive and useful to the healing process. As will be seen, however, Franklin himself, one of the founding fathers of the United States and a scholar of electricity, played a role of *expertise* in the process of discrediting Mesmerism.

Franklin and Mesmer represented two different ways of looking at the hidden forces of nature. The former used systematic observation; the latter was more prone to methodological eclecticism. Both were prestigious exponents of Freemasonry, influenced in different ways by the esotericism learned in the lodges. Franklin applied it according to the experimental method, going in systemic search of the electromagnetic forces of the Earth. Mesmer, driven by the urgency of finding an efficient cure for pathological phenomena, based his theory of animal magnetism on labile and imprecise evidence.[5] As a result, Mesmer's ideas were also used, in spite of himself, in an occultist perspective by a series of his followers, who proposed to control the obscure forces acting in nature through the practice of magnetization. The history of occultism – in all its forms (magic, mind-reading, telekinesis, spiritualism) – starting from the 18th-century Mesmerism began to run parallel to that of experimental psychology, at least until the first half of the 20th century.[6] Probably because of the dangers he saw in the magical practices, and also convinced that it was not possible to prove the existence of animal magnetism, Franklin opposed Mesmerism. To Mesmer then happened what had already happened to Gassner. In 1784, two royal commissions were created to analyze animal magnetism: composed of the most important scientists of the time, both from universities and from science academies. The first one was headed by Franklin himself, the second was composed exclusively of members of the Société Royale de Médecine.[7] Mesmer did not participate directly in the work of the commissions. The role of defender of Mesmerism was played by a dissident student of his, Charles Nicolas Deslon (1750–1786), who was part of the medical establishment in Paris. He even tried to *mesmerize* Franklin himself. The conclusions of both commissions denied the existence of animal magnetism as an authentic physical phenomenon, claiming that all evidence in support of it was due to the power of *imagination* and *imitation* (Franklin, 1837; see Turbiaux, 2009). A secret report to the king was also written, which further scuttled the possibility of the affirmation of animal magnetism, pointing out that magnetic practices would have even been morally dangerous. Erotic bonds could be easily established between the magnetizer and the magnetized because of the touches and attitudes during the sessions (Carroy, 1991). The conclusions also unmasked a certain crudely materialistic aspect of Mesmerism and credited, therefore, psychopathological and psychological phenomena cured by magnetic practices to psychological causes. The origins of the cured ailments were not thought to be the product of an obscure natural force as believed by Mesmer and his students.

The Society of Harmony

Mesmer's choice of Masonry was not accidental but the result of a political vocation that tried to spread new egalitarian ideas in the heart of Europe through magnetism. The Mozart family had a close friendship with the Mesmer family, and the Mozarts and the Mesmers were in turn at the center of a network that included leading figures from societies related to the Enlightenment, Freemasonry, and the Bavarian Illuminati.[8] An ideal foundation of Mesmerism was, therefore, the spread of a cure that could be innovative, enlightened, scientific, and able to benefit humanity in an effective, economic, and democratic way. Medicine had not yet made great progress, was far from being experimental, and, moreover, was not practiced among the majority of the population. The use of the *baquet* itself was considered by Mesmer's contemporaries to be democratic, capable of uniting around the same tub people from different social classes and of circulating energy in an interclass way (Bramani, 2005, p. 12). Mesmer wrote to defend himself:

> In France, the cure of a poor person is nothing. Four cures of bourgeoisie are not worth that of a marquis or a count: The cure of four marquises is hardly equivalent to that of a duke, and four cures of dukes are not worth

anything compared to that of a prince. What a contrast with my ideas, since I thought I would deserve the attention of the world, even if I had only cured dogs!

(Mesmer, 1781/1971, p. 198; see Rausky, 1977)

As pointed out by Darnton (1968) and Giarrizzo (1994), for the diffusion of magnetism, Mesmer founded in Paris the Société de l'Harmonie (Society of Harmony; 1783–1784), a society with rites very similar to the Masonic ones (Darnton, 1968, pp. 180–181), devoted to the change of humanity, with programs therefore comparable to those of the Enlightenment Freemasonry:

While the whole of nature ceaselessly shows, in the same principle, the harmony of the worlds and the life of all beings, man lost through the abuse of his reason still misunderstands this sublime truth. (. . .) The theory of magnetism will be for men the gospel of nature (. . .); it will show them virtue is always followed by health and happiness (. . .).

(Mesmer, 1785/1971, pp. 209–210)

Specifically, Darnton (1968) pointed out that Mesmer, with the support of the economically and culturally wealthier bourgeoisie, promised a program for the improvement of humanity, public health, and morals, thus trying to revolutionize the welfare state and health, by means of magnetic practices. He represented, therefore, an intellectual transition to the age of the Revolution. In support of this thesis, it should be noted that some mesmerists – such as Nicolas Bergasse (1750–1832), the Marquis de Lafayette (1757–1834), and Jacques Pierre Brissot (1754–1793) – actually participated in the establishment of the new French state and the events related to the Revolution of 1789. The Société de l'Harmonie achieved a certain success, gathering several hundred affiliates with a diffusion in some major cities in France (see Armando & Belhoste, 2018).[9]

From Mesmerism to induced somnambulism

Armand-Marie-Jacques de Chastenet (1751–1825), better known simply as Marquis de Puységur, also played a fundamental role in the history of Mesmerism. Initiated into Freemasonry and associated with the Société de l'Harmonie, Puységur completed the process of democratization of Mesmerism, bringing it to less affluent people, specifically peasants of the town of Buzancy, in the Picardy region, where his estates were located.

Puységur chose and *magnetized* a large elm tree (a tree that in ancient times was already considered sacred and a symbol of sleep and dreams). Through the tree, he aimed to free the peasants from their illnesses, convincing them to become their own healers. The magnetized tree represented a sort of social cure, whose therapeutic virtues all citizens could freely draw upon. Ordinary people were tied around the tree with long ropes, just as aristocrats and bourgeois were gathered around the *baquet*. Thus, mesmerism operated a sort of reversal of the doctor-patient relationship. The patients became fundamental for the elaboration of the Mesmerizers' theories, and, at the same time, they could acquire a wealth of therapeutic knowledge, in a sort of initiatory-esoteric training process, which put them on the same level as the doctor. The culture of magnetism, at least in Puységur's version, overturned and gave new meaning to the classically asymmetrical relationship of the medical clinic (Carroy, 1991; Gallini, 1983; see also Belhoste & Edelman, 2015).[10]

The patient, in turn, became a therapist, establishing a new egalitarian horizon that had never before been possible. Such an equal relationship, however, immediately seemed dangerous to some. One can speculate that academic opposition to magnetization reflected a fear of these novelties, of which magnetism was the bearer. Perhaps the 19th-century reemergence of magnetist culture in the new guise of hypnotism, which cleared away what was judged dangerous, improper, and metaphysical in magnetism, was also due to an attempt to restore traditional healing relationships, which should have remained asymmetrical.[11]

The magnetized tree seemed to be able to heal many people at the same time, harmonizing their psychophysical state. The trees of the magnetizers soon turned into the trees of liberty of the French Revolution. They were almost always elms, just like the one in Buzancy; the trees of liberty became a popular symbol of a new epoch ushered in by the French Revolution, an epoch that would definitively overcome the Ancien Régime. These trees were planted in the main squares of all the communes of France and in every place where the French model inspired revolution. The tree of liberty became the living symbol of the ideas of 1789. Puységur, however, hypothesized that magnetism was due to a specific fluid. He thought that magnetic crises were psychologically triggered by the patients' desire to heal and were attributable to an altered state of consciousness, which he began to call "induced somnambulism," because it actually resembled natural somnambulism (Puységur, 1811). With Puységur a *psychofluidic* current of Mesmerism was born, which replaced magnetism with a mental cause, linked to the imagination and to the will of the magnetized person (Méheust, 1999).

Magnetism was thus emancipated from Mesmer's theory and gradually transformed into hypnotism, through a simplification of the theory and a confinement of practices to a patient-therapist relationship, rather than referring to a great palingenetic theory, like the one advocated by Mesmer. Some illustrious names completed the transition to true hypnotism, among them José Custódio de Faria, *aka* Abbot Faria (1756–1819), Joseph Philippe François Deleuze (1753–1835), but especially Alexandre Bertrand (1795–1831).

Abbot Faria is known to have accentuated the psychological and relational component of magnetic practices, which with him began to resemble what, as will be seen, would become the suggestive relationship. Deleuze, on the other hand, was the organizer of a magnetism that, in the Napoleonic and Restoration eras, gave itself new structures and institutions, founding in 1813 the

Société du Magnétisme de Paris (Society of Magnetism of Paris) and publishing editorial series and journals, modeled on other fields of scientific research (Gauld, 1992). Before its definitive replacement by hypnotism, Alexandre Bertrand was the most important systematizer, from a theoretical point of view, of magnetism. Bertrand had initially defended a conception that was faithful to Mesmer. However, he later developed an entirely psychological idea of the magnetic relationship, which for him was certainly not due to the effects of an unproven entity such as the magnetic fluid but was the result of the magnetizer-magnetized relationship, which caused sleepwalking phenomena during an artificially induced sleep (Bertrand, 1823; see Gauld, 1992). Bertrand also began to consider dreams as means of understanding the mind, preceding psychoanalysis by about 80 years (Carroy, 1991, p. 143).

Induced somnambulism constituted the transition from magnetism to suggestive and hypnotic practices.[12] It was also considered *both* a means for the psychological investigation of the inner world of man *and* a psychotherapeutic method. This dual role remained typical of the first real psychotherapeutic practices. Psychoanalysis itself was considered by Sigmund Freud to be a method of psychological research, as well as a specific form of psychotherapy.

Carroy (1991) also pointed out that magnetic culture survived throughout the 19th century and, despite being hampered by official medicine and science, took root. In Paris, in the 1880s of the 19th century, there were about 40,000 followers of the various institutions related to magnetism, 500 magnetizing cabinets, and 20 specialized newspapers. It is possible that the magnetic culture was considered by many as a culture of compensation, which opposed the post-Napoleonic Restoration era. Along these lines, some revolutionaries of 1848 later formed the generation of great medical reformers who reused magnetism, under the new guise of hypnotism, in the halls of the great university hospitals. Bertrand, who was a physician and a member of the Charbonnerie,[13] was also an opponent of the Restoration and wrote the texts on which forty-eighters[14] such as Jean-Martin Charcot (1825–1893), Ambroise-Auguste Liébeault (1823–1904), and their successors, such as Hippolyte Bernheim (1840–1919), Charles Richet (1850–1935), and Pierre Janet (1859–1947), were formed.[15] Carroy (1991) showed that induced somnambulism/magnetism had also been disseminated in paramedical settings and, by 1870, integrated into official science by doctors at the top of their career who, "by putting their patients to sleep, no doubt, regained their lost youth" (p. 41) and the time they were trained on magnetizer texts. The advent of hypnotism through magnetic practices – the so-called late 19th-century rediscovery of magnetism – was thus also favored by the particular relational conditions that bound magnetizer to magnetized and mimicked an erotic relationship, made of proximity and touching.

This multifaceted culture of the late 19th century emerged clearly at the first International Congress for Experimental and Therapeutic Hypnotism, held in Paris in August 1889. This congress also marked the official transition of hypnotic techniques to the medical sphere: the participants, by means of a resolution later sent to the French government, demanded that only the medical and academic use of hypnotism be permitted, and that public and collective use be prohibited (Bérillon, 1890).[16]

Psychology and hypnotism

Hypnosis and suggestion were thus considered therapeutic means and research tools for psychology, a discipline that gradually tended to be represented as *scientific* and *experimental*, as opposed to speculative philosophic psychology. The devotees of the new psychology were all positivists *sui generis*. Auguste Comte (1798–1857), the founder of French positivism, considered psychology a discipline incapable of achieving the status of a true science, since the mind was both the subject and the object of investigation (lecture 45 of the *Cours de philosophie positive*; see Clauzade, 2003). Rather, human conduct should have been studied through brain physiology, as far as the individual was concerned, and through sociology, for the implications of interaction with others (see lectures 56 and 58). Other positivists, especially proponents of evolutionism, supported instead the legitimacy of psychology, thanks to its links with physiology and medicine. The best-known names associated with this approach were those of Théodule-Armand Ribot (1839–1916) and Hippolyte Taine (1828–1893) in France, Roberto Ardigò (1828–1920) in Italy, Herbert Spencer (1820–1903) and Alexander Bain (1818–1903) in England, and Wilhelm Wundt (1832–1920) in Germany (see Baker, 2012).[17] The experimental psychology of the last quarter of the 19th century, in essence, included all possible *fin de siècle* streams of research on the mind. In that sense, the term *experimental* had been accepted with a double meaning, that of laboratory experimentation, according to the German model, and that of a broader systemic study of phenomena based on experience. It is now well known that, at the end of the 19th century, French psychology presented itself as a real alternative model to the German one and promoted a different conception of the first psychological research and of the first applications. This occurred during the period of the Third Republic, characterized by the strong modernization and secularization of French society in view of a complete overcoming of the mentality and culture of the Ancien Régime and the Restoration that, until 1870, had opposed the progressive, republican, and socialist ones. Medicine was at the forefront of the modernization process, and, inspired by Ribot, the first exponents of scientific psychology were trained as philosophers and as physicians: Janet was somewhat the progenitor of a long and illustrious tradition of French intellectuals that culminated with Georges Canguilhem (1904–1995) and Michel Foucault (1926–1984).[18] From this perspective, one can also better understand a singular historiographical phenomenon: a sort of eclipse from the international historiography of French pathological psychology in favor of the history of German psychology (Carroy, 1991, 2000; Carroy et al., 2006; Danziger, 1990; Foschi, 2003a). The French approach of the second half of the 19th century differed because it took hypnosis as an experimental technique, in a laboratory setting, in which the subjects were primarily young hysterics, to explore the more hidden aspects of consciousness and to resolve its pathologies.[19] Because the use of hypnosis originated in the medical field, its history was evidently considered to be traceable more to medicine than to psychology.

Psychological schools compared

France and Germany were competing, with clearly differentiated research traditions, in the field of the treatment of mental pathologies, as in the study of the normal mind. In Germany, the path pursued was all within the normal physiology and physiopathology of the brain: the mind could be investigated in the laboratory with an appropriate adaptation of physiological methods, especially through the use of reaction time recordings and the stimulation of different sensory pathways. In Germany, moreover, psychology was constructed on the basis of the professor-student relationship: the first pole represented the observing scientist, while at the other was the observed student as a lab rat. According to Danziger (1990, pp. 68–70), in this German model, in order to describe the *normal* functioning of the mind, the poles of the research relationship were interchangeable, in contrast to the French model, which was primarily *clinical* and based on the asymmetrical doctor-patient relationship.[20]

In France, as will be seen in the following paragraphs, the hypnotic method and the *pathological* method were used above all. According to Jacqueline Carroy (1991), the conviction that hypnotism was a practice that could fall within the domain of experimental knowledge of the mind was particularly popularized by three people: the aforementioned Jean-Martin Charcot, Eugène Azam (1822–1899), and especially Henri-Etienne Beaunis (1830–1921).[21] Those who, through hypnosis, were placed in a state of immobility were considered as psychologically livable subjects who could be investigated in the laboratory through the same hypnotic situation. The so-called *pathological* method had a wide use, especially from 1870 and through the work of Taine and Ribot. Its assumption was based on a paradigmatic idea, already widely developed by French medicine: that pathology resulted from the *quantitative* alteration of normal phenomena. The parallel idea that the pathology corresponded to an experiment induced by nature could also be applied in psychology. In this perspective, the pathological fact was also the privileged object of research, with the ultimate goal of knowing the normal functioning of psychological dynamism.

The approaches, however, were not mutually exclusive. Hypnosis was also used as an experimental technique by Ribot himself, who in his first lecture on experimental psychology stated: "Hypnosis is practically the only form of psychological experimentation in France" (Ribot, 1888, p. 451). The hypnotic method, however, began to be used in France in the therapeutic field as well. In this context, suggestion made its appearance at the same time as hypnosis, to which it was always intrinsically linked. It became the bridge between hypnotic psychotherapy and psychotherapy based on words (and on the relationship between patient and therapist). Technically, suggestion was (and is) a process of psychological influence, achieved by word or gesture, which has a nonreflexive nature. The beliefs and perceptions suggested are assumed without critical elaboration by the suggested person.

The suggestive process, therefore, misleads the critical and perceptual functions of the individual. Suggestion may involve the exercise of power by the influencer over the influenced person, and the process of influencing is always psychosocial in nature. Persuasion, imitation, deception, social contagion, *placebo* effect,[22] illusion, and sleight of hand are all phenomena that can be linked to hypnosuggestion.

Hypnosis and suggestion, though related, represented two different looks at the psychological nature of the individual. Hypnotists defended the idea that hypnotizability was an alteration of the state of consciousness due to the individual qualities of people. Suggestion theorists emphasized the importance of the act of suggestion rather than the specific quality of the person being suggested. For them, hypnosis would have been nothing more than an altered state of consciousness linked to a heightened susceptibility to suggestion. Even today, experimental investigations concerning the dependence/independence of the suggestive phenomenon on the hypnotic one do not clarify the connections between the two conditions. In any case, at the origins of psychology and psychotherapy there are two techniques, hypnosis and suggestion, which also represented a different sensitivity to the dialectic between the individual and the context.

Individual or context?

As Ellenberger (1970) amply illustrated, the conception of hypnosis and suggestion became the object of dispute between two groups of French neurologists, which have gone down in history as the School of Paris and the School of Nancy. This dispute influenced an entire generation of scholars, both in experimentation and in psychotherapeutic applications. The founder of the School of Paris was Jean-Martin Charcot, leader of a host of scholars who passed through the Salpêtrière Hospital. For Charcot, it was essential to identify an objective basis of hypnotic and hysterical phenomena, and he came to the conclusion that hypnotizability was a symptom of hysteria, linked to the nervous system. Only those suffering from hysteria and who were subject to hysterical attacks would be susceptible to being hypnotized. Other symptoms would have characterized the personality of hysterics as real and permanent hysterical stigmata, like pain in the ovaries or belly, and gynecological disorders. Charcot actually used hypnosis as a clinical method to study hysteria.[23] In his opinion, every attack of hysteria could be divided into phases, the transitions of which could be hypnotically procured on command. In particular, in great hysterical attacks, according to Charcot, there were generally prodromes, the epileptoid phase (with states of tetanism), clownism (or a phase of large movements), the phase of passionate attitudes, and delirium. After these critical phases there was resolution. The phases could occur in the sequence just described, or be interspersed with temporary resolution or lethargy. Fundamental was the idea that the phases expressed the neurological condition of the patients. Hysteria was thus compared to epilepsy, which would have presented similar phases. For Charcot and the Parisian doctors, the symptoms were due to lesions of the nervous system of a *dynamic* type, that is, not localized, but able to affect the brain organ from time to time in different locations, "projecting" outside changing symptoms, and difficult to classify or understand from a neurological point of view.[24]

The School of Charcot[25] should therefore be considered fundamentally a school of clinical neurology, interested in highlighting symptoms, similarities, and differences between different diseases of the nervous system. Paris was basically a gymnasium for the training of many doctors and researchers interested in the neurological and physical study of hysteria, evaluated, as well as through hypnosis, with the use of other means. Victor Burq (1822–1884), for example, used metals for diagnosis and therapy (metal therapy), investigating how they could make hysterical symptoms appear and disappear – for example, a contracture – or transfer them from one part of the body to another (see Binet & Féré, 1885). In this sense, at the Salpêtrière, concepts of a physical and neurological kind were elaborated, which were later used, especially within Freudian theory, albeit through a metaphor (Sulloway, 1979).

For the history of psychotherapy, the role of the institutions and their relationships with their Parisian hypnotists was very important. Marie "Blanche" Wittman, Augustine Gleizes,[26] and other patients became real hospital and academic celebrities, linked to their doctor-hypnotist. Blanche was portrayed together with Charcot in a very famous painting by the painter Pierre André Brouillet, as the paradigmatic patient of the hypnotic and hysterical phases that the scholar described and passed on to his illustrious students and listeners.

The images of the patients of the Salpêtrière still illustrate how the Parisian individualist paradigm was constructed. The hypnotist assumed as real and authentic all the phenomena shown by the hypnotized woman. He did not take into account his own role of power in the relationship, nor the secondary benefits that the hypnotized Parisian woman, who came from a working-class background, would have obtained as a model patient, usable for the lessons and iconographies of the Salpêtrière. Such secondary benefits created a veritable culture of late 19th-century hysteria and the epidemic phase of the disease (Bourneville & Regnard, 1876–1880; see also Carroy, 1991, 1993; Didi-Huberman, 2004; Hacking, 1995; Hustvedt, 2011; Plas, 2000).[27]

Hippolyte Bernheim was the best known of the hypnotists associated with the so-called School of Nancy (founded by Liébeault). He was the leader of those who considered hypnosis a contextual and suggestive phenomenon rather than an individual symptomatic one. Bernheim maintained, contrary to the Parisians, that no neuropathological or psychopathological fact could be traced back to hypnosis, which should be considered instead as a product of the *relationship* between the influencer and the influenced. As for the alleged empirical demonstrations in support of the Parisian conceptions, they were in fact simulations. The characteristic phenomenon of posthypnotic suggestion – to assume, while awake, behaviors suggested in the state of hypnotic sleep – for Nancy's theorists would have demonstrated that hypnosis was only an epiphenomenon of suggestion. With Bernheim's ideas, suggestion became a concept with potentially wide application. Jules Joseph Liégeois (1833–1908), working with Bernheim himself, demonstrated that even crimes could be suggested and caused by posthypnotic suggestion.[28] The crowd, on the other hand, would also have been the product of imitative and suggestive links (Tarde, 1890). It would also have been easily conditioned by a directing instructor.[29]

The conception of suggestion proposed by the Nancy School has since that time influenced the practices of scientific psychology and psychotherapy far more than has been finally recognized by historiography (see Carroy, 1991).[30]

Healing the personality: consciousness revisited

Within French pathological psychology, personality was no longer considered an object of philosophic research connected to consciousness, but a concrete entity that could be "affected by disease." With Ribot, personality was defined as a *tout de coalition* (a whole, made of a coalition), an empirically detectable composite of physiological, affective, and intellectual states. In this way, the way was paved for the componential model on the basis of which the personality would have become the object of scientific knowledge during the 20th century, assuming new features even in culture (Lombardo & Foschi, 2002a, 2002b, 2003).

Personality became a construct to be studied scientifically when some anomalies in its functioning were noticed and described clinically, implying a discontinuity in consciousness and in the very existence of people. The phenomena of pathology of consciousness and pathology of personality, studied in France since 1870, were functional in legitimizing this new scientific and philosophical perspective. They became in fact a very effective empirical argument to oppose those who (from a spiritualist or positivist perspective) challenged the idea that consciousness was not unitary and resisted the very possibility of an experimental psychology. In any case, the study of dissociative phenomena led to investigating consciousness by means of the pathological method (see Foschi, 2003a; Hacking, 1995).

The psychological investigation of personality was therefore developed in the context of clinical and experimental research on consciousness. The pioneers of these investigations systematically described clinical cases of personality disorders and hypothesized mechanisms that regulated the normal and pathological functioning of consciousness. Thus, *multiple personality* became, next to hysteria, an exemplary pathology, undermining the idea that the individual acted by controlling his or her own behavior and making rational choices determined by consciousness. The two different personalities of the young Félida X, described by Eugène Azam, or the many personalities of the young sailor Louis Vivet, described by the doctors Henri Bourru (1840–1914) and Prosper Ferdinand Burot (1849–1921), showed all the limits of the idealist and spiritualist philosophy when it assumed consciousness as a fundamental and undivided function able to make individuals know reality (Azam, 1876a, 1876b, 1877; Bourru & Burot, 1888). Doubts were thus raised about the unitary nature of the individual. Such doubts helped to legitimize the French scientific psychology by providing it with an empirical conception of the mind as its object of study to be investigated by hypnosuggestion. The new method promised to clarify, better than the philosophic-introspective one, how consciousness realistically operates.[31]

François Broussais (1772–1838) was the key figure in the development of the pathological method, which led to the foundation in France of a positive perspective in psychology. A physiologist, Broussais was a pupil and the personal physician of Franz Joseph Gall (1758–1828). He was also an outspoken opponent of philosophic psychology. Between 1822 and 1823, Broussais theorized that the functions of the healthy man could be understood by studying the sick, a few years later he based an entire volume – devoted to the relationship between physiology and "moral pathology" – on the assumption that pathology and mental health were determined by the same principle: arousal. Normal arousal would lead to normal existence, while excessive arousal would cause irritation, the source of moral pathology (Broussais, 1828). The consequent idea that pathology resulted in continuity with normality was christened by Auguste Comte "Broussais's principle." The result was a conception of general pathology and mental pathology that contrasted with the nosographic and classificationist view of the alienists (Braunstein, 1986; Chazaud, 1992).

French experimental psychology, influenced by the principle of Broussais, studied the pathological as if it were an experiment,[32] spontaneously performed by nature, impossible to reproduce in the laboratory, but able to show the researcher the basic elements constituting psychological phenomena, which in normality function in an integrated way and in pathology are disaggregated, dividing.

It was Ribot who developed the first specific theory of personality based on the same principle. According to his conception, personality and ego-consciousness would be but the result of kinesthetic processing[33] and memory work. Ribot assumed an evolutionary perspective, whereby, on the one hand, the most complex psychological functions (memory, will, feelings) were phylogenetically formed from the simpler, in a *continuum* that led to considering pure motion as the simplest one. On the other hand, in contrast, pathology would have been determined by a regression, that is, by an inverse process on the evolutionary scale. The more complex elements of the more evolved functions would be lost first, in the less serious forms of pathology. In the more severe forms, one would progressively lose the elements of decreasing complexity, eventually leading to the loss of the functions themselves and, in extreme cases, to the preservation of only the most primitive and unconscious capacities, such as reflexes (see Innamorati, 2005).[34]

Pierre Janet, one of the main pupils of Ribot and Charcot, and grandson of Paul Janet (1823–1899)[35] (a real mandarin of the eclectic-spiritualist philosophy), was then the most consistent continuer of the French psychopathological approach. Janet made empirical the theoretical framework envisaged by his teacher: he built, therefore, in turn, a theory of personality that became fundamental for the history of psychotherapy.

Pierre Janet and psychological analysis

Pierre Janet, although he was one of the main scholars of the so-called School of Paris, can also be considered the most important systematizer of the use of hypnosuggestion for therapeutic purposes. His perspective can be considered the opposite of Sigmund Freud's, who developed the psychoanalytic setting just as a barrier to suggestion. Janet was born in Paris in 1859 to a bourgeois family of liberal orientation, and lived until the age of 87, along the entire span of the Third Republic. His scholastic and academic career was exemplary: he first studied at the Collège Sainte-Barbe in Paris, then at the Lycée Louis-le-Grand, and finally at the École Normale Supérieure. In 1883, he arrived at the lycée in Le Havre as a professor of philosophy and he spent six and a half years there (1883–1889). In Le Havre, Janet met Dr. Joseph Gilbert (1829–1899), by whom he was urged to study induced somnambulism, and he began to conduct experiments in hypnosis on young women, including Léonie and Lucie, who became his famous clinical cases. From the research begun in Le Havre, which earned him the interest of Ribot and Charcot, Janet drew his first doctoral thesis, in philosophy, which made him notable: *L'automatisme psychologique: Essai de psychologie expérimentale sur les formes inférieures de l'activité humaine* (*Psychological automatism: Essay of experimental psychology on the inferior forms of human activity*). The thesis, discussed on June 21, 1889, was immediately issued by the publisher Alcan (Janet, 1889). In 1889, he also embarked on medical studies, with many internships in hospitals in Paris (Laennec, St-Antoine, and, in particular, Salpêtrière), and devoted himself to clinical training (Ellenberger, 1970). In the same year he took part in the first International Congress of Psychology held in Paris, on the initiative of Ribot and Charcot. Charcot himself called him to direct the laboratory of psychology of the Salpêtrière. On July 29, 1893, Janet discussed his second thesis, in medicine, *Contribution à l'étude des accidents mentaux chez les hystériques*.

In 1895, Janet replaced Ribot at the Collège de France in teaching experimental and comparative psychology. Between 1897 and 1898 he was still professor of philosophy at the Lycée Condorcet, but in 1898 he obtained the complementary course of experimental psychology at the Faculty of Letters of the Sorbonne, which had already been held by Ribot. In 1900, he was secretary of the Fourth International Congress of Psychology in Paris and edited the publication of the proceedings. In 1901, he founded the Société de Psychologie; in 1902, he definitively obtained the chair of experimental psychology at the Collège de France that Ribot had by then left, and in 1903 he founded the journal *Journal de Psychologie Normale et Pathologique*. In 1910, Jules Dejerine (1849–1917), the new director of the Salpêtrière, removed him from the direction of the psychology laboratory, officially because he did not approve psychological investigation of patients. With Dejerine, the Salpêtrière returned to being primarily an institution concerned with neurology *stricto sensu*. In addition to theses in philosophy and medicine, Janet's other important monographs were *Névroses et idées fixes* (Neuroses and Fixed Ideas, 1898) and *Les obsessions et la psychasténie* (Obsessions and Psychastenia, 1903). In the course of the 20th century Janet broadened his research, devoting himself on the one hand to psychopathology and psychotherapy dynamically oriented and on the other hand to a psychology that investigated normal behavior (with the study of so-called *conduct*) and dealt with personality, memory, and intelligence according to an evolutionary and psychosocial orientation.

Pierre Janet was a tireless scholar. Until 1898, when he obtained the complementary course at the Sorbonne, he continued to teach in the schools, developing a manual of philosophy that, published for the first time in 1896, was reprinted in several editions until 1935. Especially under the methodological profile, he followed the teaching of the masters Ribot and Charcot. His fame grew especially abroad. He was particularly successful in the United States where, together with Freud, he was recognized as a luminary of psychopathology and psychotherapy. His work, however, was quickly forgotten during the 20th century, overshadowed by the success of psychoanalysis. His decision to destroy his archive, in order to respect the privacy of patients, was another obstacle to the studies of Janet. As is well known, Ellenberger (1970) was the first to rediscover the importance of his work, defining it as "a vast city buried" (ibid., p. 409). Today, his studies on the dissociation of personality, which he significantly defined as "disaggregation" (*désagrégation*), are especially re-evaluated (Bromberg, 1998). In the vision of Janet, in fact, the personality would be a psychological construction composed of variable levels of consciousness, tendencies, and energies that in the disease are decomposed (disaggregated).

To Pierre Janet we owe substantially all the tradition born from the psychopathological and psychotherapeutic conception based on the idea that pathology corresponded to an unconscious disaggregation-dissociation[36] of the personality. It would be cured through a process of reaggregation favored by the therapist, especially through hypnotic and suggestive practices. Influenced precisely by his eclectic training and the influence he received from his uncle Paul, Pierre Janet nevertheless tended to preserve part of the conception of the ego that was present in the spiritualist philosophy, adding it to that of a more empirical ego, as it resulted using the pathological method. In this sense, his psychology of personality was based on the view that consciousness appeared as unique and identical to itself. For Janet, our thoughts were united in a system, with a unitary, unique, individual, and distinct appearance. At the same time, personality would be equally a systematic organization of internal (kynesthetic) sensations, memories, and imaginations that could unconsciously autonomize.

In this conception, Janet rediscovered the *pétites perceptions* of Gottfried Wilhelm Leibniz's (1646–1716) philosophy. In short, for Leibniz there would be sensations (such as noises to which we do not pay attention) that we perceive automatically.[37] Consciousness would present different degrees to which correspond personalities of different levels of functioning. In some people the consciousness of their own personality would be precise and clear-cut, other individuals present a variation of consciousness from an automatic and basic level to an aggregate and self-conscious one.[38] Personality dissociations were then considered by Janet to be empirical evidence of the complexity and levels of consciousness. Disaggregating disorders thus highlighted elements that functioned as a unit in others (Janet, 1896).

Multiple personalities, sleepwalking, automatic writing – and all psychopathology – would have shown the way in which sensations (external or internal), memories, and imaginings existed in the same person. They excluded and alternated with one another. In particular, Janet attributed much importance to psychological trauma as the cause of hysteria and disaggregations (splits) of the personality. It should be noted, however, that as far as therapy was concerned, *trauma* and memories were treated as if they could be modified through hypnosis. The late Janet actually advocated a constructivist[39] conception of personality. The personality would be the result of a perpetual synthesis, elaboration, and assimilation of experiences and psychological functions. Therapy would then consist in the implementation of psychological processes to build a synthesis in the disaggregated and altered personality.

History of science, until very recently, has considered Janet above all as a pioneer of dynamic psychiatry. On the other hand, his research has not often been recognized by 20th-century psychologists even as fully internal to scientific psychology. Perhaps Janet's oblivion is due to an identity that cannot be framed in a simple scheme: Janet was, as we have seen, at the same time a philosopher, a theoretical psychologist (who embodied perhaps more than any other the ideal indicated by Ribot), an experimental psychologist at the Salpêtrière, and a psychotherapist.

It can be justifiably argued that he represented, together with Alfred Binet, inventor of the first intelligence test (Cicciola, 2019), the second generation of French experimental psychologists, while maintaining some ambiguities with respect to the autonomy of psychology from philosophy and medicine. Both psychologists and psychiatrists were his pupils, among the latter, at least Jean Delay (1907–1987), one of the greatest representatives of 20th-century French psychiatry, should be mentioned.

Janet's Theses

Psychological Automatism already contains a complete theory of personality, normal and pathological, and a technique of therapeutic intervention to restore the functioning of the personality itself (Janet, 1889). In the first part of the thesis, Janet described all those cases that he considered to be of total automatism, that is, the result of a completely disaggregated personality: catalepsy, alternating personalities, and the narrowing of the field of consciousness are all typical phenomena of *generalized automatism*. Janet described the disaggregation and narrowing of perception, determined by the disease or by hypnotism.

The second part of the thesis concerned *partial automatism*. Janet used several schemes to highlight that, in normality, the personality at first perceives every kind of stimulation (tactile, muscular, visual, auditory), which it then synthesizes. In the case of personality alteration and partial automatism, the ability to synthesize would be lost. Partial psychological automatism turned out to be, therefore, the theoretical model that also served to interpret all the bizarre phenomena that were observed by those who, in the same period, dealt with parapsychology. Dowsing, the explorer pendulum, mind-reading, the different forms of spiritualism, and possession would derive from the oscillation of automatism and psychological disaggregation of the subjects:

> The mental disaggregation, the formation of successive and simultaneous personalities in the same individual, the automatic functioning of these different psychological groups isolated from each other are not artificial things, the result of bizarre experimental maneuvers. They are perfectly real and natural things that experimentation allows us to study but does not create. These things show themselves naturally in all ways and in all gradations. Sometimes, a very slight separation leaves outside the mind only insignificant phenomena, incapable of acting independently and docile servants of conscious thought. They exaggerate, they modify the manifestations of normal thought, but they do not oppose them. Sometimes the second personality speaks on its own behalf, takes the name of a spirit, and highlights its reflections, but only when the first personality allows it to do so and leaves it free to act. Sometimes, finally, the normal group is rich enough in itself to oppose the attention of the subject, to disturb him and take away his freedom. But from the most insignificant subconscious act to the most terrible possessions it is always the same psychological mechanism that gradually brings about the complete dissolution of the mind.
>
> (Janet, 1889, pp. 442–443)

It should be noted that in *Psychological Automatism* was also outlined a draft *energy* model of personality. At the basis of Janet's theory of personality there was therefore what, perhaps at a stretch, could also be defined as a metapsychology.[40]

Weakness (*misery*) or moral *strength* would differentiate the pathological personality from the normal one:

> The splitting of the personality is rather the immediate consequence of this weakness of psychological synthesis, which allows psychological phenomena to exist but does not connect them to the idea of personality. We can represent to ourselves the phenomena of somnambulism and subconscious acts as secondary groupings, incidental systematizations of these neglected psychological phenomena.
>
> Things go on as if the system of psychological phenomena that forms personal perception in all men was in these individuals disaggregated and gave birth to two or more simultaneous or successive groups, most often incomplete and mutually subtracting from each other the sensations, images, and consequently the movements that normally must be brought together in one and the same consciousness and power.[41]
>
> Suggestibility itself and maladies by representation are connected with this general conception: the exaggerated development of certain ideas depends on their isolation, and this isolation is a consequence of the narrowing of the field of consciousness. The exaltation of automatic phenomena most often results from a diminution of the power of voluntary reactivity that unites present phenomena at every moment of life. It is this set of conceptions that we have designated with the name of *mental disaggregation*, and it still seems to us, on the basis of the preceding analyses, that this idea can provide the means of summarizing a large number of hysterical phenomena.
>
> (Janet, 1911, pp. 428–429)

Automatism and disaggregation would be part of this energy system, whose theory in the course of subsequent works was based on the concepts of strength (ability to sustain a psychical work for a long time) or psychological tension (psychological activation present in the personality of subjects able to synthesize mental activities effectively and in a continuous process). Indeed Janet, back in the medical thesis of 1893, continued to refine the contents discussed in the first psychological thesis. This dissertation was published extensively as the second part of a work on the mental state of hysterics (Janet, 1893–1894, 1911). The first half of this work, on *mental stigmata*, was devoted to the physical symptoms of hysteria and the narrowing of the field of consciousness, while the second half, on *mental accidents*, dealt more closely with the psychological symptoms of hysteria and fixed ideas. The medical thesis consisted, therefore, mainly in a description of hysteria, studied in the laboratory of psychology of the Salpêtrière, directed by Janet himself. In this contribution there were some details about the mechanisms already traced in *Psychological Automatism*. Namely, Janet outlined a distinction between hysteria and *psychoasthenia*, on the basis of the different personality functioning of subjects suffering from these pathologies. In hysteria the ability to synthesize seemed partial and the consciousness limited, then the ideas acted as ideational cores that in hysteria were mostly subconscious and fed the symptomatic behavior of the subjects. These ideas could also derive from forgotten traumatic memories. The difference between psychoasthenics and hysterics would have been initially a more specific weakness for the latter and the presence of fixed ideas that would have besieged instead consciously the psychoasthenics (Janet, 1903, 1911). Over the following decades, Janet then continued to clarify and went on to elaborate a grand theoretical synthesis of his conception of normal and pathologic personality (Janet, 1929; see Foschi, 2003b).

The legacy of French psychology and psychotherapy

It should be noted that French positivist psychologists followed a transformist[42] and optimistic conception of personality, influenced by Lamarckian and Spencerian evolutionism, which was different from the psychiatric and alienist model that referred instead to the hegemonic *théorie de la dégénérescence* (degeneracy theory).[43] The differences between degeneracy and transformism have often not been grasped by historiography, which has instead privileged degeneracy theory as the sole key to interpreting an entire historical period (Pick, 1993). Ian Dowbiggin (1991) has, however, highlighted how, around 1890, the political and cultural orientations operating in the Third Republic, due to an actual social crisis, had pushed to solidarity the political engagement of many scholars, including the first psychologists. This would have contributed, among other things, to a reform of medical-psychiatric knowledge that led to a critical attitude toward hereditary and fatalistic theories of madness – just like the theory of *dégénérescence* or the Lombrosian theory of atavism – and toward the assumption of a strongly interventionist approach oriented toward education with Binet and psychotherapy with Janet. In this sense, Janet's work would have represented a novelty and would have been welcomed as a vis-à-vis alternative to the moral treatment of the alienists and asylum therapies. Dowbiggin also pointed out some similarities between the instances that were active in France at the end of the 19th century and the anti-psychiatric movement that, in the 1960s of the twentieth century, characterized the Western psychiatry.[44] Both these moments were in fact marked by the criticism of psychiatric classifications and by the search for alternative therapies to the mere and impotent institutionalization of patients (on this point see also Fauvel, 2004). In this sense, the interest in Janet of the historiography starting from Ellenberger was probably also conditioned by these anti-psychiatric instances, tending to examine the aspects of history that could be used to justify those particular cultures and policies of intervention, in discontinuity with the custodialist and degenerative psychiatric tradition.

Since Ellenberger's rediscovery, a growing number of contributions have been published that reconstruct Janet's work, treating him primarily as a psychiatrist or psychopathologist who used psychological principles to treat his patients. Emphasis is thus placed on Janet's sources, psychopathological theory, and psychotherapy, especially in polemics with Freud.

Janet, since the 1880s – as well as all French psychology – had indeed developed concepts that Freudian psychoanalysis seemed then to redefine: Janet's subconscious became Freud's unconscious; the theory of real trauma became the theory of fantasy; the theory of dissociation made way for the theory of repression and so on. Freud often quoted Janet – also associating him with his uncle Paul, his brother Jules, or Binet – in reference to his observations on hysteria. On the other hand, Janet on some occasions defended psychoanalysis, while on others he claimed that it was nothing but his own *psychological analysis* in disguise. The two experienced, therefore, a long controversy whose culmination is represented by a communication by Janet in 1913, taken up extensively in his *Journal de Psychologie* (Janet, 1914). Beyond this controversy, it should be emphasized that Janet and Freud were the two most important exponents of a psychopathology based on a psychological theory and also the developers of theories of intervention that have overwhelmingly conditioned 20th-century clinical psychology and psychotherapy. Janet developed psychological analysis with the aim of reintegrating those dissociated/disaggregated components of ego and memory that acted subconsciously, producing the symptoms of psychopathology. He used hypnosis and especially suggestion to recreate a more tolerable mental reality for the patient. For these reasons, analogies can be highlighted between Janet's way of proceeding and that of current cognitive psychotherapy in relation to the use of instances that refer to the so-called cognitive unconscious and to constructivism (see Heim & Bühler, 2006).[45] About that, Ian Hacking very appropriately wrote:

> I see Freud as driven by a terrible Will to Truth, illustrated by a second contrast with Janet. Ellenberger writes that the values of Freud were those of the romantic era; Janet was an Enlightenment rationalist. That insight is partial at best. Janet was flexible and pragmatic, while it was Freud who was the dedicated and rather rigid theoretician in the spirit of the Enlightenment. (. . .) Freud (. . .) like many a dedicated theoretician, probably fudged the evidence in favor of theory. Freud had a passionate commitment to Truth, deep underlying Truth, as a value. (. . .) Janet had no such Will to Truth. He was an honorable man, and (we might say *hence*) he had no inflated sense of the Truth. He dealt with traumatically caused neuroses by convincing the patient that the trauma had never happened. He would do this by suggestion and hypnosis whenever he could. Take, for example, his early patient who at the age of six had been made to sleep beside a girl suffering terribly from impetigo on one side of the face. His patient would break out in hysterical marks, and would experience loss of sensibility, even blindness, on that side of her face. So Janet used hypnosis

to suggest to his patient that she was caressing the soft beautiful face of the girl she had lain beside at age six. All symptoms, including the partial blindness, disappeared. Janet cured his patient by telling her a lie, and getting her to believe it. He did this over and over again with his patients – got them to believe what he himself knew was a lie. (. . .) Freud was the exact opposite of Janet. His patients had to face up to the truth – as he saw it. We can have no doubt, in retrospect, that Freud very often deluded himself, thanks to his resolute dedication to theory. (. . .) But there is no evidence that Freud systematically, as a method of therapy, got his patients to believe what he himself knew to be lies. Janet fooled his patients; Freud fooled himself.

(Hacking, 1995, pp. 195–196; see also Heim & Bühler, 2006)[46]

It should be noted, however, that in spite of recent attempts at revaluation, Janet's impact on psychological sciences has been quite different from Freud's. The Parisian psychologist counts, for example, a few hundred citations in the databases of international scientific literature (PsycINFO), mostly between 1980 and today. On the other hand, if we look for the name of the Viennese psychologist in the same databases, we collect tens of thousands of citations. Notwithstanding, therefore, the recent rediscovery of Janet and French psychology, Freud remains a pivot that still attracts an enormously greater number of exegetes.

Philosophies of the unconscious and history of psychotherapy

Before meeting the key figures for the birth of dynamic psychotherapy – Freud, Adler, and Jung – it is appropriate to mention how the 19th century witnessed the flourishing of a series of philosophies for which the concept of the unconscious assumed a central role.[47] It was already the most illustrious representative of the Enlightenment, Immanuel Kant, who believed that the mind was, for the subject, effectively unknowable. In the *Critique of Pure Reason*, in fact, Kant (1781–1787) distinguished between what can be known through the a priori structure of the intellect (the phenomenon) and the world as it actually is (the thing in itself or noumenon). In this sense, the human mind itself could not be known as the thing-in-itself but only through its phenomenal manifestations.

On the one hand, Kant was followed, in a German-speaking environment, by the affirmation of Idealism, which, particularly with Hegel, saw in history the progressive and finally complete self-awareness of the Spirit. On the other hand, however, the unconscious dimension of the mind acquired an increasingly central role, in parallel with an increasingly pessimistic attitude about the possibilities of knowledge. It can be recalled how a fortunate definition, although historically questionable, has put Freud together with two 19th-century philosophers who are very different from each other, namely Karl Marx (1818–1883) and Friedrich Nietzsche (1844–1900), in a "school of suspicion" that would question the human illusions about consciousness:

> The philosopher trained in the school of Descartes knows that things are doubtful, that they are not such as they appear; but he does not doubt that consciousness is such as it appears to itself; in consciousness, meaning and consciousness of meaning coincide. Since Marx, Nietzsche, and Freud, this too has become doubtful. After the doubt about things, we have started to doubt consciousness.
>
> (Ricoeur, 1965/1972, p. 33)

Karl Marx, however, certainly did not limit himself to a critique of subjective knowledge, but constructed a critique of society, interpreted as divided between a capitalist class and a proletarian class. He imagined, consequently, a historical dialectic that would lead, through the struggle between classes, to a future communist society in which the exploitation of man on man would be abolished. Actually, there are no elements to establish an influence of Marx on Freud, who never imagined he would reform society through his own ideas. The author of *The Capital*, however, inspired psychoanalytic culture, through the so-called Freudomarxists.[48]

Nietzsche, unlike Marx, addressed his work to an intellectual elite rather than to the class of the exploited and directed his main interest at overturning the clichés of knowledge and especially morality. In *Human, All Too Human* (1878/1996) Nietzsche envisioned a future in which it would be possible to live as free spirits, abandoning the stratified and useless traditions and certainties. Nietzsche affirmed *perspectivism*, that is, the principle that every truth is formulated from a particular point of view and can never aspire to absoluteness. Moving from the perspectivism of knowledge he developed a critique of the idea of absolute ethics. In this sense, he was able to state in *Dawn* that "morality is nothing else (and, above all, nothing more) than obedience to customs" (1881/1924, p. 14). Everything that was honored by society as moral contrasted with the true tendencies of human beings, and everything that was abhorred corresponded to their secret aspirations. For example, Nietzsche wrote: "Cruelty is one of the most ancient enjoyments" of humankind (ibid., p. 25). Unconfessable feelings were in fact adaptive. In *The Gay Science*, Nietzsche observed:

> Hatred, the mischievous delight in the misfortunes of others, the lust to rob and dominate, and whatever else is called evil belongs to the most amazing economy of the preservation of the species. To be sure, this economy is not afraid of high prices, of squandering, and it is on the whole extremely foolish. Still it is proven that it has preserved our race so far.
>
> (1882–1887/1974, p. 73)

In *The Gay Science* also appeared several times the idea of the death of God, perhaps the one most commonly associated with Nietzschean thought: "God is dead; but given the way of men, there may still be caves for thousands of years in which his shadow will be shown. – And we – we still have to vanquish his shadow, too" (ibid., p. 167; see also pp. 167–181). Beginning with *Thus Spoke Zarathustra*, the free spirit was embodied in the superman, the being who, aspiring to greatness, would be able to enact the will to power (Nietzsche, 1883–1885/1969). The will to power progressively became a pivotal concept in Nietzsche's thought, defining the very essence of life. We read, in fact, in *Beyond Good and Evil*: "A living thing seeks above all to *discharge* its strength – life itself is *will to power*; self-preservation is only one of the indirect and most frequent *results*" (Nietzsche, 1886/1966, p. 21 [emphasis in original]). Fascinated by physiological psychology[49] and disgusted by philosophical psychology, Nietzsche imagined the ego not only as conditioned by largely unmentionable forces and desires but also acted by a bodily self, as is explicitly stated in *Thus Spoke Zarathustra*:

> Behind your thoughts and feelings, my brother, stands a mighty commander, an unknown sage – he is called Self. He lives in your body, he is your body. (. . .) Your Self laughs at your Ego and its proud leapings. "What are these leapings and flights of thought to me?" it says to itself. "A by-way to my goal. I am the Ego's leading-string and I prompt its conceptions."
> (Nietzsche, 1883–1885/1969, p. 62)

Nietzsche's influence on dynamic psychology can hardly be overstated. All three fathers of dynamic psychology, Alfred Adler, Carl Gustav Jung, and Sigmund Freud, were clearly influenced by it, although Freud claimed never to have read him.[50] However, Freud did not deny reading another philosopher, even mentioning it quite often, while claiming that he had developed his ideas in a way totally independent from him: Arthur Schopenhauer (1788–1860), who was also admired by Nietzsche. In his main writing, *The World as Will and Representation*, Schopenhauer described the universe as the result of a universal will that operates "completely without knowledge as an obscure driving force" (1818–1859/1966, Vol. I, p. 149), animated moreover by conflicting motivations: "Thus everywhere in nature we see contest, struggle, and the fluctuation of victory, and later on we shall recognize in this more distinctly that variance with itself essential to the will" (Vol. 1, p. 146). Moving from Kant's perspective, for which we only know the world phenomenally, Schopenhauer reached a radical epistemological pessimism, so that the entire content of the intellect is our simple representation, a pure illusion. The epistemological pessimism was also reflected in an existential pessimism. The very famous paragraph 58 of the *World* begins as follows:

> All satisfaction, or what is commonly called happiness, is really and essentially always *negative* only, and never positive. It is not a gratification which

comes to us originally and of itself, but it must always be the satisfaction of a wish. For desire, that is to say, want, is the precedent condition of every pleasure; but with the satisfaction, the desire and therefore the pleasure cease.

(Vol. 1, p. 319)

As will be seen, there are clear assonances with Freud's principle of pleasure/unpleasure.[51] Freud actually affirmed, in a mature work: "We have unwittingly steered our course into the harbor of Schopenhauer's philosophy" (1920/1955a, pp. 49–50).

Certainly Freud could look at Schopenhauer as a philosopher who had anticipated many of his ideas not only about the unconscious but also about sexuality, dreams, and death drive, to the point of including, in several of his works, crypto-citations of the philosopher from Frankfurt (Assoun, 1976). One particular idea deserves to be mentioned here: the link between memory and madness, in which Freud (1914/1957) saw a first theory of repression (though not admitting a direct drift of his ideas from those of Schopenhauer): "real soundness of mind consists in perfect recollection" wrote, for example, Schopenhauer, while madness was "the *broken* thread of this memory which nevertheless continues to run uniformly" (Schopenhauer, 1818–1859/1966, Vol. 2, p. 399). Moreover, Schopenhauer specified:

The description of the origin of madness given in the text will become easier to understand, if we remember how reluctantly we think of things that powerfully prejudice our interests, wound our pride, or interfere with our wishes; with what difficulty we decide to lay such things before our own intellect for accurate and serious investigation; how easily, on the other hand, we unconsciously break away or sneak off from them again; how, on the contrary, pleasant affairs come into our minds entirely of their own accord, and, if driven away, always creep on us once more, so that we dwell on them for hours. In this resistance on the part of the will to allow what is contrary to it to come under the examination of the intellect is to be found the place where madness can break in on the mind.

(Vol. 2, p. 400)

Having established that it would be more proper to link these words to the etiology of neurosis than to that of madness, one cannot but be amazed by their sharpness.

In addition to Nietzsche and Schopenhauer, a reflection on the unconscious runs through the thought of several other philosophers of the 19th century, such as Friedrich Schelling (1775–1854), Carl Gustav Carus (1789–1869), and Eduard von Hartmann (1842–1906), author of a work entitled *Philosophy of the Unconscious* (1869/1884). While these three thinkers may have been unknown to Freud, they were repeatedly mentioned by Carl Gustav Jung as theorists, before him, of the collective unconscious (see, e.g., Jung, 1932/1976, 1936/1968a, 1954/1968b). Freud, however, was familiar with the thought of Johann Friedrich Herbart (1776–1841) (Andersson, 1962), who for two reasons could be said to be an advocate of a dynamic conception of the psyche: the idea that, because of the struggle between reason and appetite, men have a *double ego*; the belief that there is a threshold of consciousness, separating conscious from unconscious representations and sensations on the basis of their intensity and/ or repetition; and that furthermore unconscious ideas could be, and often are, active agents in a threshold conflict (Herbart, 1813; see Whyte, 1960). The question of the unconscious was eventually discussed extensively by both Wilhelm Wundt (1832–1920) and Franz Brentano (1838–1917), fundamental leaders of German psychology. Both, however, ended up ruling it out. At least Brentano's lectures were followed by Freud, who nevertheless felt its influence (Araujo, 2012; Merlan, 1945, 1949).

The role of Freud

The creation of psychoanalysis by Sigmund Freud is certainly the event that coincided with the real birth of psychotherapy in today's sense of the term, because it combined for the first time the two fundamental features that define it. Freud in fact (a) did not use (or at least did not intentionally use) suggestion in an attempt to heal patients, as in the case of hypnotists; (b) did not entrust physical activity and training of a sick person with a significant part of the cure, as in the case of alienists who applied moral treatment. Whatever evaluation of Freud's work one may propose today, surely the emergence of psychoanalysis can be seen as the origin of a new scientific paradigm in the Kuhnian sense (Kuhn, 1962), which crystallized in a different overall form a number of already existing paradigmatic ideas. The most important of these ideas was certainly that of the unconscious. We could see, at least in passing, how the concept of the unconscious went through a long history to become particularly central and controversial in philosophical, psychological, and neurological thought at the end of the 19th century. Only in Freud, however, the unconscious clearly took on the connotations of a part of the psyche characterized by a "play of forces" that conditioned the conscious life. The forces represented divergent impulses and motivations. A person could simultaneously desire something for the possible pleasure that he would get from it but refrain from trying to get what he wanted for, say, reasons of social convenience. Such a conflict, in Freud's view, could take place on a conscious level but much more often on an unconscious level. Even the expression "dynamic psychology," which is still used today to identify theories derived directly or indirectly from Freud's, expresses precisely the concept of the mind as a play of forces and reveals at the same time a metaphor taken from physics. From chemistry had finally originated another metaphor that was expressed in the very name psychoanalysis that Freud imposed on his own theory, supposing that neurotic psychopathologies could be both traced back to their first components (i.e., also explained from the causal point of view) and dissolved (analysis means etymologically "dissolution"), that is, resolved in their problematic nature for the patient.

The 19th-century sciences had outlined a deterministic conception of the universe, according to which every phenomenon was traceable to specific causes (even if not necessarily knowable in the immediate term). This was reflected in Freud's physical determinism, which remained in the background of his thought, but in his opinion constituted the foundation of any scientific conception of the world and any discipline that one wanted to define as scientific. According to physical determinism, every phenomenon had to have its physical causes – even, therefore, the mind. Above all, however, *psychical determinism* was fundamental for Freudian psychoanalysis: every psychological phenomenon had in turn psychological causes. This was translated into the general principle that every conscious manifestation of the psyche had essentially unconscious origins. It was precisely this basic idea that substantiated the principle by which even psychical epiphenomena, which were generally considered insignificant (such as dreams, slips missed acts in general), could not be considered accidental, but referred back to specific unconscious causes.

In apparent contradiction with Freud's physical determinism was the concept of psychical trauma, the notion of which had recently been developed in France. In this concept was made explicit the idea that an event could be considered traumatic even if it had not caused damage to the body of a person: the damage could also be simply on a mental level. The Freudian conception of *psychical trauma* varied greatly over time. Initially Freud (1888/1966a) adhered to Charcot's perspective of trauma as *agent provocateur*: a single triggering event that had to be favored by a specific physical predisposition. Later Freud believed that the single event could cause pathology per se. Finally, the trauma became rather traceable to a series of events, following the general principle of over-determination (no mental fact had its own single cause), which became one of the theoretical bases of Freudian thought. Freud, however, did not postulate the independence of physical reality from psychological reality and indeed emphasized that, ideally, science should come to an identification of the physical causes of psychopathology. Psychological reality as such, however, could not be denied: psychological events could in turn affect the physical level. The paradigmatic idea of continuity between normal and pathological acquired with Freud a very special meaning. At least since *The Interpretation of Dreams*, it was clear that every human being was to some extent neurotic and that the so-called normality was determined by a quantitative, rather than a qualitative, threshold (Freud, 1900/1953a). The main motivational factor was sexuality, and psychical energy had in any case a sexual nature. Mental health depended on a more or less effective use of this energy, called "libido." Any use of libido, unrelated to sexuality, would still have been the result of a repression of the original drives. Civilization persisted at the price of such repression and was therefore, as such, neurotic. It should be emphasized, however, that the suppression of sexuality constituted for Freud a necessary evil, while it will be seen that other theorists (such as Reich and Marcuse) hoped for full sexual liberation as a necessary precondition for a desirable revolution of common feeling. The continuity between normality and pathology implied for the normal individual the presence of pathological aspects and in pathology the presence of aspects of normality. Perversion was not the result of a deviant behavior. The child, in the early stages of its development, for Freud was necessarily a polymorphous pervert, in the sense that it was motivated to seek pleasure from parts of the body (erogenous zones) other than the genitals, or in other ways than their use as genitals. The perverse adult was therefore the one who had not been able to successfully overcome a phase that every human being goes through. Phenomena, which were attributable to neurosis and psychosis by their nature, characterized the daily life of all. Dreams, as hallucinatory satisfactions of desires, could be considered "micropsychotic" phenomena, and slips and missed acts could be interpreted as "microneurotic" phenomena. All this, however, is the result of an evolution of Freudian thought, which will be described in the following paragraphs.

Freud's scientific training and early years

The future father of psychoanalysis trained in Vienna as a neurologist, while also cultivating philosophical interests. On the one hand, in fact, he chose as a point of reference Ernst Brücke (1819–1892), a leading exponent of the Physicalistic Circle of Berlin, which was a group of physiologists united by the intent to explain the vital phenomena only in materialistic terms. On the other hand, however, he followed the lessons of Franz Brentano, finding himself even fantasizing about becoming a doctor of philosophy (Freud, 1990). In fact, however, Freud soon focused on neurological research, achieving results that earned him the esteem of his mentors, even if it left him very unsatisfied. Biographers, moreover, describe him as being in search of a significant scientific discovery that would give him notoriety (Gay, 1988; Jones, 1953–1957). This eagerness to succeed, however, led him to a misstep: after conducting some research on cocaine, Freud recommended its use as an anesthetic in a book, praising its lack of side effects such as addiction and suggesting a possible use on a large scale (Freud, 1885/1974).

This proved to be a serious mistake, which attracted the heavy criticism of having introduced "the third scourge of humanity" after morphine and alcohol (Erlenmayer, 1886, p. 483). Among the neurological writings, deserving of particular mention is a book on aphasia, in which Freud (1891/1953b) opposed the localizationist tendency, that is, the tradition of research that attributed specific disorders (in this case of language) to specific lesions of the brain. In his opinion, in fact, aphasias had to be traced back to functional disorders (i.e., systemic problems). The approach is noteworthy because in this field localizationism had just obtained its first indisputable successes, thanks to Paul Pierre Broca (1824–1880) and Carl Wernicke (1848–1905). Although Freud did not present new material (it was based mainly on studies of the Anglo-Saxon area), the book is still of some interest because it shows how the author maintained a materialist approach but had already abandoned what could be considered the mainstream of German-speaking neurology. The need to find a working arrangement made Freud abandon the dream of dealing with pure research, to open instead a private medical practice. Before starting his own practice, however, he was able to take advantage of a scholarship for a stay in Paris in 1885. This became the turning point that marked his career. Freud began attending Charcot's lectures at the Salpêtrière, developing a keen interest in the phenomenology of hysteria.

His colleague Joseph Breuer (1842–1925) had already told him in 1883 about the course of hysteria of one of his patients, who became known as Anna O. (Bertha Pappenheim [1859–1936], who later became one of the protagonists of the women's emancipation movement). Breuer noted that all of his patient's symptoms had gradually appeared at specific moments in her life, which Anna O. could not remember, except under hypnosis. However, when she could recall the episodes linked to the onset of the symptoms, the symptoms themselves disappeared. For example, Anna O. could not drink water and could only quench her thirst by eating fruit. Hypnotized by Breuer, she was able to remember when her housekeeper (whom she hated) had made her dog drink water from a glass, arousing in her a deep disgust. Once Anna O. had recalled the episode, she was able to drink plenty of water and awoke from hypnosis with the glass in her hand, no longer feeling repulsion. Freud had not initially attributed a particular importance to the case recounted by Breuer, but the Parisian experience convinced him to take an interest in hypnosis.

If it was Charcot who attracted Freud's attention on this subject, the work of Bernheim interested him more and more, because it promised therapeutic efficacy. Freud, in fact, translated into German works by both Charcot and Bernheim. However, the latter, like Janet, used hypnosis as a therapy essentially through suggestion. Freud, on the other hand, taking his cue from Breuer's experience, used it primarily as a means of exploration (Breuer & Freud, 1893–1895/1955). At the origin of hysteria would have been a psychical trauma (which no longer had the pure and simple role of *agent provocateur*, according to Charcot), whose effects would be more or less severe depending on three factors: (a) the intensity of the trauma itself; (b) the subjective predisposition to hysterical pathology; (c) the possibility of reacting to the trauma in an adequate way (physically and/or verbally). The trauma was actively forgotten – that is, it was repressed – because the memory was not bearable by the consciousness. The result was a block of psychical energy (for now Freud used the expression *sum of excitation*). Thanks to hypnosis it would have been possible, by recovering the memory, to carry out that reaction to the trauma (*abreaction*) that had not originally been possible, and it would be this reaction that would bring about the fundamental therapeutic effect. The method could be defined as *cathartic*, due to affinity with the catharsis that, according to Aristotle, was reached by the Greek spectator after watching a tragedy. The show had aroused in him intense feelings of emotional participation and then evoked a sense of liberation after the end.[52] Breuer and Freud did not exclude, however, especially in the first part of the *Studies on Hysteria* (*Preliminary Communication*), that suggestion could also achieve a certain success. In fact, Freud had used a technique very similar to Bernheim's in the treatment of the first of the cases he described, that of Emmy von N. (Baroness Fanny Moser [1848–1925]) (Breuer & Freud, 1893–1895/1955, pp. 48–105).

The abandonment of hypnosis and the new therapeutic technique

Despite the relative optimism shown in *Studies on Hysteria*, neither the treatment of Anna O. nor that of Emmy von N. and other patients treated by Freud with hypnosis were totally satisfactory. Freud, however, was already convinced that an alternative method to hypnosis had to be found for several reasons: (a) the nonhypnotizability of some patients; (b) the unwillingness of other patients to be hypnotized; (c) the conviction Freud reached that it was possible to recall apparently forgotten events even without hypnosis (Breuer & Freud, 1893–1895/1955); (d) the side effects of hypnosis, such as the possible awakening of the sexuality of female patients (Freud, 1925/1959a). It should also be noted that the patients hypnotized by Freud and the Parisian patients had different social backgrounds. The Parisians were hospitalized and belonged to a disadvantaged social class, whereas in Vienna they were mainly upper-middle-class patients (see Edelman, 2003). This probably resulted in a greater hypnotizability of the Parisian patients, who tended to trust the doctor *meneur de femmes*, while Freud had a more difficult and reasoned relationship with his Viennese patients. According to Carroy (1991), these differences also influenced Freud in the construction of a new method.

A new technique was applied for the first time in the case of Elisabeth von R. (a young woman from an affluent Hungarian family). It was developed from the observation that, if the patient was encouraged to remember the first occasion of the onset of hysterical symptoms, he seemed to get results, albeit with great effort: "The situation led me at once to the theory that *by means of my psychical al work I had to overcome a psychical al force in the patients which was opposed to the pathogenic ideas becoming conscious (being remembered)*" (Breuer & Freud, 1893–1895/1955, p. 268; emphasis in the text). The representations evoked feelings of shame, pain, and annoyance, in other words, it seemed as if a force was defending the secret, even to themselves. Inevitably, the thread of memories was broken and Freud proposed proceeding in this way:

> I inform the patient that, a moment later, I shall apply pressure to his forehead, and I assure him that, all the time the pressure lasts, he will see before him a recollection in the form of a picture or will have it in his thoughts in

the form of an idea occurring to him; and I pledge him to communicate this picture or idea to me, whatever it may be.

(p. 270)

Obviously, it was not a miraculous procedure, and Freud did not propose it as such: it could be considered instead a pure and simple attempt to surprise the person in a defensive attitude. The pathogenic representation was hardly ever obtained at once. More frequently an "intermediate link" (ibid., p. 271) was reached between the mental content that had induced the patient to stop and the content that the defense was covering. That is, it was understood in which direction, so to speak, research should proceed. Nor did Freud insist on spectacular results from the therapeutic technique he had inaugurated. Very realistically, he purposed to transform "hysterical misery into common unhappiness" (p. 304). He added that it would be easier to defend oneself from unhappiness with a "nervous system that has been restored to health" (after 1925, however, Freud replaced the words "nervous system" with "mental life"). In 1895, Freud was still convinced of the possibility of explaining neurotic mechanisms on the basis of neurophysiological functioning, as will be seen in the next paragraph.

The birth of psychoanalysis

While Breuer was rapidly losing interest in the treatment of hysteria, Freud was expanding his studies into other forms of psychopathology. The main Freudian interlocutor had become Wilhelm Fliess (1858–1928), a Berlin doctor who was developing, for his part, some strange theories about biorhythms, the role of the nasal cavity in determining diseases of various kinds, and especially about the fundamental bisexuality of the human being. Freud ended up appropriating this last idea and talked openly about it with another of his acquaintances, Otto Weininger (1880–1903), who in turn used it as the basis of a book that gave him immediate international fame, *Sex and Character* (1903/2005). Since Weininger's book was issued before Fliess could publish anything on the matter, the circumstance constituted a reason for a break between Fliess and Freud (Kerr, 1993).

The letters and the *Drafts* addressed to Fliess (Freud, 1985), however, especially those of the last five years of the 19th century, constitute a valuable testimony of the period of incubation of Freudian psychological theories. If the letters contain a sort of chronicle of Freud's work in progress, the *Drafts* are already quite clear sketches of the ideas that were being born and that would later see the light in Freud's publications of the following years. Among the material sent to Fliess, however, a separate position is occupied by the *Project for a Scientific Psychology* (Freud, 1895–1950/1966b), which remained unpublished (until 1950) but reveals the author's intent to build a general psychological theory, linking its contents to the functioning of the brain. The *Project* was immediately shelved, but the ideas contained therein would retain a subterranean interest for Freud

(Sulloway, 1979). In this sense, the recent presentist reinterpretation of Freud as the founder of a neuropsychoanalysis is understandable (Kaplan-Solms & Solms, 2000; Solms & Turnbull, 2003).

Abandoning the *Project's* ambitions, Freud would deal exclusively with psychical reality, beginning to call *psychoanalysis* the discipline he progressively constructed (Freud, 1896/1962a, 1896/1962b). Psychoanalysis was intended to develop as (a) a general theory of the human mind and motivation; (b) a theory of psychopathology; (c) a method of treatment based on the above theories. To these three aspects should actually be added, despite the protests of Freud himself (1932/1964a), (d) a general worldview. Indeed, Freud would not fail to use the tools of psychoanalysis to interpret the meaning of civilization (Freud, 1930/1961a, 1932/1964c), the origin of religion (Freud, 1913/1955b, 1927/1961b, 1939/1964b), and the meaning of art and literature (e.g., Freud, 1907/1959b, 1908/1959c, 1914/1955c). The fascination and influence of his writings were certainly also related to the extraordinary breadth of the heuristic horizon opened by them.

In the years following *Studies on Hysteria*, a general theory of psychopathology was born that identified sexuality as the sphere of origin of all neuroses and at least some psychoses. In this sense, Freud distinguished between psychoneuroses and actual neuroses. Among the former, Freud included phobias, obsessive neurosis, and defense hysterias (at this stage Freud was still convinced that some hysterias had a hereditary origin). They would have had a distant traumatic origin and could have been cured by the cathartic method, thanks to the liberation of blocked psychical energy. The latter (anxiety neurosis and neurasthenia) would derive from harmful sexual practices carried out in adult life (respectively from *coitus interruptus* and excessive masturbation).

The traumatic origin of psychoneurosis went through, according to the Freud of this period, two phases: originally the person was initiated into sexuality at too early an age by an adult. The child, however, did not possess notions about the nature of the acts in which he had participated. The future neurotic, therefore, went through a period of apparent mental health. Only with the maturation of the genital organs would the infantile episode begin to exert its influence as a trauma. Its memory would be placed in the unconscious and its presence would be felt only through the symptoms. Thus, in summary, "The traumas of childhood operate in a deferred fashion as though they were fresh experiences; but they do so unconsciously" (Freud, 1896/1962b, p. 167 footnote). Instead, analytic therapy was supposed to allow for the recovery of the memory itself.

In its first formulation, the concept of defense referred to a condition of the conscious personality in the face of unwanted mental content (representations), which led to the effort to cancel, forget, or consider as nonexistent such content: "But it amounts to an approximate fulfilment of the task if the ego succeeds *in turning this powerful idea into a weak one*, in robbing it of the affect – the sum of excitation – with which it is loaded" (Freud, 1894/1962c, p. 48). The origin of defensive hysteria, phobias, and obsessions would have had the same root. The different outcome would have depended on the different fate of the "sum of excitation." In the case of hysteria, for example, there was a conversion into a somatic symptom, linked to an organ affected by the trauma on a symbolic level (such as Anna O.'s hydrophobia, linked to her disgust at the sight of the dog drinking from the glass).

The concept of defense was destined to be an important development and is still considered the most widely accepted theoretical contribution of psychoanalysis in the other "psy" sciences. The idea of neurosis as the result of an infantile seduction, however, lost importance in Freud's eyes within a few months. Writing to Fliess in a letter from 1897, Freud stated that he no longer believed in this theory, and for several reasons. First of all, he was recording an excessive number of therapeutic failures; then he was beginning to think that, in the unconscious, it was difficult to distinguish between real memory and fantasy; finally, in his opinion, it would be necessary to assume too many cases of seduction of children (Freud, 1985, pp. 297–299). In fact, the infantile sexual trauma would have been, logically, a necessary but not sufficient condition to induce neurosis (and if there were already many cases of neurosis, the violence toward children should have been even more). Freud therefore began to assume that the alleged traumas were actually fantasies of neurotics and that the infantile onset of sexuality had an endogenous origin.

Between the end of the 19th and the beginning of the 20th century Freud began, therefore, to definitively develop psychoanalysis. So it made its entry into Western culture at the end of a century that had led many European states to new institutional arrangements, based on forms of participation in political life of the bourgeois and popular classes. In this new historical context, on the way to the most complete participatory democracy and the consequent modernization of society, the contemporary "psy" sciences took their cue.

The other psychotherapy: Paul Dubois

If we want to trace a genealogy of psychotherapy, we must not forget that in the field of mental hygiene, parallel to Freud, some other pioneers were trying to develop therapies of the mind that were new and opposed to the theories of psychopathology whose causes were exclusively imagined as neurological. Hugo Munsterberg (1863–1916), author of *Psychotherapy* (1909), Morton Henry Prince (1854–1929), Boris Sidis (1867–1923), James Jackson Putnam (1846–1918), and John G. Gehring (1857–1932) all sought to create a community of psychotherapy pioneers in the United States. These scholars were mostly influenced by the French hypnosuggestion culture introduced to the United States by William James (1842–1910) (Caplan, 1998; Harris & Stevens, 2020). All of these early psychotherapists were overshadowed, however, by the powerful rise of Freudian doctrine.

After all, before psychoanalysis, even in Europe psychotherapy was mostly based on hypnosuggestion and, at the beginning of the 20th century, commonly practiced by doctors who had elected psychology as their main field of interest (like Sante De Sanctis [1962–1935] in Rome). In the European context, however, it is necessary to specifically describe the psychotherapy of Paul Charles Dubois (1848–1918), a Swiss neurologist and psychotherapist who is today an almost forgotten author and who, between the end of the 19th and the beginning of the 20th century, was a famous European pioneer of psychotherapy. It is even likely that the term "psychotherapy" was popularized precisely by his works (that widely circulated among doctors at the beginning of the 20th century), as opposed to Freudian psychoanalysis.

From 1902 Professor of Neuropathology at the University of Bern, Dubois began to deal with the treatment of diseases that would later be defined as psychosomatic and then as neurotic, using a persuasive technique that had similarities with modern cognitive techniques, based on critical discussion of the solution of their symptoms (see Del Corno & Lang, 2008), so much so that Albert Ellis himself cited it as a historical precedent of his own "rational emotional behavior therapy [REBT]."[53]

Dubois made use of logic and reasoning to deconstruct the beliefs connected to the states that disturbed his patients. His technique, in some ways, was not unlike awake suggestion, but he was certainly uninterested in hypnotic techniques or unconscious causes of mental disorders. Dubois used the relationship between doctor and patient and dialogue as a therapy, to the point of being considered one of the greatest international experts in the field. His great innovation was the systematic use of the interview with the patient as if it were a medical, physical, or pharmacological intervention.

For Dubois, the therapeutic interview had to become a sophisticated technique of medicine, as were all the other systems in use in psychiatry, which did not necessarily imply an interview with the patient. The work of this Swiss doctor thus undermines the historiographic common view, according to which psychoanalysis would have been the first psychotherapy based on the interview: a refinement of hypnosis and suggestion, which had no intermediate psychotherapeutic models. Actually, at the time of the crisis of hypnosis and suggestion, and at the same time as psychoanalysis, other psychotherapeutic methods were developed that made use of persuasion and that were connected to the traditional moral treatment.[54] Among these, Dubois's model – which he called "rational psychotherapy" – was probably the most paradigmatic and the one that, around turn of the century, was the most successful.

His most famous book was *Les psychonévroses et leur traitement moral* (*Psychoneuroses and Moral Treatment*, 1904), in which the author described and categorized all the areas of use of psychotherapy. His other main works were *De l'influence de l'esprit sur le corps* (*The Influence of the Mind on the Body*, 1901) and *L'éducation de soi-meme* (*The Education of Oneself*, 1908), which were translated into many languages, reprinted several times, and published in England and the United States of America. Dubois thus became one of the most accessible points of reference for psychiatrists and practicing doctors who wanted to deal with psychotherapy. He was also one of the first systematic critics of the idea of unconscious and sexuality as the major causes of mental disorders. For Dubois, disorders stemmed from faulty reasoning and could be corrected with the support of the therapist by focusing therapy on the illogicalities and false beliefs held by the patient (Dubois, 1904).

For Dubois, the mental processes could result in neurological and somatic changes. Psychotherapy could be a tool for treating physical illnesses, because they too, in part or entirely, were psychological in origin. In this conception, psychotherapy became the most viable alternative to the traditional physical and chemical treatments of medicine and psychiatry. The ultimate goal of psychotherapy was to make the individual capable of self-management through the exercise of reason. In this sense, the moral influence of the therapist altered the mental state of the patient, replacing disturbing ideas with more adaptive thoughts, attitudes, and behaviors (Dubois, 1904).

Reflected in the title *Psychoneuroses and Moral Treatment* (1904) are the elements of continuity of Dubois's psychotherapeutic model with the psychiatric tradition of moral treatment. Significantly, the introduction to the first edition of this work was written by his friend Jules Dejerine, who, as we have seen, inherited at the Salpêtrière the chair of the Clinic of diseases of the nervous system that had been Charcot's and who removed Janet from the Parisian hospital. Dubois was certainly closer than Janet to Dejerine's line. His ideas probably represented the most coherent outcome of a path that had begun with moral treatment and that through the new anatomical and physiological means of research would have led to clarifying the links between the psychological and the physical. These links were highlighted by the effectiveness of a psychotherapy that did not make use of notions distant from those traditionally medical and that did not stray from Aristotelian logic, nor did it use a heterodox epistemology, marginal to the academic one. Dejerine (1904) defined Dubois's therapy as a refinement of moral treatment, which in his view was now neglected by psychiatrists and alienists in favor of the exclusive use of physical and chemical methods for the treatment of any mental or psychosomatic pathology (see Shamdasani, 2017).

On the other hand, Dubois considered as useful a particular regimen characterized by relaxation, massage, rest, overfeeding, isolation from the family, and anything else that could distract the patient from recovery. Indeed, such a treatment had been proposed by Silas Weir Mitchell (1829–1914) in Philadelphia. Mitchell's rest cure was based on isolation in the psychiatric hospital, forced bed rest, and overfeeding on milk, butter, and carbohydrates for many weeks in order to recover from psychopathologies considered to be a kind of nervous breakdown (see Harris, 2016). Dubois (1904, pp. 310–325) believed that his psychotherapy represented the completion of the rest cure.

Dubois (1904), however, beginning with the history of psychopathology from the perspective of histopathology and neurology, and then with the history of hypnotism in Paris and Nancy's suggestion, drew a sharp critique of the other methods of psychiatry contemporary with him, arguing that a psychotherapy based on "rational suggestion" could profitably replace the drugs then in use (p. 26). In contrast, Dubois appreciated Pinel's moral treatment, which in his opinion had represented the real beginning of a psychotherapy, aimed at educating the patient to take care of him/herself. In essence, Dubois's psychotherapy was based on the "education of the will" (p. 28), which would be the prerequisite for any psychotherapeutic approach not meant for giving importance to the unconscious. Dubois described his intervention as a pedagogy or moral orthopedics, aimed at dismantling autosuggestions, at the basis of some psychogenic diseases that he analyzed (p. 81), and at making individuals responsible to the point of an educational use even of judicial repression. He claimed that "in a quarter of an hour" it was possible to realize the illogicalities of a patient's thinking and to plan a treatment that would allow him to recover from this basic reasoning problem. Rational psychotherapy would thus have supplanted the puerilities of hypnosis and suggestion, replacing them with a primarily educational technique (pp. 109–114). The therapist would have to stubbornly convince the patient, "inculcating in him the fixed idea that he will get well" (p. 272).

On the other hand, Dubois's was essentially an attempt to enhance a psychotherapy that was possible in the context of psychiatric hospitals. He thus described cases in which, after a short period of rest cure, rational psychotherapy alone (i.e., the therapist's activity in convincing the patient of the illogicality of his or her own behavior and the thoughts underlying the symptoms) proved effective within six weeks (pp. 452–455). In the concluding part of his treatise, Dubois also highlighted the effectiveness of rational psychotherapy administered even without the aid of traditional psychiatric care and the rest cure itself.

Dubois, far from representing, like Janet, a "lost continent" in the field of psychotherapy, was above all a pioneer and systematizer of a psychotherapy aimed at curing the patient by means of hospitalization, and of a "mental orthopedics" that would bring the patient back to rationality, using also the suggestive power of the doctor (p. 66). The continuity with the moral treatment elevated Dubois to the rank of the greatest opponent of the early depth psychotherapies that used instead particular techniques such as hypnosuggestion or the analysis of the unconscious components of the personality.

Significant, in this regard, was the story of Sergej Kostantinovic Pankeev (1886–1979), the famous Freudian case of the Wolf Man. Pankeev, who before meeting Freud had been diagnosed as depressed by Kraepelin, represented a paradigmatic case of psychoanalysis in which the patient resolved his symptoms on the basis of analytic interpretation (in particular of a dream in which the protagonists were wolves), which was able to reveal to the patient the meaning of his oedipal fantasies related to the "primary scene" (witnessing or fantasizing about sexual intercourse between his parents) (Freud, 1918/1955d). The reliability of the story told by Freud has been questioned, since many years after his psychoanalysis, Pankeev was interviewed and had the opportunity to tell his version of events (see, e.g., Borch-Jacobsen & Shamdasani, 2012). Pankeev, however, after having tried all sorts of physical therapy, had considered both a psychotherapy with Freud and one with Dubois. Having decided to undertake the psychoanalytic treatment in Vienna by Freud first, he did not enter the latter (see Muller, 2002, 2003). In the eyes of the Russian notable Pankeev, only depth psychotherapies represented the novelties of the new century, a true point of rupture with the medical-psychiatric and philosophical traditions. Pankeev was a man in search of a radical transformation, reflecting a changing world that wished to be modernized and secularized and that was not satisfied with a shrewd reinterpretation of a medical therapy of the past. From this point of view, Freud seemed in step with the times, while Dubois no longer appeared so.

Notes

1 In this regard, the story of *tarantism*, in which truth and fiction were mixed, is specifically interesting. It was widespread in the south of Italy, namely in Puglia. According to popular opinion, it was caused by the spider, taranta or tarantula (*Lycosa tarantula*), which, on biting, would cause a crisis that could be resolved only with the achievement of an altered state of consciousness similar to a hypnotic trance. This could be reached after hours of dancing (pizzica). Medical treatises were dedicated to this spider and related phenomena by observers from all over Europe, some of which were the exclusive product of the imagination of the doctors who dealt with them (Lüdtke, 2008). In the Mediterranean area, tarantism was also referred to by different names (pizzica in Salento, tarantella in Naples, San Vito's dance in Germany, the argia dance in Sardinia, etc.) and was clearly an attempt to use music with a cathartic and exorcistic function, effective in regulating passions, especially those of young people.

2 In the magical-religious tradition of folk therapies, women had a double role. They were identified as healers, capable, through special rites, of removing the psychophysical "evil" that affected people (for example, the evil eye), chasing it away from the unfortunate. On the other hand, they could be easily possessed by evil and, therefore, in specific need of being freed through various practices and rites, especially musical ones (see De Martino, 1959, 1961; Gallini, 1988).

3 Actually, exorcism has never definitively disappeared from the religious world. In the course of the last decades, on the contrary, a collaboration of exorcists with Catholic psychiatrists has arisen, aimed at distinguishing with an alleged scientific method the cases of *true* from those of *false* possession. The process of secularization of the Devil, therefore, has not yet ended (see Innamorati et al., 2018, 2019).

4 See Ch. 5, pp. 171–177.

5 On science and Freemasonry see Cicciola, 2018.

6 Such different filiations from the same strand of Mesmerism and magnetization are now the subject of numerous studies in the history of psychology (see Mülberger, 2016; Plas, 2000). Indeed, Mesmerism was the first form of what later was called "hypnosis," which became the object and method of investigation of experimental psychology, and marked the birth of psychotherapy. But it was also used as a practice of stage entertainment. It became also part of the so-called "occult sciences," and was the object of exploitation by artists. Eventually, it marked a culture in which the magnetized saw the possibility

of emancipating themselves from a masculinist and patriarchal context (Carroy, 1991; Gallini, 1983); thus, it also had political importance, possibly not credited enough in historiographical circles.

7 In this commission also participated Antoine-Laurent Lavoisier (1743–1794), who in the same period demonstrated the nonexistence of *phlogiston*.

8 The term "Bavarian Illuminati" is often used to refer to circles whose historical reality is doubtful. In the case of the circles frequented by Mesmer and Mozart, reference is made instead to political exponents of Enlightenment who were members of lodges that operated both within Freemasonry and within the Illuminati, which was a society born from the German Freemasonry with political, radically secular aims (see Bramani, 2005; Giarrizzo, 1994; on the role of Freemasonry in the Enlightenment see Jacob, 1991).

9 On Mesmerism and the French revolution see *Le Mesmerisme et la Révolution française,* monographic number of the *Annales historiques de la Révolution française*, n. 391, 2018.

10 The Catholic Church opposed Mesmerism, officially because it was considered *immoral* and compromised with magic and occultism, but perhaps also because it brought novelty with respect to a conservative representation of nature and relationships. At first, a position prevailed in the Church that tended to recognize magnetism as being acceptable if distinct from occultism. Then, in 1856, the Holy Inquisition promulgated a clear official condemnation by means of an encyclical letter, addressed to all Catholic bishops (see Armando, 2009, 2013; Gallini, 1983).

11 Moreover, the issue of the popular use of magnetization and hypnotism, which led to the acquisition by patients of the title of therapist-magnetizer, was the initial moment of what soon became the *vexata quaestio* of the possibility of "non-doctors" practicing psychotherapy. Only recently, and after a very long conflict, has the figure of the non-doctor clinical psychologist been introduced into the pantheon of liberal professions alongside the psychiatrist (see Reisman, 1991; see *infra*, Vol. 2, Ch. 6, pp. 4–5).

12 However, the word *hypnotism* was introduced in 1843 by James Braid (1795–1860).

13 The Charbonnerie or Carboneria was an initiatory society very active in the 19th century, similar to the Freemasonry, from which it was distinguished by its symbolism, related to the charcoal burner trade and not masonry, but also by its explicit political values, democratic-radical, promoted in society by its adherents.

14 The Forty-Eighters were the revolutionaries who participated in the European democratic uprisings of 1848.

15 It is also certain that Bertrand's psychological theories influenced philosopher Maine de Biran (1766–1824), who in turn was an essential source for Janet's psychological automatism (see below) (see Carroy, 1991, pp. 143–145).

16 We should briefly recall some peripheral experiences with respect to the French hypno-suggestive culture such as those promoted by the Belgian Joseph Delboeuf (1831–1896), and especially by the Swiss Théodore Flournoy (1854–1920). Delboeuf criticized the naivety of suggestionists because they were not aware of the simulations they induced and developed the original idea of the co-construction of the experimental situation by the hypnotist *and* his or her suggested subject, who was no longer considered a *puppet* (Carroy, 1991; Delboeuf, 1886). Flournoy, with his studies with the sleepwalker and medium Hélène Smith, pseudonym of Élise-Catherine Müller (1861–1929), demonstrated the creative, rather than merely pathological and negative, potentialities of the unconscious (Carroy, 1991; Flournoy, 1900; Plas, 2000). Hélène Smith told Flournoy about her experiences as a medium, her encounters with spirits of famous people, her interplanetary travels, and her knowledge of Martians and their language. The case described by Flournoy thus marked the end of an era in which sleepwalkers and spiritual or paranormal phenomena were used as if they were experimental and useful to the real scientific understanding of the mind. He believed that these fantastic tales were just an artifact of Hélène's creativity, but tried to give them a psychological meaning. It

was probably the refusal to deal with clinical psychology that relegated Flournoy to the margins of the history of psychotherapy (Shamdasani, 1994).

17 From a historiographical point of view, it is still unclear why, next to an orthodox positivism that excluded psychology from the classification of sciences, another positivism developed, which was instead open to psychological demands. With regard to France, reference has been made to the eclectic *milieu* from which Ribot-like positivism emerged, influenced by Spencer and Lamarckian evolutionism. Such "other" positivism is also deeply related to the idea of the educability of the individual (see Brooks, 1998; Innamorati, 2005).

18 It is little known that Foucault, before becoming a philosopher, had trained as a psychologist, precisely in the tradition of *psychologie pathologique*.

19 On early French psychopathology, see also Innamorati, 2005.

20 As Danziger (1990, pp. 72–73) points out, there was a third tradition of empirical research: the Anglo-American one, based, from the beginning, on another asymmetrical relationship, that of the trader-customer. Francis Galton inaugurated his research suggesting his practices were useful to the subjects, thus charging for the service that actually came in handy for himself and not for his unsuspecting "clients." The foundation of this tradition was the statistical and correlational study of a more or less representative sample of the population. It developed more or less simultaneously with the French and German traditions.

21 Beaunis, in the wake of Bernheim, advocated the experimental use of suggestion and investigated related psychophysiological facts – including the bizarre phenomenon of vescification. He was the founder and first director of the Sorbonne Psychology Laboratory. Alfred Binet (1857–1911) was his pupil.

22 The *placebo* effect corresponds to a perception of improvement of symptoms by patients, in the presence of an inert drug therapy and administered exclusively with the sole purpose of understanding the real efficacy of an experimental therapy of comparison. There can also be the *nocebo* effect, which is a worsening of symptoms in the presence of an inert treatment (on the placebo effect see Benedetti, 2012).

23 Charcot was a formidable clinical neurologist (on the clinical method see supra, Ch. 1, pp. 27–29). He studied the symptomatic pictures of neurological pathologies, and attempted to describe typical and atypical symptoms (*formes frustes*) of nosographic pictures (Goetz et al., 1995).

24 On the metamorphoses of hysteria in the history of psychopathology see Edelman, 2003.

25 Charcot should also be remembered for his proposal of a physiological conception of the unconscious (an idea that was also shared by Ribot: see Gauchet, 1992; Innamorati, 2005).

26 Two films have recently been dedicated to "Augustine," one by Alice Winocour and the other by Jean-Claude Monod and Jean-Christophe Valtat. Her story has thus been used to reinterpret the context of the Paris School with different results.

27 Alfred Binet too, until the 1890s, was a member of the Salpêtrière school and shared Charcot's theory of hypnosis. Moreover, in 1885 he used hypnosis, together with the application of metals and magnets, to understand some psychological phenomena (metalloscopy or magnetoscopy). Binet and Féré described in various articles of those years and in the 1887 volume on magnetism the experiences of transferring symptoms by magnet. This is a bizarre episode in the history of science: On the basis of experiments conducted on hysterics, the most famous of which was Blanche Wittman, it was shown that hypnosis and the application of magnets could transfer the symptoms of hysteria from one side to another of the body, and make them migrate on the body surface. This technique was believed to act directly on the functioning of the brain, to change the personality from joyful to unhappy, as well as to make one hemicorpus feel joy and the

other unhappy, etc. The term that was used for these phenomena, which were considered experimental by the Parisians, was *transference*. That of transference was therefore a pre-psychoanalytic concept, whose original meaning was the dynamic transfer of symptoms that could be moved, modified, eliminated, or produced by techniques inherent in magnetism (Binet & Féré, 1885; see Foschi & Cicciola, 2006).

28 The criminologists who referred to the School of Nancy also contrasted the Lombrosian criminal anthropology, on the basis that they considered predominant the contextual causes rather than the individual and genetic ones of the criminal fact.

29 The dictators of the 20th century adopted this idea of crowd psychology spread by the French Gustave Le Bon (1841–1931). Mussolini, for example, studied Le Bon and succeeded in embodying the *meneur des foules* (leader of the masses), considering the crowd as a hysteric person to be trained (De Felice, 1965).

30 Among the main heirs of the suggestive psychotherapy of the School of Nancy is Emile Coué (1857–1926) (see Walker, 1957). In Italy, the systematic study of hypnosis and suggestion in the experimental and psychotherapeutic field is related to the name of Vittorio Benussi (1878–1927), who nevertheless approached these problems several decades after the French scholars (Benussi, 1905–1927).

31 See Danziger, 1990; Foschi, 2003a; Hacking, 1995; Innamorati, 2005; Lombardo & Foschi, 2003. On the importance of multiple personality inquiry in the history of psychotherapy see also Crabtree, 1993.

32 To use the words of Galileo Galilei (1564–1642), the experiment can be considered a combination of "sensible experiences" and "necessary demonstrations" (Galilei, 1615). An initial moment of formulating hypotheses based on observations should be followed by an experimental demonstration based on experiences, created ad hoc by the scientist, to accept or refine the hypotheses. In this sense, the experiment is not spontaneous, but enacted by the researcher.

33 Kynesthesia is the complex of perceptions, including automatic ones, through which the brain detects the body in space. There are special nerve pathways that promote kynesthetic processing.

34 The idea of pathology as regression and regression as the inverse of evolution originated in the English neurological tradition, and in particular with John Hughlings Jackson (1835–1911).

35 Paul Janet (1823–1899) was an influential professor of philosophy at the Sorbonne. He was a follower of Hegel and a pupil of Victor Cousin (1792–1867), the greatest representative of 19th-century French spiritual eclecticism.

36 Janet initially used the word *dissociation*, which he later changed to *disaggregation* for the sake of clarity. Just as he initially used the term *unconscious*, which he later replaced with *subconscious,* again for theoretical reasons (see Carroy & Plas, 2000). The term *disaggregation* was then translated *tout court* to *dissociation* or *splitting*. This translation actually led to a confusion between dissociation as a pathological process that, according to Janet, affects the conscience and the self and dissociation/splitting as a defense mechanism or mode of functioning of the mind, systematized by Melanie Klein (1882–1960) in the schizo-paranoid position (see infra, Ch. 5, pp. 191–192).

37 For Leibniz, the *petites perceptions* are the simplest elements from which knowledge evolves. The small perceptions are plenty and do not reach the threshold of consciousness, even though they are part of the perceived whole. For example, noise is composed of many small noises that reach consciousness only as a single whole noise.

38 Janet's automatic conception of the unconscious was also influenced by Maine de Biran (1766–1824), whom he cited explicitly and who was one of the sources of French spiritualism (see Brooks, 1998, pp. 189–190).

39 In the course of the volume, terms such as *construction* and *construct* will often recur, referring respectively to constructionism and constructivism. The term *constructionism* refers

to a large set of epistemological theories based on the criterion that reality is the result of a more or less likely and socially shared construction. Constructivism, on the other hand, is oriented towards understanding how the subject knows reality through internal constructs that favor its cognitive representation. The two terms, however, are often used equivalently, especially because in English *constructivism* is preferred to mean a broad epistemological and psychological domain. It is therefore necessary to keep in mind that, although constructionism and constructivism are similar terms, we must inevitably contextualize them in the thought of the authors who use them.

40 The word *metapsychology* was used by Freud to indicate those theoretical points of view of psychoanalysis (energetic, topical, structural, evolutionary) that made use of notions derived from other scientific disciplines to describe the dynamics of the mind. Janet did not use this word. However, the notions of strength and misery of the personality, automatism, disaggregation, narrowing of the field of consciousness, and the function of synthesis are all theoretical concepts that sketch an alternative model to Freud's metapsychology.

41 Janet is quoting himself here (Janet, 1889, p. 364).

42 See Ch. 1, footnote 24, p. 35.

43 The degeneration theory was first formulated by Bénédict Augustin Morel (1809–1873) and revised by Valentin Magnan (1835–1916) and was a huge success in 19th-century psychiatry. According to this theory, the origin of mental illnesses derives from the transmission of a hereditary "taint" in which it was not possible to intervene and which indeed worsened from generation to generation. Therefore, degeneration could mark the existence of members of an entire family and was considered the cause of the pathologies and behaviors studied by psychiatrists (Coffin, 2003). This theory left no room for the optimistic transformationism of other French positivists and psychologists who referred to a trustful praxis in changing and improving generations through clinical and educational intervention (see Ch. 1, pp. 30–33). The theory became popular in the French cultural world, to the point of inspiring Zola's novels based on family epopees.

44 See infra, Vol. 2, Ch. 7, pp. 81–85.

45 Reference is made to the more recent cognitivist schools, which integrate some of the concepts of dynamic psychology by referring primarily to automatisms, trauma, dissociation, and Janetian constructivism. Such theories will be discussed in the last chapter of Vol. 2.

46 However, as we will see in the following chapters, one of the last Freudian texts, *Constructions in analysis* (1937/1964d), marks a change in Freud's relationship with the "truth" of interpretation. In this essay Freud attached much importance to the effects of the coherence of the construction of the analyst on the patient's belief, rather than merely on the veridical contents of what is interpreted by the analyst (see Ch. 4, pp. 148–154).

47 This theme can only be touched upon here. For further reference, see specific studies on the history of the unconscious such as Ellenberger, 1970; Tallis, 2002; and Whyte, 1960.

48 See Ch. 4, pp. 158–166; Ch. 5, pp. 213–215; Vol. 2, Ch. 7, pp. 76–78.

49 Nietzsche was among other things a great admirer of Ribot: see the letter of 4/8/1877 to Malwida von Meysenbug (Nietzsche, 2015).

50 The concept of the will to power was explicitly taken up by Alfred Adler (1870–1937), who made it the core of human motivation. The interest in Nietzsche was so explicit on the part of Carl Gustav Jung (1875–1961) that he called Zarathustra one of what he considered to be his two personalities (Jung, 1961). Moreover, Jung (1934–1939) devoted to *Thus Spoke Zarathustra* years of seminars, the transcript of which constitutes the most extensive edited commentary on a Nietzschean text (perhaps on any philosophical text). In contrast, Freud never admitted to having been influenced by Nietzsche and even explicitly stated that he denied himself the pleasure of reading him for a long time in order not to let himself be influenced by his reading (Freud, 1925/1959a). Actually, in his

letters to his friend Eduard Silberstein, Freud (1990) had explicitly written that he had read Nietzsche.
51 See Ch. 3, pp. 90–91.
52 See Ch. 1, pp. 58–59.
53 See Vol. 2, Ch. 7, pp. 70–75.
54 See Ch. 1, pp. 29–30.

References

Andersson, O. (1962). *Studies in the prehistory of psychoanalysis*. John Gach Books.

Araujo, S. D. F. (2012). Why did Wundt abandon his early theory of the unconscious? Towards a new interpretation of Wundt's psychological project. *History of Psychology, 15*(1), 33–49.

Armando, D. (2009). Scienza, demonolatria o 'impostura ereticale'? Il Sant'Uffizio romano e la questione del magnetismo animale [Science, demonolatry or 'heretical imposture'? The Roman Holy Office and the question of animal magnetism]. *Giornale di Storia, 2*, 1–13.

Armando, D. (2013). *Spiriti e fluidi. Medicina e religione nei documenti del Sant'Uffizio sul magnetismo animale (1840–1856)* [Spirits and fluids. Medicine and religion in the documents of the Holy Office on animal magnetism (1840–1856)]. In M. P. Donato, L. Berlivet, S. Cabibbo, R. Michetti, & N. Nicoud (Eds.), *Médecine et religion: Compétitions, collaborations, conflits (XIIe-XXe siècles)* [Medicine and religion: Competition, collaboration, conflict (12th-20th centuries)] (pp. 195–225). Editions de l'Ecole française de Rome.

Armando, D., & Belhoste, B. (2018). Le mesmérisme entre la fin de l'ancien régime et la révolution: Dynamiques sociales et enjeux politiques [Mesmerism between the end of the old regime and the revolution: Social dynamics and political issues]. *Annales Historiques de la Révolution Française, 391*, 3–26.

Assoun, P. L. (1976). *Freud, la philosophie et les philosophes*. PUF.

Azam, E. (1876a). Amnésie périodique, ou doublement de la vie [Periodic amnesia, or doubling of life]. *Revue Scientifique, 10*(47), 481–489.

Azam, E. (1876b). Le dédoublement de la personnalité. Suite de l'histoire de Félida X★★★ [The split of the personality. Continuation of the story of Félida X ★★★]. *Revue Scientifique, 11*(12), 265–269.

Azam, E. (1877). Le dédoublement de la personnalité et l'amnésie périodique. Suite de l'histoire de Félida X★★★ – Relation d'un fait nouveau du même ordre [Split personality and periodic amnesia. Continuation of the story of Félida X ★★★ – Relation of a new fact of the same order]. *Revue Scientifique, 13*(25), 577–581.

Baker, D. B. (Ed.). (2012). *The Oxford handbook of the history of psychology: Global perspectives*. Oxford University Press.

Belhoste, B., & Edelman, N. (2015). *Mesmer et mesmérismes* [Mesmer and mesmerisms]. Omniscience.

Benedetti, F. (2012). *L'effetto placebo* [Placebo effect]. Carocci.

Bérillon, E. (Ed.). (1890). *Premier congrès international de l'hypnotisme expérimental et thérapeutique* [First international congress of experimental and therapeutic hypnotism]. Doin.

Bertrand, A. (1823). *Traité du somnambulisme et des différentes modifications qu'il présente* [Treatise on sleepwalking and the various changes it presents]. Dentu.

Binet, A., & Féré, C. (1885). L'hypnotisme chez les hystériques [Hypnotism in hysterics]. *Revue Philosophique, 19*, 1–25.

Borch-Jacobsen, M., & Shamdasani, S. (2012). *The Freud files: An inquiry into the history of psychoanalysis*. Cambridge University Press.

Bourneville, D. M., & Regnard, P. M. L. (1876–1880). *Iconographie photographique de la Salpêtrière* [Photographic iconography of the Salpêtrière]. Delahaye.

Bourru, H., & Burot, P. F. (1888). *Variations de la personnalité* [Personality variations]. Baillière.

Bramani, L. (2005). *Mozart massone e rivoluzionario* [Mozart freemason and revolutionary]. Bruno Mondadori.

Braunstein, J. F. (1986). *Broussais et le matérialisme* [Broussais and the materialism]. Klincksieck.

Breuer, J., & Freud, S. (1955). Studies on hysteria. In *The standard edition of the complete psychological works of Sigmund Freud, Volume 2 (1893–1895)*. Hogarth Press. (Original work published 1893–1895)

Bromberg, P. M. (1998). *Standing in the spaces: Essays on clinical process, trauma, and dissociation*. Analytic Press.

Brooks, J. I. (1998). *The eclectic legacy: Academic philosophy and the human sciences in nineteenth-century France*. University of Delaware Press.

Broussais, F. J. V. (1828). *De l'irritation et de la folie* [Irritation and madness]. Librairie polymathique.

Caplan, E. (1998). *Mind games: American culture and the birth of psychotherapy*. University of California Press.

Carroy, J. (1991). *Hypnose, suggestion et psychologie* [Hypnosis, suggestion and psychology]. PUF.

Carroy, J. (1993). *Les personnalités doubles et multiples. Entre science et fiction* [Double and multiple personalities. Between science and fiction]. PUF.

Carroy, J. (2000). L'invention du mot psychothérapie et ses enjeux [The invention of the word psychotherapy and its challenges]. *Psychologie Clinique, 9*, 11–30.

Carroy, J., Ohayon, A., & Plas, R. (2006). *Histoire de la psychologie en France* [History of psychology in France]. La Découverte.

Carroy, J., & Plas, R. (2000). La genèse de la notion de dissociation chez Pierre Janet et ses enjeux [The genesis of the notion of dissociation in Pierre Janet and its challenges]. *Évolution Psychiatrique, 65*, 9–18.

Chazaud, J. (1992). *F.J.V. Broussais. De l'irritation à la folie* [F.J.V. Broussais. From irritation to madness]. Ères.

Cicciola, E. (2018). Scienza e massoneria: storia e storiografia [Science and Freemasonry History and historiography]. *Physis, 53*, 213–253.

Cicciola, E. (2019). *La scoperta dell'intelligenza. Alfred Binet e la storia del primo test* [The discovery of intelligence. Alfred Binet and the history of the first test]. Fefè.

Clauzade, L. (2003). Auguste Comte et Stuart Mill. Les enjeux de la psychologie [Auguste Comte and Stuart Mill. The challenges of psychology]. *Revue d'histoire des sciences humaines, 8*, 41–56.

Coffin, J.-C. (2003). *La transmission de la folie: 1850–1914* [The transmission of madness: 1850–1914]. Harmattan.

Crabtree, A. (1993). *From Mesmer to Freud: Magnetic sleep and the roots of psychological healing*. Yale University Press.

Crabtree, A. (2008). The transition to secular psychotherapy. In E. R. Wallace & J. Gach (Eds.), *History of psychiatry and medical psychology* (pp. 555–586). Springer.

Danziger, K. (1990). *Constructing the subject: Historical origins of psychological research*. Cambridge University Press.

Darnton, R. (1968). *Mesmerism and the end of the enlightenment in France.* Harvard University Press.

De Felice, R. (1965). *Mussolini il rivoluzionario* [Mussolini the Revolutionary]. Einaudi.

Dejerine, J. (1904). Préface [Foreword]. In P. Dubois (Ed.), *Les psychonévroses et leur traitement moral* [Psychoneuroses and moral treatment] (pp. V–VI). Masson.

Delboeuf, F. J. (1886). De l'influence de l'education et de l'imitation dans le somnambulisme provoqué [On the influence of education and imitation in induced somnambulism]. *Revue Philosophique, 22,* 146–171.

Del Corno, F., & Lang, M. (2008). *Elementi di psicologia clinica* [Outlines of clinical psychology]. FrancoAngeli.

De Martino, E. (1959). *Sud e magia* [South and magic]. Feltrinelli.

De Martino, E. (1961). *La terra del rimorso. Contributo a una storia religiosa del Sud* [The land of remorse. Contribution to a religious history of the South]. il Saggiatore.

Didi-Huberman, G. (2004). *Invention of hysteria: Charcot and the photographic iconography of the salpêtrière.* MIT Press.

Dowbiggin, I. (1991). *Inheriting madness: Professionalization and psychiatric knowledge in nineteenth-century France.* University of California Press.

Dubois, P. (1901). *De l'influence de l'esprit sur le corps* [The influence of the mind on the body]. A. Francke.

Dubois, P. (1904). *Les psychonévroses et leur traitement moral* [Psychoneuroses and moral treatment]. Masson.

Dubois, P. (1908). *L'éducation de soi-même* [The education of oneself]. Masson.

Edelman, N. (2003). *Les métamorphoses de l'hystérique* [The metamorphoses of the hysterical]. La Découverte.

Ellenberger, H. F. (1970). *The discovery of the unconscious: The history and evolution of dynamic psychiatry.* Basic Books.

Erlenmayer, A. (1886). Über Cocainsucht. Vorläufige Mitteilung [About cocaine addiction. Preliminary communication]. *Medizinal-Zeitung, 7,* 483–484.

Fauvel, A. (2004). Aliénistes contre psychiatres. La médicine mentale en crise (1890–1914). *Psychologie Clinique, 17,* 61–76.

Flournoy, T. (1900). *Des Indes à la planète Mars, étude sur un cas de somnambulisme avec glossolalie* [From India to Mars, study on a case of sleepwalking with glossolalia]. Eggimann et Alcan.

Foschi, R. (2003a). L'indagine sulla personalità alle origini della psicologia scientifica francese (1870–1885) [The study of the personality at the origins of French scientific psychology (1870–1885)]. *Physis, 40,* 63–105.

Foschi, R. (2003b). La psicologia sperimentale e patologica di Pierre Janet e la nozione di personalità (1885–1900) [Pierre Janet's experimental and pathological psychology and the notion of personality (1885–1900)]. *Medicina e storia, 3,* 45–68.

Foschi, R., & Cicciola, E. (2006). The notion of 'double consciousness' in Alfred Binet's psychological experimentalism. *Physis, 43,* 363–372.

Franklin, B. (1837). *Animal magnetism.* Perkins.

Freud, S. (1953a). The interpretation of the dreams. In *The standard edition of the complete psychological works of Sigmund Freud, Vols. 4–5.* Hogarth. (Original work published 1900)

Freud, S. (1953b). *On aphasia; a critical study.* International Universities Press. (Original work published 1891)

Freud, S. (1955a). Beyond the pleasure principle. In *The standard edition of the complete psychological works of Sigmund Freud, Volume 18* (pp. 1–64). Hogarth. (Original work published 1920)

Freud, S. (1955b).Totem and taboo. In *The standard edition of the complete psychological works of Sigmund Freud,Volume 13* (pp. 7–162). Hogarth. (Original work published 1913)

Freud, S. (1955c).The Moses of Michelangelo. In *The standard edition of the complete psychological works of Sigmund Freud,Volume 13* (pp. 211–238). Hogarth. (Original work published 1914)

Freud, S. (1955d). From the history of an infantile neurosis. In *The standard edition of the complete psychological works of Sigmund Freud,Volume 17* (pp. 7–122). Hogarth. (Original work published 1918)

Freud, S. (1957). On the history of the psycho-analytic movement. In *The standard edition of the complete psychological works of Sigmund Freud, Volume 14* (pp. 1–66). Hogarth. (Original work published 1914)

Freud, S. (1959a).An autobiographical study. In *The standard edition of the complete psychological works of Sigmund Freud* (Vol. 20, pp. 3–74). Hogarth. (Original work published 1925)

Freud, S. (1959b). Delusions and dreams in Jensen's Gradiva. In *The standard edition of the complete psychological works of Sigmund Freud,Volume 9* (pp. 1–96). Hogarth. (Original work published 1907)

Freud, S. (1959c). Creative writers and day-dreaming. In *The standard edition of the complete psychological works of Sigmund Freud,Volume 9* (pp. 141–153). Hogarth. (Original work published 1908)

Freud, S. (1961a). Civilization and its discontents. In *The standard edition of the complete psychological works of Sigmund Freud, Volume 21* (pp. 57–145). Hogarth. (Original work published 1930)

Freud, S. (1961b).The future of an illusion. In *The standard edition of the complete psychological works of Sigmund Freud, Volume 21* (pp. 1–56). Hogarth. (Original work published 1927)

Freud, S. (1962a). Heredity and aetiology of neuroses. In *The standard edition of the complete psychological works of Sigmund Freud, Volume 3* (pp. 141–156). Hogarth. (Original work published 1896)

Freud, S. (1962b). Further remarks on the neuro-psychoses of defence. In *The standard edition of the complete psychological works of Sigmund Freud, Volume 3* (pp. 157–185). Hogarth. (Original work published 1896)

Freud, S. (1962c).The neuro-psychoses of defence. In *The standard edition of the complete psychological works of Sigmund Freud, Volume 3* (pp. 45–61). Hogarth. (Original work published 1894)

Freud, S. (1964a). New introductory lectures on psychoanalysis. In *The standard edition of the complete psychological works of Sigmund Freud, Volume 22* (pp. 5–182). Hogarth. (Original work published 1932)

Freud, S. (1964b). Moses and monotheism. In *The standard edition of the complete psychological works of Sigmund Freud, Volume 23* (pp. 1–138). Hogarth. (Original work published 1939)

Freud, S. (1964c).The acquisition and control of fire. In *The standard edition of the complete psychological works of Sigmund Freud, Volume 23* (pp. 187–193). Hogarth. (Original work published 1932)

Freud, S. (1964d). Constructions in analysis. In *The standard edition of the complete psychological works of Sigmund Freud, Volume 23* (pp. 257–269). Hogarth. (Original work published 1937)

Freud, S. (1966a). Hysteria. In *The standard edition of the complete psychological works of Sigmund Freud, Volume 1* (pp. 39–59). Hogarth. (Original work published 1888)

Freud, S. (1966b). Project for a scientific psychology. In *The standard edition of the complete psychological works of Sigmund Freud,Volume 1* (pp. 281–391). Hogarth. (Original work published 1895–1950)

Freud, S. (1974). *Cocaine papers*. New American Library. (Original work published 1885)

Freud, S. (1985). *The complete letters of Sigmund Freud to Wilhelm Fliess*. Bellknap.

Freud, S. (1990). *The letters of Sigmund Freud to Eduard Silberstein, 1871–1881*. Harvard University Press.

Galilei, G. (1953). Lettera a madama Cristina di Lorena [Letter to Madame Cristina of Lorena]. In F. Flora (Ed.), *Opere di Galileo Galilei* [Writings of Galileo Galilei] (pp. 1013–1015). Ricciardi. (Original work published 1615)

Gallini, C. (1983). *La sonnambula meravigliosa* [The wonderful sleepwalker]. Feltrinelli.

Gallini, C. (1988). *La ballerina variopinta. Una festa di guarigione in Sardegna* [The Colorful dancer: A healing feast in Sardinia]. Liguori.

Gauchet, M. (1992). *L'inconscient cérébral* [The unconscious brain]. Seuil.

Gauld, A. (1992). *A history of hypnotism*. Cambridge University Press.

Gay, P. (1988). *Freud: A life for our time*. Dent & Sons.

Giarrizzo, G. (1994). *Massoneria e illuminismo nell'Europa del Settecento* [Freemasonry and enlightenment in eighteenth-century Europe]. Marsilio.

Ginzburg, C. (1980). *The cheese and the worms: The cosmos of a sixteenth century miller*. Routledge and Kegan Paul.

Goetz, C. G., Goetz, B. G., Bonduelle, M., & Gelfand, T. (1995). *Charcot: Constructing neurology*. Oxford University Press.

Hacking, I. (1995). *Rewriting the soul: Multiple personality and the sciences of memory*. Princeton University Press.

Harris, B. (2016). Therapeutic work and mental illness in America, c. 1830–1970. In W. Ernst (Ed.), *Work, psychiatry and society, 1800–1950* (pp. 55–76). Manchester University Press.

Harris, B., & Stevens, C. J. (2020). Practicing mind-body medicine before Freud: John G. Gehring, the "Wizard of the Androscoggin". *Journal of the History of the Behavioral Sciences, 56*(2), 75–98.

Heim, G., & Bühler, K. E. (2006). Psychological trauma and fixed ideas in Pierre Janet's conception of dissociative disorders. *American Journal of Psychotherapy, 60*, 111–129.

Herbart, J. F. (1813). *Lehrbuch zur Einleitung in die Philosophie* [Introductory textbook of philosophy]. A. W. Unzer.

Hustvedt, A. (2011). *Medical muses: Hysteria in nineteenth-century*. W. W. Norton & Company.

Innamorati, M. (2005). *Il meccanismo intimo dello spirito. La psicologia di Théodule Ribot nel suo contesto storico* [The intimate mechanism of the spirit. The psychology of Théodule Ribot in its historical context]. FrancoAngeli.

Innamorati, M., Taradel, R., & Foschi, R. (2018). Psicopatologia e demonologia. La 'diagnosi' di possessione nel corso del xx secolo [Psychopathology and demonology. The 'diagnosis' of possession during the twentieth century]. *Psicoterapia e Scienze Umane, 52*(1), 31–46.

Innamorati, M., Taradel, R., & Foschi, R. (2019). Between sacred and profane: Possession, psychopathology, and the Catholic church. *History of Psychology, 22*(1), 1–16.

Jacob, M. C. (1991). *Living the enlightenment: Freemasonry and politics in eighteenth-century Europe*. Oxford University Press.

Janet, P. (1889). *L'Automatisme psychologique. Essai de psychologie expérimentale sur les formes inférieures de l'activité humaine* [Psychological automatism: Essay on experimental psychology and the inferior forms of human activity]. Alcan.

Janet, P. (1893–1894). *État mental des hystériques, Vol. 1: Les stigmates mentaux; Vol. 2: Les accidents mentaux* [État mental des hystériques, Vol. 1: Les stigmates mentaux; Vol. 2: Les accidents mentaux]. Rueff.

Janet, P. (1896). Résumé historique des études sur le sentiment de la personnalité [Historical summary of studies on the personality]. *Revue Scientifique, 5*(4), 97–103.

Janet, P. (1898). *Névroses et idées fixes, vols. 2* [Neuroses and fixed ideas]. Alcan.

Janet, P. (1903). *Les obsessions et la psychasténie, vols. 2* [Obsessions and psychastenia]. Alcan.

Janet, P. (1911). *L'état mental des hystériques* (2nd ed.) [The mental condition of hysterics]. Alcan.

Janet, P. (1914). La psychoanalyse [Psychoanalysis]. *Journal de Psychologie, 11*, 1–130.

Jones, E. (1953–1957). *The life and work of Sigmund Freud* (3 vols). Basic Books.

Jung, C. G. (1961). *Memories, dreams, reflections*. Pantheon.

Jung, C. G. (1968a). The concept of the collective unconscious. In *Collected works of C. G. Jung, Vol. 9, part 1* (2nd ed., pp. 42–53). Princeton University Press. (Original work published 1936)

Jung, C. G. (1968b). Archetypes of the collective unconscious. In *Collected works of C. G. Jung, Vol. 9, Part 1* (2nd ed., pp. 3–41). Princeton University Press. (Original work published 1954)

Jung, C. G. (1976). The hypothesis of the collective unconscious. In *Collected works of C. G. Jung, Vol. 18* (pp. 515–516). Princeton University Press. (Original work published 1932)

Kaplan-Solms, K., & Solms, M. (2000). *Clinical cases in neuro-psychoanalysis. Introduction to a depth neuropsychology*. Karnac.

Kerr, J. (1993). *A most dangerous method: The story of Jung, Freud, and Sabina Spielrein*. Knopf.

Kuhn, T. S. (1962). *The structure of scientific revolutions*. University of Chicago Press.

Lombardo, G. P., & Foschi, R. (2002a). The European origins of "personality psychology". *European Psychologist, 7*(2), 134–145.

Lombardo, G. P., & Foschi, R. (2002b). *La costruzione scientifica della personalità* [The scientific construction of personality]. Bollati Boringhieri.

Lombardo, G. P., & Foschi, R. (2003). The concept of personality in 19th-century French and 20th-century American psychology. *History of Psychology, 6*(2), 123–142.

Lüdtke, K. (2008). *Dances with spiders*. Berghahn Books.

Méheust, B. (1999). *Somnambulisme et mediumnité (1784–1930), Vol. 1* [Sleepwalking and mediumship (1784–1930), Vol. 1]. La Découverte.

Merlan, P. (1945). Brentano and Freud. *Journal of History of Ideas, 6*, 375–377.

Merlan, P. (1949). Brentano and Freud – A sequel. *Journal of History of Ideas, 10*, 451.

Mesmer, F.-A. (1779). *Mémoire sur la découverte du magnétisme animal* [Thesis on the discovery of animal magnetism]. P. Fr. Didot le jeune.

Mesmer, F.-A. (1971a). *Précis historique des faits relatifs au magnétisme-animal jusques en avril 1781* [Precise history of facts relating to animal magnetism until April 1781]. In R. Amadou (Ed.), *Le Magnétisme animal. Œuvres* [Animal magnetism. Writings] (pp. 93–194). Payot. (Original work published 1781)

Mesmer, F.-A. (1971b). Règlements des Sociétés de l'Harmonie Universelle [Regulations of the societies of the universal harmony]. In R. Amadou (Ed.), *Le Magnétisme animal. Œuvres* [Animal magnetism. Writings] (pp. 203–227). Payot. (Original work published 1785)

Midelfort, H. E. (2005). *Exorcism and enlightenment*. Yale University Press.

Mülberger, A. (Ed.). (2016). *Los límites de la ciencia: Espiritismo, hipnotismo y el estudio de los fenómenos paranormales (1850–1930)* [The limits of science: Spiritualism, hypnotism and the study of paranormal phenomena (1850–1930)]. Consejo Superior de Investigaciones Científicas.

Müller, C. (2002). *Paul Dubois (1848–1918)*. Schwabe.

Müller, C. (2003). Paul Dubois, pionnier de la psychothérapie [Paul Dubois, pioneer of psychotherapy]. *Psychothérapies, 23*(1), 49–52.

Münsterberg, H. (1909). *Psychotherapy*. Moffat, Yard & Co.

Nietzsche, F. (1924). *The dawn of day*. Allen & Unwin. (Original work published 1881)

Nietzsche, F. (1966). *Beyond good and evil*.Vintage Books. (Original work published 1886)

Nietzsche, F. (1969). *Thus spoke Zarathustra*. Penguin. (Original work published 1883–1885)

Nietzsche, F. (1974). *The gay science*.Vintage Books. (Original work published 1882–1887)

Nietzsche, F. (1996). *Human, all too human*. Cambridge University Press. (Original work published 1878)

Nietzsche, F. (2015). *Briefwechsel, Band 6.2: Juli 1877 – Dezember 1879* [Letters, Vol. 6.2: July 1877 – December 1879]. De Gruyter.

Pick, D. (1993). *Faces of degeneration: A European disorder, c. 1848–1918*. Cambridge University Press.

Plas, R. (2000). *Naissance d'une science humaine, la psychologie: les psychologues et le "merveilleux psychique"* [Birth of a human science, psychology: psychologists and the "psychical wonder"]. PUR.

Puységur, A.-M.-J. (1811). *Recherches, expériences et observations physiologiques sur l'homme dans l'état de somnambulisme naturel et dans le somnambulisme provoqué par l'acte magnétique* [Research, experiments and physiological observations on man in the state of natural sleepwalking and in sleepwalking caused by the magnetic act]. Dentu.

Rausky, F. (1977). *Mesmer ou la révolution thérapeutique* [Mesmer or the therapeutic revolution]. Payot.

Reisman, J. M. (1991). *A history of clinical psychology*.Taylor & Francis.

Ribot, T. H. (1888). La psychologie contemporaine [Contemporary psychology]. *Revue Scientifique*, *41*, 449–455.

Ricoeur, P. (1972). *Freud and philosophy: An essay on interpretation*.Yale University Press. (Original work published 1965)

Schopenhauer, A. (1966). *The world as will and representation* (2 vols). Dover. (Original work published 1818–1859)

Shamdasani, S. (1994). Encountering Hélène:Théodore Flournoy and the genesis of subliminal psychology. In T. Flournoy (Ed.), *From India to the planet mars: A case of multiple personality with imaginary languages* (pp. XI–LI). Princeton University Press.

Shamdasani, S. (2017). Psychotherapy in society: Historical reflections. In G. Eghigian (Ed.), *The Routledge history of madness and mental health* (pp. 363–378). Routledge.

Solms, M., & Turnbull, O. (2003). *The brain and the inner world*. Other Press.

Sulloway, F. J. (1979). *Freud, biologist of the mind*. Harvard University Press.

Tallis, F. (2002). *Hidden minds: A history of the unconscious*. Arcade Publishing.

Tarde, G. (1903). *The laws of imitation*. Henry Holt. (Original work published 1890)

Traetta, L. (2007). *La forza che guarisce. Franz Anton Mesmer e la storia del magnetismo animale* [The force that heals. Franz Anton Mesmer and the history of animal magnetism]. Edipuglia.

Turbiaux, M. (2009). À l'occasion de deux expositions sur le tricentenaire de la naissance de Benjamin Franklin, Benjamin Franklin (1706–1790), Antoine Mesmer (1734–1815) et le magnétisme animal [On the occasion of the third centenary of the birth of Benjamin Franklin. Benjamin Franklin (1706–1790), Antoine Mesmer (1734–1815) and animal magnetism]]. *Bulletin de psychologie*, *499*(1), 51–65.

Von Hartmann, E. (1884). *Philosophy of the unconscious, 3 vols*.Trübner & Co. (Original work published 1869)

Walker, N. (1957). *A short history of psychotherapy*. Routledge.

Weininger, O. (2005). *Sex and character*. Indiana University Press. (Original work published 1903)

Whyte, L. L. (1960). *The unconscious before Freud*. Basic Books.

3

The 20th century and the rooting of psychotherapy

Psychoanalysis and the interpretation of dreams

In 1899, two fundamental texts for the history of psychotherapy saw the light of day, but they had very different fates: *From the Indies to Planet Mars* by Théodore Flournoy and *The Interpretation of Dreams* by Freud. Both books were published with a date of 1900, to project them into the new century. Flournoy's text, which mainly described the mental life of a patient in an imaginary world, had extraordinary immediate success and then ended up in almost total oblivion. *The Interpretation of Dreams*, on the other hand, was initially read almost exclusively by Viennese physicians but was to become the symbolic text of psychoanalysis and perhaps the most famous psychological book in history. Its success obscured over time the work of another pioneer of the study of dreams, Sante De Sanctis, who also published in 1899, his *I sogni. Studi clinici e psicologici di un alienista* (*Dreams. Clinical and Psychological Studies of an Alienist*).[1]

Freud's masterpiece made a deep mark on the 20th-century forms of psychotherapy, thanks to the use of an apparently unprecedented and rigorous technique.[2] Before *The Interpretation of Dreams*, in fact, it would have been difficult for any reader to understand the originality of psychoanalysis: Janet himself (1913/2004) considered *Studies on Hysteria* (Breuer & Freud, 1895/1955) no more than a confirmation of his theses. The gestation of the book was slow and meditated, as it is possible to infer from Freud's correspondence with Wilhelm Fliess. The intuition that a dream consisted of the realization of a desire had already appeared in the then unpublished *Project of a Psychology* (Freud, 1895/1966). *The Interpretation of Dreams* proposed the same principle but broadened the basis: the dream basically tried to satisfy a desire (present or childish) by hallucinatory means and through compromise-formations. In September 1897, after having confessed to Fliess that he had abandoned his own convictions regarding the theory of infantile seduction (Masson, 1985, p. 297), Freud informed him of a new idea, which he would never abandon. It was the conviction that the fundamental desire of the male child consisted of taking over the father next to the mother. Freud had recognized this desire in his own self-analysis, that is, by applying to himself the examination of thoughts,

DOI: 10.4324/9781003252405-3

fantasies, and dreams that he normally conducted with his patients. He also believed he saw it veiled in Sophocles' *Oedipus Rex*, where Oedipus becomes King of Thebes by killing his father Laius and marrying his mother Jocasta. The driving force of Sophocles' tragedy had always been considered destiny, because Oedipus thought that his real parents lived in Corinth and went to Thebes precisely to escape an oracular response that wanted him to murder his father and marry his mother. However, according to Freud, myths, like dreams, were formed by hiding a desire behind transformations that seemed to overturn its meaning (ibid, p. 298). Thus was born the idea that would crystallize into the concept of the "Oedipus complex."

Dream interpretation seemed to be a new way to understand the unconscious contents of the mind, namely the decisive contents: the most intense and less confessable desires. *The Interpretation of Dreams* theorized how the transformation of the original, authentic contents of the dream (*latent content*) assumed the form remembered upon awakening (*manifest content*). According to Freud, the deformation (*dream-work*) was carried out by a *censorship*. It worked, unconsciously, in the same way as the censorship enacted by totalitarian political regimes against the spread of news which was potentially dangerous to the established order. Dream-work operated through (a) *condensation*, whereby several elements of latent content are unified (e.g., several people become one character in the dream); (b) *displacement*, in order to place the decisive elements of the latent content in the background; (c) *consideration of representability*, so that the original thought was converted into a story; and the (d) use of *symbols*,[3] in order to mask objects, especially those related to sexuality. Through this last mechanism, for example, elongated objects such as bell towers and poles replaced the male sexual organ. Hollow objects such as caves and bottles replaced the female sexual organ.

Dream-work using only these procedures, however, would have led to a chaotic result: through (e) *secondary elaboration*, instead, the modified elements of the dream were reorganized into a somehow narratable story.

The contents of a dream were not entirely traceable to the dreamer's wishes: first, because references to a real event that had recently occurred to the dreamer (day residues) would often be interpolated into the dream, and second, because, according to Freud, the human being dreams also to keep on sleeping. For this purpose somatic stimuli perceived during sleep would be incorporated into the dream: it could be endosomatic stimuli (often the origin of distressing feelings in the dream) or external stimuli (e.g., the sound of a doorbell could produce the feeling, during the dream, of hearing a distant bell). It should be noted that, while the discussion on the possible psychological meaning of dream activity is still alive today, the idea that dreams preserve sleep has been completely abandoned by neurophysiological research, after the discovery of rapid eye movement (REM) sleep (Aserinsky & Kleitman, 1953). We now know with certainty that instead of dreaming in order to sleep, people sleep in order to dream; and that dream deprivation can damage the human physique even more than sleep deprivation (Arkin et al., 1978).

Freud believed that he had legitimately reconstructed the mechanisms that induce dream formation by subjecting dreams to an analytical procedure. He started from the single elements of the dream and suggested that the dreamer make free associations. Spontaneous associations led the interpreter to identify hidden desires. In fact, in Freud's opinion, it would have been possible to trace these desires to a relatively limited set of themes, of which sexuality was the most common (although not the only one, as Freud was keen to point out).

The Interpretation of Dreams was not only a fundamental contribution to the history of psychotherapy, it also proposed a model of the mind and a theory of human motivations – little less than a complete new psychological paradigm. The "topography" divided the mind into consciousness, the preconscious, and the unconscious. The consciousness corresponded to what was immediately present in the mind of a human being. The preconscious consisted of the mental contents that were not conscious but could become so without difficulty: the memories retained by an adult of their elementary school teacher are a Freudian example, memories that, however neglected for decades, would be evoked, in general, with the greatest ease. The unconscious consisted of content that was not accessible to the consciousness. The mechanism of repression banished this content from the consciousness, and censorship made any attempt to return directly to them impossible. Compared to *Studies on Hysteria*, the concept of repression had definitely changed: forgetting due to repression was no longer influenced by conscious will. The contents of the unconscious could only be deduced from their indirect manifestations, what would later be called *compromise-formations*. Dreams were actually typical examples of the activity aimed at rising above the threshold of consciousness, made possible since censorship was less strong during sleep.

Conscious thoughts were for Freud only a minimal part of the mental world: consciousness was comparable to the tip of an iceberg, because the activity of the mind would take place essentially in the unconscious. Unconscious mental activity, moreover, was different from the conscious. In the conscious world rationality and the principle of noncontradiction dominated: Freud called conscious mental processes the secondary processes, to distinguish them from the primary processes that took place in the unconscious. There, in fact, contradiction and chaos would be the rule rather than the exception. The paradoxical feature of dreams was in some way a testimony to this.

The theory of motivation outlined by Freud in his contributions prior to *The Interpretation of Dreams* was based on the principle of constancy. According to this principle, the mind tended to maintain a state as far as possible free from stimuli. When some form of arousal occurred, an essentially motor activity tended to restore the state of quiet as soon as possible. In this new (still provisional) conception, the principle of constancy was still considered a valid explanatory model, but only for the very first part of human life. An infant would soon find that the condition of perpetual quiet was less satisfactory than its restoration after excitement due to a stimulus. The sucking of breast milk to appease hunger was certainly a satisfying moment for a child. The experience of gratification was therefore associated with the condition of need. Each time the need recurred, the child would try to reproduce the perception that had led to the gratifying experience. If the actual perception could not be actualized, they would try to reproduce it in a hallucinatory way. This process would continue throughout life: the first compelling needs corresponded to desires, and their satisfaction to the fulfillment of those desires. In other words, there would no longer be the principle of constancy at the basis of the functioning of the human mind, but the unpleasure principle (Freud, 1900/1953a, p. 600) or, as it would be called later, the pleasure principle (Freud, 1911/1958a).

In *The Interpretation of Dreams* Freud already proposed the idea of the mind as conditioned by a play of forces. Desires tended to be satisfied, but censorship (linked to the sociocultural situation and individual educational experience) tended to repress them. From this perspective, as mentioned earlier, Freud's can be called a "dynamic psychology." The forces could also be evaluated in terms of intensity: psychical life would be characterized by a certain amount of energy, used partly at an unconscious and partly at a conscious level. The more energy that was invested in the unconscious desires and drives (essentially of a sexual nature), the more energy would be used by the censorship to block them (and less energy, conversely, would be left for the conscious life, for its own purposes). In the neurotic mind, the amount of energy used to block the repressed impulses would be so significant as to make a person's conduct clumsy, lacking in naturalness. The blockage of energy induced a behavior that appeared artificial, forced, and unnatural. The purpose of psychoanalytic psychotherapy was to bring unconscious impulses to consciousness so that the energy used by censorship could be unlocked and become usable for the conscious psyche. In normal human development, Freud would clarify, the sexual nature of psychical energy was largely modified (through *sublimation*). At the dawn of history this would allow the birth of civilization and would have caused every human being to become part of it.

The theory of drives

The Freudian conception of dreams led psychoanalysis to adhere to the paradigmatic idea of continuity between normal and pathological. This idea was supported in the late 19th century by French psychologists and British neurologists such as John Hughlings Jackson (1835–1911), who Freud knew and cited on several occasions. The dream was a daily experience for every human being, yet it corresponded to a micropsychotic phenomenon, characterized as it was by events similar to hallucinations. Latent oneiric thoughts could be traced back to the desires present in a normal person, as well as in a neurotic. The fact, noted earlier, that Freud mainly analyzed his own dream world in *The Interpretation of*

Dreams was further implicit confirmation of Freud's conviction that the under-lying themes were the same. Freud remained convinced that there was no quali-tative difference between the condition of normality and that of neurosis.

From this point of view, Freud's essays on slips, missed acts (Freud, 1901/1960a), and witticisms (Freud, 1905/1960b) completed the picture. According to Freud, every mental event was significant. His adherence to physical determinism was never in question: every event in the physical world had a specific cause(s) and nothing happened by chance. Freud extended this perspective to his own conception of the mind, also supporting psychical determinism. If it was not possible to identify the causes of a mental event with the certainty and precision of physics, then the circumstance was due to the *principle of over-determination*. To say that a psychical event was overdetermined was to recognize that it had multiple causes that were traceable to a much more articulated dynamic than a physical event. Such an approach explained why some aspects of human behav-ior remained inaccessible to analysis, although this never corresponded, on Freud's part, to a renunciatory attitude.

Slips and parapraxis in general (i.e., the daily occurrences of small errors, in linguistic expression or behavior) were, in Freud's interpretation, the result of pressure from the unconscious impulses, which were contrary to the conscious will. These clamored to be realized and were generally blocked by censorship. On some occasions the impulse was partially realized, according to the same logic of compromise formation. Thus, the chairperson of an assembly could declare a meeting closed when they should have opened it (betraying their desire to end it as soon as possible), a person who wanted to hypocritically manifest a desire for more frequent meetings with someone else could express the wish to finally see them more infrequently, or someone who found a task particularly unpleas-ant could "forget" to carry it out. These daily microneurotic acts were certainly a source of interest to Freud, offering in his view tangible evidence of the exist-ence of the unconscious. However, they also became important within psycho-therapy, pointing out the issues through which a patient indirectly manifested underlying unconscious problems. To commit a slip of the tongue and deny an interpretation could be, on the contrary, a confirmation. Forgetting to recount a significant event could conceal an unexpected unconscious attitude toward the event itself. The unconscious processes of the formation of slips and missed acts were similar to the mechanisms of the condensation and displacement in dreams, just as would happen in the jokes, which were, however, voluntary. The play on words invented by the French when Napoleon III seized the Orléans' property was certainly an example of condensation: "le premier vol de l'aigle" can mean both "the first flight of the eagle" and "the first theft of the eagle." An example of displacement was the response offered by a less-than-clean person who was asked if they had "taken a bath," claiming with feigned innocence that they "didn't know there was one missing."

Drive theory, but especially the developmental theory related to it, was a fur-ther step by Freud in adopting the principle of continuity between normality and pathology. Freud presented his third and final model of motivation in the *Three Essays on Sexual Theory* (Freud, 1905/1953c), a work that fixed for the first time some concepts destined to remain an undisputed cornerstone of psychoanalytic theory well after the death of its founder.

The *drive* was defined as a concept on the border between the psychical and the somatic or, more specifically, as the psychical representation of a continuous flow of stimuli of an endosomatic nature (external stimuli, however, could not have continuity). The drive was characterized by its *source* (the organ at the origin of the flow), *aim* (the satisfaction of the stimulus through the discharge of tension), and *object* (that which enables the discharge). The sexual drive was perceived as necessary, like the need to eat food to survive. If the latter was expressed through what language usually designates as hunger, then the sexual drive, Freud noted, was not correlated with a corresponding term, which he therefore proposed to designate with the Latin *libido*. Since the drive sought its own satisfaction, libido was understood as the energy of that drive. The concept of drive did not coincide with that of instinct. The latter was normally understood as the predisposition to a standardized behavior identical for all members of the species (as opposed to the drive), and its origin was ascribed to heredity (it was therefore only somatic in itself).

Defining the concept of "the object" was particularly problematic. Freud later wrote that the object is the "most variable" element of the drive and "is not originally connected with it, but becomes assigned to it only in consequence of being peculiarly fitted to make satisfaction possible" (Freud, 1915/1957d, p. 122). When the abstract concept of the object is replaced with the concrete human being who embodies it, in adult sexuality, we understand how, in the Freudian conception, the fundamental aspect was composed of the satisfaction of the impulse, while the identity of the other assumed an ancillary role. Any Freudian attempt to respond to criticism was always vitiated by an approach that foresaw the other as a means and not as an end. Much post-Freudian psychoanalysis, as will be seen, was fundamentally characterized by a different theory of the role of the object in the relationship.

The conception of drives had multiple consequences for a theory that wanted to explain the relationship between normality and neurosis. It must be emphasized that, although Freud showed himself willing in principle to admit different types of drives, he did not consider it necessary to postulate them except for the types not reducible to others. The drives strictly necessary for the theory were finally limited to two: those for self-survival and sexual drives. Sexuality thus acquired a feature that was no longer only central (as in the model of desire) but almost exclusive.

The theory of transference

The theory of transference was born in parallel to the theory of drives, as one of the key concepts of psychoanalytic psychotherapy. The expression had been used, in a relatively generic way, in *Studies on Hysteria*, to identify the peculiar nature of the relationship between therapist and patient. A therapy interrupted by a hysterical patient under Freud's care offered the cue for a substantial deepening: such was the fate of the clinical case of Dora (Freud, 1905/1953b), published shortly before the *Three Essays*. It is likely, in fact, that Dora's case, although resulting in a substantial therapeutic failure, inspired Freud's "seeds of psychoanalytic knowledge that would flower afterward in Freud's scientific development – aggression, narcissism (. . .) defense organization (. . .) and the theory of analytic technique" (Mahony, 1996, p. 149).

Freud (1905/1953b, p. 116) considered transference to be the "new editions or facsimiles of the impulses and phantasies which are aroused and made conscious during the progress of the analysis," in which, however, the person who had originally solicited these impulses and fantasies was replaced by the figure of the analyst. As a result, the patient relived past psychical experiences within the relationship with the therapist. The patient developed feelings toward the therapist that they had previously felt toward another person, while at the same time attributing to them the thoughts and feelings originally felt by the latter. These feelings could be more or less unconscious. Sometimes, perfectly conscious impulses were experienced, but their repetitive nature was completely unconscious to the patient. In the case of erotic transference, the open physical attraction felt toward the therapist, it would have been difficult for the person analyzed to understand either that the analyst was the object of love only because of the role they played or that the attraction had a completely unrealistic aspect, given the therapeutic situation (Freud, 1915/1958f).

Freud also explicitly stated that transference was a necessary requirement of any analysis, that it could not be avoided and that its resolution was one of the objectives to be achieved during treatment (Freud, 1905/1953b): after all, the pathologies treatable with psychoanalysis would later be defined as *transference neurosis* (Jung, 1907/1960a), as opposed to *actual neurosis* (caused by harmful sexual behavior), but especially to psychosis. The formation of transference was thus defined as the essential requirement for analytic therapy (although this did not imply that the phenomenon was easy for the therapist to understand and manage). This principle has long remained an undisputed cornerstone of the theory of technique in psychoanalysis. It is only in relatively recent times that the principle that psychodynamic therapy can also find application in the treatment of psychosis has been confirmed. It has now also been recognized that the psychotic can, in certain particular cases, establish a transference toward their analyst.

It soon became clear that the transference of the patient could be matched by a *countertransference* of the analyst (Freud, 1910/1957a). That is, the analyst could find themselves in the position of responding to the feelings of the person analyzed with complementary feelings. Freud tried to make it clear that the analyst's position should not lose neutrality, especially in the face of the transference-love. The position of a male analyst toward a female patient was particularly delicate: the therapist had to

> recognize that the patient's falling in love is induced by the analytic situation and is not to be attributed to the charms of his own person; so that he has no grounds whatever for being proud of such a "conquest", as it would be called outside analysis.

On the other hand, the patient "must relinquish psycho-analytic treatment or she must accept falling in love with her doctor as an inescapable fate" (Freud, 1915/1958f, pp. 160–161).

Freud and the dawn of the psychoanalytic movement

Freud's collaboration with Breuer definitely ended with the publication of *Studies on Hysteria*. His friendship with Fliess was completely compromised at the turn of the century. Freud found himself virtually without points of reference when one of his first patients suggested that he organize periodic meetings to discuss psychoanalytic issues with interested people. The patient in question was Wilhelm Stekel (1868–1940), and his proposal was accepted by Freud: thus were born in 1902 the "Wednesday Psychological Evenings," weekly meetings whose tradition was quickly consolidated, and did not fail until Freud's old age. The meetings were initially attended – with Stekel – by Alfred Adler, Max Kahane (1866–1923), and Rudolf Reitler (1865–1917). The group expanded slowly but steadily. If at first the members of the group only listened to Freud, within a few years their speech were of sufficient interest that the decision was taken to keep a record of their contents. This happened in 1906, and the task of secretary (with a small salary) was entrusted to Otto Rank (1884–1939), a character destined to play a key role in the movement. Rank carried out his task with continuity and diligence until 1915. The minutes he left offer elements of considerable interest with which to understand the evolution of the movement. Rank himself and Alfred Adler were certainly the members of the group who emerged before the others for their originality. The first was a philosopher, initially interested in using psychoanalysis as a tool to interpret myth and culture. The second was a doctor, politically committed as a socialist, who tended to consider individual conflicts a reflection of social conflict. Soon Stekel also gained importance. His influence, as mentioned earlier, was decisive for Freud, who began to consider the use of symbols as one of the mechanisms of dream work.

Despite the fact that *The Psychopathology of Everyday Life* and *Jokes and Their Relation to the Unconscious* met with a certain success, the entire group of Freud's followers was initially made up only of Viennese Jews. In 1906, however, important signs of interest came from the research group at the Burghölzli Hospital in Zurich, led by Eugen Bleuler (1857–1939). In particular, one of Bleuler's assistants, Carl Gustav Jung, had developed an *association experiment* that seemed to confirm the hypotheses of the unconscious formulated by Freud (Jung, 1906/1973a). Jung officially took a stand in favor of Freud at a psychiatric congress in Baden Baden, responding to Gustav Aschaffenburg (1866–1944), a well-known German psychiatrist who had in turn criticized psychoanalysis (Jung, 1906/1961a): this was the first official defense of Freudian ideas in an institutional setting.[4]

Freud and Jung began a close correspondence that established a relationship of cordiality and collaboration between them. Although the Swiss did not accept all of Freud's ideas (and in particular the concept of the libido as sexual energy), the father of psychoanalysis began to consider him a kind of ideal collaborator and the person who could contribute most to the affirmation of psychoanalysis in the world. Jung and Freud met for the first time in 1907, and later other students of Bleuler from Zurich went to visit Freud in Vienna, destined for a fruitful collaboration with the psychoanalytic movement: Max Eitingon (1881–1943), Sándor Ferenczi (1873–1933), Karl Abraham (1877–1925), and Ludwig Binswanger (1881–1966). From across the Channel came Ernest Jones (1879–1958), who became one of Freud's most important collaborators, and also his first biographer (Jones, 1953–1957).

International interest in psychoanalysis grew rapidly. In 1909 both Freud and Jung were invited to Clark University, in the United States, for a series of lectures. The number of Freud's students and of people willing to use psychoanalysis professionally as a therapeutic technique grew to the point of suggesting the establishment of journals that would be the organ of the movement and of specific international congresses. So the *Jahrbuch für psychoanalytische und psychopathologische Forschungen* (*Yearbook for Psychoanalytic and Psychopathological Research*) was created, of which Freud became the director and Jung the editor: it became the journal in which the most important theoretical-clinical essays by Freud and his students were published. Later the *Zentralblatt für Psychoanalyse* and *Imago* were founded, the latter intended to accommodate studies on the cultural world based on critical tools offered by psychoanalysis. At the beginning of the 20th century, Freud's closest collaborators founded the *Wednesday Psychological Society*, which later became the *Vienna Psychoanalytical Society*. The first congress of a society organized by Jung was held in 1908 in Salzburg which was later remembered as the first international congress of psychoanalysis. The participants expressed the idea of an international society, which was founded later. The International Psychoanalytic Association (IPA) was actually founded on the occasion of the 1910 congress, which was held in Nuremberg. Jung was its first president, while Adler assumed the presidency of the Vienna Society.

The problem of the psychoanalytic movement was not only refuting the criticisms of its opponents but also isolating those who, with misguided enthusiasm, believed they were applying Freudian theories in medical practice, even though they did not understand them well (*wild psychoanalysis*) (Freud, 1910/1957b).

With the increasing establishment of psychoanalysis, however, came the first disagreements. Alfred Adler was developing a theory increasingly independent of psychoanalysis. In *individual psychology*, unconscious sexual desires lost their importance, the main motivation of human actions was the desire for power, and the cause of psychopathology always originated from a sense of inferiority linked to the presumed or real inadequacy of one or more organs of the body. Adler left the psychoanalytic movement in 1911 following repeated invitations from Freud to do so and was immediately considered an outsider. Carl Gustav Jung did not abandon his idea that the libido was not essentially sexual and began to develop the theory of a trans-personal unconscious. The main reason for his now inevitable break with Freud, however, was the proposal, made at the Psychoanalytic Congress of Munich (Jung, 1913/1971b), that different theories were possible within the field of depth psychology, corresponding to different *psychological types* (of their creators as well as of potential patients). In 1914, as will be seen, Jung also left the psychoanalytic movement for good.

In the meantime, Freud had created a secret committee of his most faithful collaborators: Ferenczi, Rank, Jones, and Abraham (to all of whom he gave a ring) would help him to preserve the orthodoxy of psychoanalysis.[5] Not only the adversaries of his own theory, but also the self-styled allies who did not accept it in its entirety were in Freud's eyes victims of *resistance*, like the patients who did not accept interpretations that he considered true. It would have been the unconscious that pushed all of them to perceive as dangerous for their own conscious balance the deep truths of which psychoanalysis was the bearer. This attitude continued to characterize the Freudian environment for a long time and made the dialogue with the external scientific world very difficult.

The codification of psychoanalytic technique

The idea of writing a manual on psychoanalytic technique had occurred to Freud, before his trip to the United States. Several letters to Abraham, Ferenczi, and Jung attested to the intention, a postponement, and then the drafting of a text that seems to have eventually been lost. Presumably, Freud ultimately thought it inappropriate to publish a volume, the reading of which physicians could consider sufficient in itself to practice psychoanalysis on their own. The possibility that public knowledge of the technique might influence poten-tial patients also probably prompted his caution. Perhaps, however, the most important scruple was related to the risk of over-standardizing a procedure that by necessity had to remain elastic (Freud, 1913/1958d). Finally, Freud imple-mented a compromise: a sequence of short essays that he published individu-ally in the *Zentralblatt* between 1911 and 1914, and reissued later in various forms. Usually they are referred to as *Papers on Technique*. Here Freud had the opportunity to define as the *fundamental rule* something that had been indicated as a pillar of psychotherapy since *The Interpretation of Dreams*: that the patient must communicate without criticizing it, everything that comes to their mind

(Freud, 1912/1958c). However, Freud also made explicit the counterpart of the same rule from the point of view of the therapist:

> [He] must put himself in a position to make use of everything he is told for the purposes of interpretation and of recognizing the concealed uncon-scious material without substituting a censorship of his own for the selec-tion that the patient has forgone.
>
> (Freud, 1912/1958b, p. 115)

To this end, the basic principles consisted of (a) not taking note of anything in particular that the patient said and (b) using the *evenly suspended attention*, a mode of listening characterized by the absence of influences of consciousness and the intent to memorize (one relied on what Freud called unconscious memory). The result of suspended attention, according to Freud, was that details of what the analyst had heard from the patient emerged from the analyst's memory as soon as the patient produced material which could be traced back to these details. Nor, again according to Freud, was the analyst likely to be subject to confusion between different patients, and indeed, if a patient disputed whether or not some detail had been communicated, it would almost always be the therapist who was on the side of reason.

Although the training of analysts was still an informal process, Freud believed that, in addition to a knowledge of theory, knowledge of one's own uncon-scious was an indispensable requirement for the potential therapist. It was essential that the process of listening to and recalling the material produced by the patient was not influenced by unresolved personal issues in the analyst's unconscious. If the father of psychoanalysis limited himself at the Nurem-berg Psychoanalytic Congress (1910) to suggesting self-analysis, then starting with the *Recommendations to Physicians Practicing Psychoanalysis*, he began to pre-scribe a real analysis of the analyst as an indispensable requirement. It should be noted that this was ascribed to the "merits of the Zurich School of analysis" (1912/1958b p. 116), Jung's school, to have suggested such a solution. The modalities and timing of the training analysis (or didactic analysis) were later the subject of increasingly articulated codifications, which will be examined in the remainder of this work.

Other requirements were necessary for the therapeutic process to be defined as psychoanalysis. First, the analyst had to be "opaque to his patients and, like a mirror, should show them nothing but what is shown to him" (p. 118). This meant both avoiding the temptation to reveal, even with the best of intentions, aspects of one's own life, and personality, and avoiding suggestive interventions that, although effective in the short term, would not allow for stable results. Equally basic to Freud was the rule of not indicating objectives to the patient and avoiding any kind of instruction on the therapeutic process (including the reading of psychoanalytic writings). In fact, the analysis had to avoid any effort of attention or will on the part of the patient, precisely because the best results for the emergence of unconscious contents would be obtained by observing the fundamental rule of free association.

The framework of the treatment (which was later called "the setting") acquired a particular importance in Freud's eyes: rhythm, timing, payment, and the position of the patient and the analyst in the office where the therapy was carried out were specifically codified. Some of the rules established by Freud have remained almost unchanged features of analytic treatment to this day. First of all, it was appropriate to use a short preliminary period in order to make a diagnosis: since only neurosis and not psychosis could be treated effectively, it was better not to take on psychotics, for the twofold reason of avoiding their delusion and not discrediting the analytical treatment. Relatives or friends would also be excluded, since the treatment would inevitably condition their relationship with the known person. Each patient was assigned fixed hours in the therapist's schedule which had to be paid even if apparently force majeure circumstances meant the patient could not keep the appointment. In general, according to Freud, absences were more often determined by resistance to treatment and as such would be limited by such an obligation. The definition of the fee and its payment at fixed and relatively short intervals was also important:

> An analyst does not dispute that money is to be regarded in the first instance as a medium for self-preservation and for obtaining power; but he maintains that, besides this, powerful sexual factors are involved in the value set upon it.
>
> (Freud, 1913/1958d, p. 131)

On the other hand, Freud insisted, in bourgeois society hypocrisy and prudery habitually accompanied speeches concerning both sexuality and money, so it was logical that the therapist invited people to use the same sincerity on both issues. Free treatment was unadvisable, in any case, in Freud's eyes, not only for the obvious reason that this would have represented an economic loss for the analyst, but also because experience had taught him that the absence of payment generated new problems in the treatment:

> [I]n young women, for instance, the temptation which is inherent in their transference-relationship, and in young men, their opposition to an obligation to feel grateful, an opposition which arises from their father-complex and which presents one of the most troublesome hindrances to the acceptance of medical help.
>
> (p. 137)

One suggestion, which has become almost emblematic of classical psychoanalysis, was to have the patient lie on a couch during the session, with the analyst placed behind the patient. This had historical significance, in that it harkened back to hypnotic treatment, from which psychoanalysis derived. Second, however, Freud cited practical reasons, related both to the therapist's tranquility (they could avoid the fixed gaze of the patients for several hours a day) and to the possibility that the person being analyzed would be distracted by the analyst's expression when they were exercising the evenly suspended attention.

The treatment originally conceived by Freud included sessions every day, except Sundays and holidays. Even the Sunday break itself entailed a difficulty in resuming work, which Freud jokingly called "Monday crust" (p. 127). Only in less serious cases or for the more advanced stages of treatment could the number of weekly sessions be reduced to three. This applied to treatments that extended between six and twelve months, however. A relative decrease in the weekly rhythm meant that the times of therapy would later lengthen, as the title of a late Freudian text, *Analysis Terminable and Interminable* (Freud, 1937/1964a), indirectly testifies. The best method to encourage the emergence of unconscious contents, from Freud's point of view, was not to fix a specific starting point. The beginning of the treatment coincided with the invitation: "Before I can say anything to you I must know a great deal about you; please tell me what you know about yourself'" (Freud, 1913/1958d, p. 134). The patient's freedom of expression was to be total, except of course in respecting the fundamental rule, avoiding omitting thoughts that seemed unimportant or even nonsensical, because it was precisely those thoughts that comprised the possible manifestations of unconscious material. Their omission was therefore a typical example of resistance. Freud's suggestion was to invite the patient to behave in their thoughts like "a traveller sitting next to the window of a railway carriage and describing to someone inside the carriage the changing views" (p. 135). It was inadvisable for the patient to prepare the material to be discussed before the session in order to avoid resistance: the lack of spontaneity would have prevented the expression of unconscious associations. The patient should also avoid discussing the course of therapy outside the analytic sessions, because there was a great risk that the most significant material would emerge far from the therapist's presence.

For their part, the therapist could begin to interpret, that is, to communicate to the patient the meaning of the contents emerging from the unconscious, only when the transference had been established. In fact, only after the bond with the therapist had been strengthened could the patient listen to what repression had pushed back into the unconscious, precisely because it was unacceptable. With respect to *Studies on Hysteria*, therefore, Freud had abandoned the belief that the mere knowledge of unconscious dynamics was in itself an effective factor for the recovery from neurosis. In fact, he had realized that psychological illness also presented, paradoxically, practical advantages for the sick person (Freud, 1908/1959), and finally defined this phenomenon as a *primary and secondary gain from illness* (Freud, 1913/1958d). A psychoneurosis could, for example, make it impossible for a person to work and force their social environment to provide for their livelihood: while paying a very high price (mental health), they obtained legitimate abstention from work. It was precisely the reluctance to deprive oneself of the benefits of continuing psychoneurotic problems that induced resistance.

In essence, then, the will to overcome the suffering induced by neurosis was the prime mover of therapy, but it had to struggle against other forces: "Every single association, every act of the person under treatment must reckon with the resistance" (Freud, 1912/1958c, p. 103).

The will would not, therefore, be able to lead the patient to recovery, both because, obviously, the patient did not know the way to recovery on their own, and because the patient lacked the necessary energy. Analytic treatment, in Freud's conception, remedied both deficiencies: the energy required to overcome resistance was supplied by mobilizing the energies available for transference; and timely interpretations indicated the paths on which the patient should direct such energy (Freud, 1913/1958d). Simply mentioning the resistances was not enough for letting them disappear:

> One must allow the patient time to become more conversant with this resistance with which he has now become acquainted, to *work through* it, to overcome it, by continuing, in defiance of it, the analytic work. [. . .] Only when the resistance is at its height can the analyst, working in common with his patient, discover the repressed instinctual impulses which are feeding the resistance.
>
> (Freud, 1913/1958e, p. 153; emphasis in the original)

On the one hand, resistance found its most intense form of expression through transference. It was precisely the presence of transference, however, that allowed victory over resistance (Freud, 1912/1958c). The therapy would be concluded when, having torn away the veil of repression, the transference, too, was finally resolved.

Before dealing with the further development of Freud's thought, it will now be appropriate to follow the parallel work of Adler and Jung, in order to understand their role in both the accession and the detachment from the main trunk of the psychoanalytic movement. Among other things, it will be possible to see how both Adler and Jung had already set off on the paths that would lead them to found, respectively, individual psychology and analytical psychology, before meeting Freud. It would therefore be reductive to qualify one or the other as dissident students. Paradoxically, it would be more logical to be surprised that a relatively prolonged collaboration could have been born between such different characters. Certainly Freud, Adler, and Jung had a common polemical goal in the academicism and therapeutic pessimism of psychiatry at the time. On the other hand, a similar motivation would drive Harry Stack Sullivan (1892–1949) to initially adhere to classical psychoanalysis, despite the underlying misgivings that would later drive him to actually found what Greenberg and Mitchell (1983) called the relational/structure model of psychoanalysis.[6]

Alfred Adler and the birth of individual psychology

Although Adler and Freud were both Jewish and educated in Viennese medical circles, they came from families with very different geographical and social roots. Freud, who had spent his early childhood in Galicia, had witnessed anti-Semitism as a young boy. Adler's family came from Burgenland (on the border between Austria and Hungary), where his ethnic group had enjoyed a better status (both legal and social) than in the rest of the Austro-Hungarian Empire. This corresponded to a much more limited identification with Judaism on Adler's part. In contrast to Freudian writings, Adler's works do not seem to show any particular influence from Jewish culture and do not contain any reference to anti-Semitism (Ellenberger, 1970). On the other hand, despite the economic problems his father went through, Freud basically lived in a middle-class environment, while Adler spent his childhood in the poorest suburbs of Vienna. This is reflected by the fact that Adler's social commitment was much more pronounced than that of Freud. Another difference in family life seems likely to have had consequences on their respective theoretical structures: Freud, although he was the favorite of his parents, grew up under relatively strict discipline, while Adler spent his childhood without too many constraints and was involved in frequent fights and physical confrontations with other boys. As a matter of fact, Freudian theory of development focused on the relationship with parents, whereas for Adler the relationship with peers was certainly more important. It is not surprising that Adler's stance in favor of women's emancipation and against the idea of sexuality as the fulcrum of all psychopathological problems was reflected by a youth characterized by uninhibited social contact with the opposite sex (Parenti, 1987).

Adler initially adhered to Marxism during his (not particularly brilliant) medical studies[7] but soon distanced himself from it, perplexed by the renunciation of individual freedom imposed by the revolutionary communist position. Adler then moved to a social democratic and reformist position, which he maintained throughout his life, actively engaging in politics. As has been observed: "Adler's psychological doctrine, centered on respect for the unique and unrepeatable individual and on the demands of social harmonization, proves what was the genuine matrix of his inner instances" (Parenti, 1987, p. 16). In his early years, which coincided with the end of the 19th century and the beginning of the new century, Adler worked on occupational medicine and the effect of social conditions on individual health. His first work was a *Health Manual for the Tailoring Trade* (Adler 1898/2003a), which documented his interest in the relationship between medicine, work, and social conditions, proposing, among other things, the abolition of piecework and the construction of council houses (Ellenberger, 1970). His following political and publicistic activity was aimed at promoting public hygiene by involving doctors not only in the care of the poorest (social medicine) but also in the function of educators (Adler, 1902/2003b, 1903/2003c, 1903/2003d, 1904/2003e). His conversion to Protestantism dates to 1904: it seems that Adler tried to adhere to faith in a God who was neither restricted to a small ethnic group (like the Jewish god) nor subject to strict religious authorities (like the Catholic one) (Bottome, 1939). If Freud tended to increasingly emphasize his own identity as a Jewish atheist, Adler assumed an ecumenical attitude and proposed his own ideas as compatible with any religious belief (Parenti, 1987).

Adler's psychoanalytic period

The meeting between Adler and Freud took place in 1902, in circumstances that cannot be documented (various versions of the event have been denied by historical research). In fact, however, Adler was one of the first four participants of the Wednesday evenings promoted by Freud, and for a long time remained the most active participant.

Adler's first important writing, the *A Study of Organ Inferiority* (Adler, 1907/2003f), was born within the psychoanalytic movement and was already a landmark in the history of psychotherapy. It was undoubtedly the first work that manifested a certain originality compared to Freud, written by a member of his Viennese circle. Its presentation immediately aroused perplexity and attacks from other pupils of Freud, although it seemed to attract the interest of Jung, who defended it, albeit with caution. Freud, for his part, appeared to consider it a sort of complement to his ideas on the physiological level. Adler, in fact, implemented a sort of compromise between three different instances: (a) medical training, to which he was still fully attached; (b) psychoanalysis, of which he understood the historical importance; and (c) a nascent doctrine, already headed in a rather personal direction. Linked to the first was the belief that constitutional factors and physical disease were responsible for the emergence of many neuroses. Indeed, Adler's central idea was that psychopathology resulted from the inferiority of an organ, which could be developmental or functional, absolute or relative, but typically generated a subjective focus on the organ itself. This attention translated into an attempt to compensate for its inferiority. There is no doubt that Adler's personal experience might have suggested this idea to him. During his early years, Adler had been frail and scrawny, and had been forced into immobility while his peers played freely. When he had recovered from his difficult condition, he took up very intense sporting activity, which would lead him to be a good swimmer and an agile mountaineer.

Adler was also convinced that the predisposition to organic inferiority was related to heredity, as was the focus on the potentially diseased organ and the drive for a necessary compensation. Typical examples include the cases of painters from families predisposed to eye diseases or musicians with a family frequency of hearing disorders. By taking this position Adler, compared to Freud, moved closer to the French theorists of degeneration.[8]

The concept of compensation was destined to become one of the cornerstones of Adlerian psychology. On the other hand, at least two central ideas in

A Study of Organ inferiority could still place Adler within psychoanalytic theory. In fact, he argued that concentration on the inferior organ could trigger the neurotic process, especially if the corresponding body surface was an erogenous zone. Above all, however, the idea that there could be no organic inferiority without sexual inferiority seemed relatively reassuring to Freud with regard to Adler's loyalty.

The Aggression Drive in Life and in Neurosis (Adler, 1908/2003g) had placed its author, if not virtually outside the psychoanalytic movement, then on a very eccentric orbit with respect to Freud. Adler postulated the idea that aggression was a drive that could not be traced back to the sexual libido. In other words, he expressed a principle that Freud would adopt many years later (Freud, 1920/1955), but that was unacceptable to him for the time being.[9] If even Otto Rank was beginning to think of a sadomasochistic drive, Adler went further and, at Wednesday meetings, "claims [as his discovery] having separated sadism from sexuality and having placed the former above all other drives" (Nunberg & Federn, 1962, p. 400; modified translation).

Freud's attitude toward Adler, after the initial appreciation, passed from a relative tolerance to an increasing insufferance. In a letter to Jung in 1909, Freud, alluding to his own alleged "school," stated that he would certainly not want to be held responsible for Adler's writings (or Stekel's or Sadger's) (McGuire, 1974, p. 201). Freud also expressed strong misgivings toward a lecture on psychical hermaphroditism (Adler, 1910/2003h) in a letter to Ferenczi in early 1910:

> The genesis of neuroses is supposedly as follows: the child suffers from its inferiority, which it takes to be feminine; from that there develops an uncertainty about the gender role, which is the original basis for all later doubt, it attempts a masculine defense, and when that fails, neurosis results – a bad speculation!
>
> (Haynal, 1992, p. 146)

Freud later wrote to Ferenczi that he had decided to appoint Adler president of the Vienna Psychoanalytic Society:"not out of inclination or satisfaction but because he is the only [prominent] personality and because in this position it will perhaps be necessary for him to share the defense of the common ground" (p. 155). The belief that Adler's charisma partly compensated for his heterodoxy was also overshadowed in a letter to Jung, who described a contribution by Adler intended for the *Jahrbuch* as the only one (among those available) that was acceptable "without censure, though not without criticism" (McGuire, 1974, p. 291). Adler also assumed the co-editorship of the *Zentralblatt* in 1910, but retained his position for only a few months. Between late 1910 and early 1911 Freud revealed to his intimates that he considered him a neurotic who was dangerous for the movement, and that he was just waiting for the right opportunity to remove him (Paskauskas, 1993; McGuire, 1974; Haynal, 1992). A series of Wednesday sessions between January and February 1911 featured a report by Adler and its discussion. The report centered on the idea that the attempt to compensate for the sense of inferiority was essentially implemented in the form of a *masculine protest*, that is, an attempt to reassert the neurotic's masculine dignity. In view of a theoretical incompatibility now too marked, Freud first asked for and obtained the resignation of Adler from the presidency of the Society and then from the co-editorship of the journal. Finally Adler abandoned the psychoanalytic movement entirely (Adler, 1911/2003i). Freud, who greeted such events with satisfaction in his letters to Jung, commented on Adler's final defection as follows: "The damage is not very great. Paranoid intelligences are not rare and are more dangerous than useful" (McGuire, 1974, p. 428).

Individual psychology as an independent discipline

The first systematization of Adler's ideas after the break with Freud was published in *The Neurotic Character* (Adler, 1912/2002). This was the first occasion in which Adler presented his own thought as *individual psychology* (after briefly adopting the expression "free psychoanalysis"). It would be difficult to overestimate the importance of this work in the evolution of Adlerian doctrine. It is a true manifesto, which contained a series of decisive turning points, both with respect to Freud's work and to Adler's previous writings, the main points of which involved a completely new perspective.

Adler, as he pointed out in his 1922 *Preface* to the book, had definitively excluded the idea that neurosis was necessarily linked to an "organic substratum" or at least to an organic predisposition, even in the sense of a particular "cellular structure of the brain." On the contrary, psychopathology was determined by the "attitude toward the absolute logic of human coexistence," and more specifically "because of an inferiority feeling acquired in a difficult situation in childhood" (ibid., p. IX). The principle according to which the inferiority feeling could be linked to the weakness of an organ was not abandoned, but the consequences of this weakness were considered exclusively on the level of psychical life, in the light of the comparison that the child had made between themselves, the other members of their family (not only their parents but also their brothers and sisters) and the group of peers. In other words, subjective inadequacy was reflected in a failure to adapt to the environment.

Compared to Freud's position, whose work Adler nonetheless defined as "fruitful and valuable" (p. XVI), the reservations were clear and precise. Individual psychology first of all excluded the idea that the sexual libido was at the origin of neurosis: the main motivational factor was in fact the "will to power" (an expression openly borrowed from Nietzsche), with respect to which sexuality was subordinate. Above all, the role of infantile desires of an incestuous nature was denied by Adler. Neurosis, moreover, was not simply determined by causes, but rather aimed at an end. This end consisted ultimately of the "*elevation of the feeling of self-worth*, the simplest form of which may be recognized in the exaggerated '*masculine protest*'(ibid.; emphasis in the original).The neurotic started from an attempt to seek an important goal that would make life bearable: what transformed this activity into pathology was the incessant effort, the exaggerated tension, the continuous attempt to prevent any obstacle that separated the neurotic from a result that tended to be fictitious. From this perspective, Adler was explicitly indebted to *The Philosophy of "as if"* (1911/2021) of Hans Vaihinger (1852–1933), who had described human life as dominated by fictions, that is, basic assumptions that were false but considered true, which served as powerful motivators for social action. To affirm, for example, that all men were created equal was, according to Vaihinger, a pure fiction, but had led to genuine political upheavals. Individual pathology was characterized, in Adler's conception, by a similar dynamic: the neurotic pursued their own goal on the basis of erroneous assumptions, but they were no less effective in terms of motivation. Adler also acknowledged a debt to Pierre Janet: "His emphasis on the 'sentiment d'incomplétude' of the neurotic in particular agrees with the results that I have brought forward to such a degree that I may consider my own work as an expansion of this most important basic fact from the psychical life of the neurotic" (1912/2002, p. 1).

If the origin of suffering was the feeling of inferiority, then neurosis and psychosis were "attempts at compensation" (p. 257), rather than compromise-formations as in the psychoanalytic perspective. Compared to Freud, Adler also lacked the aspiration to develop a scientific theory: "Only a crank would want to try to capture the human psyche in a scientific laboratory. In the end, Individual Psychology is an artistic feat" (p. 256).

The neurotic character was expressed as a series of immutable routines that were intended to defend a person from an awareness of reality and keep them focused on their own fictions. The therapeutic strategy suggested by Adler in *The Neurotic Character* was to make people understand the meaning of these routines. For Adler, as for Freud, the patient resisted change, but for different reasons: "One will always find in neurotics that they cling tenaciously to their safeguarding patterns. Their resistance will become even greater when the patient anticipates his defeat, a sense of being 'below,' or an emasculation in the disengagement from his patterns and in the change of direction of his plan of life under influence of someone else." In the face of resistance, the therapist should strive to "the removal of the neurotic prejudice" (p. 258).

The writings immediately following *The Neurotic Character* seemed marked by a radicalization, probably due to the intent to regain ground compared to the psychoanalytic movement, in the struggle for visibility within medical circles (Alexander & Selesnick, 1966). In fact, Adler stated: "Every neurosis can be interpreted as caused by a culturally failed attempt to free oneself from the feeling of inferiority so as to gain a feeling of superiority" (Adler, 1913/2003j, p. 134), and "all the will and all the tendencies of the neurotic are subject to his policy of prestige" (p. 135), that is, to conduct aimed at obtaining consideration from others.

Adler believed that neurosis should be considered in a broader context than the person. In fact, it consisted of a reaction to the constraints of society that resulted in a counter-constraint (a limitation of oneself in order to react to the limitations imposed from outside). Among the various neurotic aspects of society, there was, according to Adler, the greater appreciation of characteristics considered typically masculine compared to those of women. This could affect both the man, who did not feel adequate with respect to the masculine ideal, and the woman, who could tend to accentuate their masculine traits (Adler, 1914/2003o).

The different psychopathological pictures retained a common trait, in spite of their differences: they "can be fashioned to serve the individual as pretexts" (Adler, 1913/2003j, p. 134), while "curing a neurotic and psychotic requires an alteration in his upbringing, correcting mistakes made, and his eventual unconditional return to human society" (p. 135). The framework of conditions for the development of a neurosis gradually expanded to include "organ inferiority, family, pressures, pampering, rivalry, a family history of neuroses "(Adler, 1913/2003k, p. 125). On the other hand, it became clear that in Adler's view, as in Freud's, the early years of life could be crucial to the development of a neurosis (Adler, 1914/2003o). The use of interpretation continued to be the essential tool for psychotherapy: "The most important aspect of therapy is to uncover the neurotic system or life plan" (Adler, 1913/2003k, p. 124). Dreams continued to represent, as they did for Freud, an important element in understanding a patient's psychology. The dream, however, did not constitute wish fulfillment, but an attempt to predict and solve a problem by enacting the ways in which the dreamer hoped events would unfold. The unintelligibility of the dream was not due to censorship but to its being "an accompanying manifestation, a reflection of powers, a trace and proof that the body and the mind have made an attempt at foreseeing" (Adler, 1913/2003m, p. 188). Even the idea that Adler had dispensed with the concept of the unconscious, raised by Freud himself (1914/1957c), was contradicted by Adlerian writings (Adler, 1913/2003l). Some of the conditions of the setting turned out to be similar to those of the Freudian treatment: establishing in advance the frequency and the time of the sessions, guaranteeing discretion, assuming a neutral attitude, not fixing a duration of the treatment in advance, and avoiding asking for favors from the patient.

It is striking, however, that Adler (in keeping with his militancy for social medicine) specifically acknowledged the possibility of free treatment (Adler, 1913/2003k), which was officially taboo in psychoanalysis. Equally peculiar was the idea that the development of neurosis could be prevented by education (Adler, 1914/2003n; 1914/2003o). Individual psychology soon began to propose its own specific educational theory (Adler, 1918/2003p, 1930/2015). In the Adlerian movement, in fact, the foundation of schools was given a specific place, active above all during the Weimar Republic (1918–1933), according to a pedagogical model inspired by social-democratic principles, which attributed great importance to children's experiences in order to prevent neurosis. Adler promoted, then, first in Europe and then in America, to which he emigrated after the advent of Nazism, the spread of a network of schools, consultants for the training of parents and teachers according to the principles of individual psychology. In this sense, we can say that Adler strongly influenced the psychotherapy movement of the 20th century, and all those who in the decades to follow believed that psychology should deal with educational problems, social and preventive medicine, and political issues, with psychological intervention aiming to build a more just society.

Carl Gustav Jung and the birth of analytical psychology

The son of a Protestant pastor, Jung undertook his schooling without ever displaying the particular brilliance that had led Freud to be consistently at the top of his class. Although he was pleased in his autobiographical recollections (Jaffé, 1961/1989) to describe himself as a person who had remained isolated for a long time, Jung must have demonstrated a certain influence on his fellow students if he assumed the presidency of an association (the Zofingia) that brought together many students from the University of Basel. There, in fact, Jung studied medicine successfully, to the point of a possibly lucrative career as an internist. Although his speeches at the Zofingia in the years 1896–1899 (Jung, 1983) showed a wide range of interests and a remarkable open-mindedness, no one could have predicted that he would specialize in psychiatry.

The choice of his thesis was a testimony to the outsider's courage that would characterize Jung's entire subsequent career. A cousin claimed to be a medium, and Jung decided to attend the séances and to study the phenomena. Although it emerged that the girl actually simulated trance and all the mediumistic activity, the young scholar did not lose heart and changed the perspective of his observation. He then wrote *On the Psychology and Pathology of So-Called Occult Phenomena*, which, presented as a thesis in 1900, was published two years later (Jung, 1902/1957). From the historical point of view, the writing's interest lies mainly in the bibliography, which turned especially to French psychology and psychiatry, and in particular to Pierre Janet. The mediumistic phenomena were in fact interpreted as a form of psychological automatism. It should be noted, however, that Jung already demonstrated knowledge of both Freud's *Studies on Hysteria* and *The Interpretation of Dreams*.

Jung's career in psychiatry began with an excellent opportunity: he was accepted as an assistant by Eugen Bleuler, head of the Burghölzli Hospital in Zurich, one of the most important European psychiatric institutions. Bleuler directed Jung toward the first decisive step of his career, which was to carry out research on verbal association. The idea of studying which words were associated with others, which was a stimulus, was linked to the tradition of associationist psychology: it had been employed sporadically by authors such as Ribot and Francis Galton (1822–1911). More recently, it had been systematically used by the father of German scientific psychology, Wilhelm Wundt (1832–1920), by Gustav Aschaffenburg and finally also by Eugen Bleuler himself. It was Bleuler, in fact, who compiled the list of 156 stimulus words used by Jung for his first experiences, however, the latter gradually modified the form, until the final structure reached in 1909 (Jung, 1910/1973b; see Cohen, 1974).

Despite the amount of effort and the importance of the scientists involved, none of the illustrious predecessors had obtained significant results with this technique. Compared to them, Jung made a fundamental improvement, realizing the need to study the association on normal individuals in order to obtain a benchmark against which to compare the results obtained by people suffering from mental illness. This was a decisive insight, which would later prove essential for the construction of all types of psychological tests. The fact that it is not usually ascribed to the Swiss psychologist is just one of many examples of the ungenerous oblivion into which he was relegated by the scientific world.

The Association of Normal Subjects, Jung's first and most important contribution on the subject (Jung & Riklin, 1904/1973), showed a rigorous attitude on the methodological level and a subtle one on the epistemological level. Jung meticulously described how he had tried to avoid systematic errors and conditioning in the experimental context; how he had introduced disturbing variables (background noise, etc.); how differences in results obtained by more or less cultured, female or male individuals could be interpreted; what kind of inferences were to be considered legitimate from the results obtained, and so on. Once all possible verifications had been carried out, Jung could legitimately describe a very important phenomenon: when confronted with certain stimulus words, one found a certain difficulty in carrying out the task of finding words that could be associated with them. These difficulties tended to occur constantly for groups of words related to particular common themes (e.g., clusters of words, the meaning of which could be related to sexuality, or to family, etc.). Said otherwise, difficult associations were "caused by definite constellation, referring to relatively new, subjective, possibly emotionally charged experiences" (Jung & Riklin, 1904/1973, p. 80). Such a circumstance could not be accidental, in Jung's perspective, since he was – at least at this stage – a convinced and explicit proponent of psychic determinism, like Freud. Jung reiterated this in a footnote: "We know, of course, that no reaction is fortuitous, but that each one, even the most objective, is caused by definite constellation" (p. 80n).

The constellations, according to Jung, identified the presence of a *complex*, that is, in the first definition offered by Jung, "the sum of ideas referring to a particular feeling-toned event" (p. 72n). Jung would later specify that the complex was a psychical unit superior to single representations. Moreover, if one examined all the psychical material obtained through the associative experiment, one would find that almost every association was ascribable to one or the other complex. The concept of complex immediately acquired a particular relevance, since Jung attributed to it, as a pole of attraction of representations, the capacity for autonomous action in the mind, independent of consciousness. This was all the more evident since the ego itself was identified as a complex. In a normal person it would be the strongest and most solid complex, which controlled the activity of the mind and constituted the personality of the individual.

The theory of complexes, in Jung's view, could be usefully linked to the Freudian theory of neurosis, from which he drew a coherent theoretical background, constituting a significant enrichment. Jung could indeed believe that his research was a true experimental confirmation of psychoanalysis. Since Bleuler was also interested in Freudian theories, Jung was able to present his results in this way without any difficulties within his own institution. Jung, at this point, entered into correspondence with Freud and became his main collaborator for a few years, despite the theoretical differences that, initially in the background, gradually led to a cooling of relations, and then the final estrangement between the two (Jaffé, 1961/1989).

Freud and Jung: collaboration and detachment

The period of collaboration between Freud and Jung was relatively short. A few years passed between Jung's first official defense of psychoanalytic theory (1906/1961a) and Jung's resignation from the International Psychoanalytic Association (in 1914) marked by good agreement at the organizational sphere, but by increasingly deep disagreement on the theoretical level. From the beginning, Jung did not accept the concept of the libido as exclusively sexual: what convinced Freud, at his first meeting with Jung, of the possibility that the Swiss could really join the psychoanalytic movement was the latter's belief that transference represents "the alpha and omega of the analytical method" (Jung, 1946/1966f, p. 172). Jung had proposed distinctions from psychoanalysis in *The Psychology of Dementia Praecox*, and in particular with respect to the ubiquity of the libido and the possibility that psychoanalysis was the only possible form of psychotherapy (Jung, 1907/1960a). Freud, obviously, did not appreciate this position: although the letter sent to Jung after receiving his book has been lost, it is easy to deduce its content from the response of Jung himself, who began: "I am sincerely sorry that I of all people must be such a nuisance to you. I understand perfectly that you cannot be anything but dissatisfied with my book, since it treats your researches too ruthlessly" (McGuire, 1974, p. 13). The father of psychoanalysis also proved himself unconvinced by Jung's argument that a complete and unconditional adoption of the Freudian point of view would make the book unpalatable to German-speaking psychiatrists. Jung's lectures on psychoanalysis (Jung, 2012a) during his second American trip (1912), containing several criticisms of Freud, marked a further distancing. Until the first part of the essay, whose original title was *Transformations and Symbols of the Libido* (Jung, 1912/2019), however, the theoretical differences between the two were still sustainable and Freud could openly praise the writing in the first version of the first part of *Totem and Taboo* (Freud, 1912/1987) for the ability shown by Jung to leave the narrow clinical field, illustrating symbolic material with elements taken from the history of mythology. Jung's attempt, in fact, took its cue from the fantasies of a patient of Théodore Flournoy ("Miss Miller"), concerning a hero she herself created, and baptized Chiwantopel. Miss Miller's fantasies were compared with a rich harvest of mythological material that she could not have known: the fact that he had never even seen the patient assured Jung that he could not have influenced her in any way. Jung was thus able to show numerous affinities between Flournoy's accounts of the patient and mythologies distant in space and time, in order to arrive at a theoretical proposal that he himself would later largely develop. A mode of expression existed in the mind that was different to that of rational daytime thinking. The dreams and fantasies of adults, the thoughts of children, the fantastic-mythological production of antiquity and the mode of expression of populations still untouched by civilization in Western eyes derive from this mental activity. The affinity of contents proposed by so many different sources would be the proof of the existence of unconscious information common to human beings through space and time, which Jung later called the *archetypes of the collective unconscious*.

Once openly assumed that the unconscious had a trans-personal dimension, the proverbial die was cast. In the second part of *Transformations and Symbols of the Libido* Jung questioned the primacy of sexuality sustained by Freud, to the point of arguing that the very sexuality recounted in myth (and in the clinical observation) could be *the symbol of something else*. In the case of Miss Miller, for example, sexual fantasies were a symbol of the activity of the libido separated from its parents for independent conquest. Perhaps, initially, Jung was still under the illusion that he could turn his own conception of the libido into a theoretical proposition acceptable even to Freud. However, by the time he outlined a theory of development that included, among other things, a pre-sexual phase, any room for dialogue was clearly precluded.

In the meantime it had become progressively clear that the Jungian conception of the dream diverged from the Freudian one in a decisive way, and not only as a consequence of their different conceptions of libido. Jung did not exclude the idea that the dream could represent the fulfillment of a desire, but he preferred to describe its content as compensatory to the daily conscious life. In other words, the dream would typically contain what the dreamer lacked in the present, whether it was sexuality or a more exciting existence. The major interest of the dream life would in fact have consisted, according to Jung, of its reflection of the dreamer's present psychological condition. Often, moreover, rather than looking to the past, as according to Freud, the dream turned toward the future: the *prospective function* would have consisted of suggesting an upcoming turning point in the life of the individual. The apparent cryptic nature of the dream, then, would not have been the result of a process of masking but rather of its peculiar mode of expression (the same, as we have seen, of mythology) (Jung, 1909/1961b, 2012a). The reflection on the dream, however, accompanied Jung throughout his life: while Jung never wrote a work comparable in bulk to Freud's *Traumdeutung*, he nevertheless returned to the theme in several essays (Jung, 1916–1948/1960d, 1945–1948/1960e), held no less than two cycles of seminars on the subject (one for his pupils [Jung, 1984] and one at the University of Zurich [Jung, 2012b], and structured his entire *Psychology and Alchemy* (Jung, 1944/1953d) as a commentary on a series of dreams by the physicist Wolfgang Pauli. An undated Jungian manuscript contains a list of seventy-eight authors of books on dreams, published mainly between the eighteenth and nineteenth centuries, a kind of initial core of a natural history of the dream world (Shamdasani, 2003, p. 135).

The cooling of relations with the father of psychoanalysis culminated in an explicit "Declaration of Independence" by Jung (McGuire, 1974, p. 500). This is in fact the expression that Freud himself used to define a Jungian letter claiming the right to an autonomous theoretical path, culminating with a quotation from Nietzsche's *Thus Spoke Zarathustra* which begins with the words: "One repays back a teacher badly if one always remains only a pupil" (quoted in McGuire, 1974, p. 491). Jung's speech (1913/1971b) at the Psychoanalytic Congress in Munich was the final push toward the end of his collaboration with Freud. Here Jung made a move that must have been sensational for the psychoanalytic movement, putting Freud's theory on the same level as the theory of the newly ostracized Adler. It was not, however, an impromptu idea on the part of Jung, who had long expressed interest in Adler's theory, despite the caution hitherto observed toward Freud in this regard. Jung had witnessed a talk by Adler on the occasion of his first attendance at one of the Wednesday psychological evenings (March 6, 1907), and had openly stated that the criticisms made on that occasion of Adler's theory of organic inferiority were far too harsh. Instead, this theory appeared to him to be "a brilliant idea" (Nunberg & Federn, 1962, p. 144).

Jung now started from the observation that both Freud and Adler proposed a coherent, and, in his own way, convincing vision of psychopathology. Each of the two systems found successful therapeutic application. It was therefore a question of understanding whether the successes were only apparent, or imagining a form of coexistence between psychoanalysis and the emerging individual psychology. The Swiss psychologist was therefore the first to formulate a question that the subsequent proliferation of psychotherapeutic theories and practices would make more and more pressing (without finding, to date, a definitive answer): how is it possible to explain the coexistence and success of different models? The answer offered by Jung in Munich and deepened in later texts (Jung, 1921/1971a) was articulated as follows:

1. human beings are characterized by different personalities, which can be traced to a number of *psychological types*;
2. each psychological theory reflects the interests, conflicts, and personality characteristics of its originator;

3. although the creator may succeed in formulating a generalizable theory, they cannot succeed in transcending the characteristics of their own psychological type (and offering a psychology of his own type must be considered a success);
4. the possibility of constructing a theory that takes into account the different types is the task of the psychology of the future.

There were initially only two types described by Jung: *introvert* and *extrovert*. An introvert tended to develop a greater interest in their own inner world than in interpersonal relationships, while an extrovert favored contact with other human beings. The psychology of the introvert was best explained, according to Jung, by the Adlerian model, that of the extrovert by Freudian psychoanalysis. The psychopathology of the introvert could justifiably be conceived as originating from a sense of organic inferiority. The extrovert developed problems that could instead be traced back to sexuality. It could be argued that the explanatory model was a bit too primitive, and that Adler's and Freud's theories were being forced into the scheme. The limitations of the Jungian attempt, however, does not invalidate its extraordinary historical importance: for decades no one would have proposed an alternative explanation. In fact, almost no one would even consider the Jungian hypothesis sketched in 1913 and refined in 1921. It was not until the 1970s that a book from a psychoanalytic environment again proposed to trace psychodynamic theories back to the psyche of their respective authors. *Faces in a Cloud* by Atwood and Stolorow (1979) indeed acknowledged Jung's attempt at a similar path, but only mentioned his first attempt.[10]

The fact that Jung was now considered foreigner within the psychoanalytic movement is certainly entirely understandable. From this point on, his theoretical contributions were systematically ignored (or at best distorted) by Freud and his orthodox followers. Jung was thereafter mentioned by psychoanalysts only as a negative paradigm. Having left the psychoanalytic movement in 1914, Jung soon cut ties with Bleuler as well, abandoning his post at the Burghölzli and devoting himself to private practice. Many of his early companions (such as Ferenczi and Eitingon) remained close to Freud, while Binswanger maintained his independence from both. The following years saw the maturation of Jungian thought in a situation of relative isolation, exacerbated by the parallel outbreak of World War I.

Psychological types and collective unconscious

After his speech at the Munich Congress *A Contribution to the Study of Psychological Types*, Jung also publicly assumed an attitude of independence toward Freudian thought. The words contained in a conference shortly afterward were unmistakable: "This is not the place for a critical discussion of Freud's psychology of dreams. But I will try to give a brief summary of what may be regarded as more or less established facts of dream psychology to-day" (Jung,

1914/1920a, p. 322). In fact, however, Jung would always recognize the merits of Freud, attributing to him the rightful role of founder of depth psychology (Jung, 1917/1920b; 1943/1953a). Conversely, the psychoanalytic movement immediately began the total ostracism of Jungian thought. Jung resigned from the International Psychoanalytic Association immediately after the publication of *On the History of the Psychoanalytic Movement* (Freud, 1914/1957c), which represented little less than an indictment of him. All of Freud's pupils and collaborators, moreover, seemed delighted to see the "crown prince" leave the scene. They even competed to criticize him (Ferenczi, 1913/2005, 1914/1990; Abraham, 1914/1955; Fichtner & Pomerans, 2003, pp. 147–149). The contempt toward him soon became such that Edward Glover (1888–1972), a student of Abraham and author of *Freud or Jung?*, considered it legitimate to propose a comparison between the two without bothering to read firsthand the Jungian writings (Glover, 1950).[11]

Jung spent the next few years developing his own theory, which he began to call analytical psychology, a term that was born as a synonym for psychoanalysis and that soon acquired an independent meaning. The central questions from which Jung's elaboration started were those presented in *A Contribution to the Study of Psychological Types* (Jung, 1913/1971b) and *Transformations and Symbols of the Libido* (Jung, 1912/2019). If in Munich Jung had problematized the possible legitimacy of Adler's theory as well as Freud's, then in the previous work he had assumed the existence of a trans-personal unconscious. Both issues presupposed the need to extend the territory explored by psychoanalysis. Jung developed both of them, arriving at problematic theoretical proposals, however, such as to constitute a premise for profound changes in clinical technique compared to classical psychoanalysis.

Jung's speech at the Munich Congress had closed by indicating that the creation of a psychology that would be "equally fair to both types" was a "difficult task" for the future (Jung, 1913/1971b, p. 509) – that is, the extrovert (like Freud) and the introvert (like Adler). In the following years, Jung (1916/1953c, 1917/1920b) seemed convinced that he could build a theory capable of absorbing both psychoanalysis and individual psychology. This optimism, however, had waned with the publication of what was perhaps Jung's capital work, *Psychological Types* (Jung, 1921/1971a). Here the Swiss psychologist set out a theory of types that in the meantime had been greatly enriched. The psychological type, in Jung's ultimate vision, was qualified, first of all, always by their fundamental attitude toward existence, or by the mode of investment of libido, that is, by introversion or extroversion:

> The introvert's attitude is an abstracting one: at bottom, he is always intent on withdrawing libido from the object, as though he had to prevent the object from gaining power over him. The extravert, on the contrary, has a positive relation to the object He affirms its importance to such an extent that his subjective attitude is constantly related to and oriented by the

object. The object can never have enough value for him, and its importance must always be increased.

(p. 330)[12]

Secondly, however, the type was also defined by the prevailing function in the relationship with reality. Four functions were described: thinking, feeling, sensation, and intuition. Using the terms in a very idiosyncratic way, Jung called the first two functions rational because they were characterized in his opinion by the use of judgments, unlike the second two, which were therefore called irrational functions. Only thinking would be based on what is normally called rationality, since it overlapped with the traditional concept of intellect. Thinking was described as the activity of "following its own laws, brings the contents of ideation into conceptual connections with one another" (p. 481). Feeling, according to Jung, judged by establishing connections based on the pleasantness or unpleasantness of an object or mental state: "a process that imparts to the content a definite value in the sense of acceptance or rejection ('like' or 'dislike')" (p. 434). Sensation "is the psychological function that mediates the perception of a physical stimulus. It is, therefore, identical with perception [and] related not only to external stimuli but to inner ones, i.e., to changes in the internal organic processes" (p. 461). Finally, intuition "mediates perceptions in an unconscious way," whether they are internal objects, external objects or connections between objects: "In intuition, any content is presented as something complete without us being able to indicate or discover in what way this content has been realized." In other words, intuition "is a kind of instinctive apprehension, no matter of what contents" (pp. 453). In summary, Jung redefined the functions as follows a few years after the publication of *Psychological Types*: "The essential function of sensation is to establish that something exists, thinking tells us what it means, feeling what its value is, and intuition surmises whence it comes and wither it goes" (Jung, 1936/1971c, p. 553).

The combination of the "choice" of one of the four possible functions and one of the two possible attitudes (extroverted or inverted) would give rise to eight possible types, which, however, would rarely be pure. In most people, it would not be possible to use only one function, and sometimes two or even three are used. Jung only excluded that thinking and feeling or sensation and intuition could coexist in a type (regardless of which function was the main one). The number of possible permutations (and possible psychological types) was thus very high, allowing Jung to predict the possibility of the future emergence of many other possible theories in the field of psychology. Such a prediction, in fact, has largely come true, and this book is a (only partial) testimony to it.

If awareness of the typological problem still seemed to Jung a sufficient tool with which to found a *super partes* psychology in *The Psychology of Unconscious Processes* (Jung, 1917/1920b), the conclusions of *Psychological Types* led him to a more problematic and relativistic position. The perspective of one's own type became an unavoidable presupposition for every psychologist. The same typology built by Jung, therefore, could be relativized: another author could legitimately build a different and equally well-founded theory (Jung, 1921/1971a). It was a conviction, moreover, that the Swiss showed he had not abandoned until the very last of his writings (Jung, 1961/1977a). Under these conditions, the "future psychology" originally envisioned by Jung became a sort of regulative ideal (to put it in Kantian terms): it was possible to strive for it, but also difficult to hope to see it realized. At this point Jung began to call complex psychology the project of theory that would have to take into account all the others, identifying his own analytical psychology as one of the perspectives that this project would have to unify.

The content of the collective psyche (Jung would later use the term *collective unconscious*) was first identified with the lower functions of the mind, which according to Janet acted when phenomena of psychological automatism occurred. Quickly, however, Jung was convinced that the collective unconscious could be traced back to two fundamental orders of content. The first was the instincts, or the "all-or-none-reactions" that were not the result of learning (according to a definition shared by biologists of the time). The constant possibility of running into "exaggerated reactions" compared to the stimulus would testify to the presence of instincts even in civilized people (Jung, 1919–1948/1960c, p. 135). The second type consisted of true representative contents common to all humankind, the *archetypes*. The existence of archetypes was demonstrated by the presence of mythological nuclei (mythologems) and very similar images in cultures distant in time and space, for which it was therefore impossible to imagine the influence of one on the other. Jung seemed decidedly uncertain on the nature of archetypes, however. In *The Psychology of Unconscious Processes*, he wrote that he did not confirm in any way the heritability of representations, but only the heritability of the possibility of representation, which he thought was quite different (Jung, 1917/1920b). In the same work, however, he also argued that the collective unconscious contained historical images of the world at large in the form of original images (*Urbilder*) or mythological motifs. Jung never solved this epistemic uncertainty, caught between the fascination of the hypothesis of true universal contents and the possible consequent accusation of Lamarckism. Only by adhering to Lamarck's evolutionism, which in the 1910s had already been discredited, was it possible to assume the existence of a shared memory of human experiences dating back to the dawn of humanity.[13]

The structure of the psyche and the nature of Jungian therapy

If it was already possible, especially after Freud, to hypothesize the existence of conscious and unconscious elements of the psyche, the hypothesis of a collective psyche allowed the theorization of four classes of mental contents: both conscious and unconscious contents could be classified as personal and impersonal. Based on this distinction, the structure of the psyche theorized by Jung included (a) the individual conscious personality (the ego); (b) an individual unconscious; (c) the collective unconscious; and (d) a segment of the collective psyche with which the individual tends to identify, accepting the instances of society (the urge to assume a role and always behave in accordance with it), namely the *persona* (Jung, 1916/1953c, 1917/1920b). The individual unconscious comprised first of all what the individual had removed over the years. Jung identified in it the *Shadow*, which was what one did not want to be but was still part of one's personality. There was also a counter-sexual dimension, that is the feminine part of the man (*Anima*) and the masculine part of the woman (*Animus*), and, finally, a nucleus that could be defined as projectual (the *Self*). The Self was in fact, according to Jung, the aspect of personality present in potency, toward which the individual would tend in the course of a maturative and self-fulfilling path that Jung defined as the *individuation process*.

The life of an individual could be defined as the result of the individual and collective tendencies of their psychological development. The first step toward the complete development of one's potential was the dissolution of the persona that is, overcoming identification with it, which would lead to a confrontation with both the personal and the collective unconscious. Jung emphasized that the contact with the unconscious was not without risks, but it was not the unconscious itself that was dangerous: the source of its dangerousness was instead the disagreement with the unconscious (Jung, 1917/1920b). The confrontation should produce a synthesis, through a psychical process which Jung proposed should be called the *transcendent function* (Jung, 1916–1958/1960b). In this sense he could consider the theories of Freud and Adler as cauterizing tools to be used 'locally', as they are destructive and reductive (Jung, 1917/1920b). On the other hand, Jung would always continue to maintain that in some analyses he could be heard using Adler's language, in others Freud's (Jaffé, 1989). Later on, Jung matured the conviction that, independent of the theory he was referring to, the main therapeutic instrument was the personality of the therapist (Jung, 1929/1966d, 1935/1966a, 1935/1966b, 1945/1966e).[14]

The analytical path, according to Jung, was not always necessary and sometimes could even be counterproductive: he came to say that the psychologist had to understand when it was appropriate to *close the door of the unconscious* rather than open it. Each human being could have decidedly different needs, even with regard to the depth to which an analysis should be conducted.

The ideal goal of analysis was individuation, corresponding to the full realization of one's potential through the creative use of unconscious contents. Nor was individuation without risk, however, since "individuation and collectivity are a pair of opposites, two divergent destinies" (Jung, 1916/1977b, p. 452). Only authentically creative people can achieve it: "Individuation remains a pose so long as no positive values are created. Whoever is not creative enough must re-establish collective conformity with a group of his own choice. otherwise he remains an empty waster and windbag" (*ibidem*). Conversely, even neurosis should not be considered an evil in itself, because "neurotic symptoms (. . .) are also endeavours towards a new synthesis of life." Even if they are failed endeavors, they "represent the germinal striving which has both meaning and value. They are embryos that failed to achieve life, owing to unpropitious conditions of an internal and external nature" (Jung, 1917/1920b, p. 411).

One's psychological type would, according to Jung, heavily affect the course of psychotherapy. For example, the mode of conducting free association would have been very different:

> In sensation and intuitive types the associations are not of an explanatory character but are coincidents or coexistences, things which are in the same picture. For example, if it is a question of the wall, the sensation or intuitive type might associate that chair with it, which is just coexistent. This is an irrational type of association. With the rational type we get explanatory associations. If the rational type tries to have irrational associations they are always false, they do not fit, so I ask them just to tell me what they think about it.
>
> (Jung, 1984, p. 162).

Above all, however, the contents of the personal unconscious, linked to the inferior function (the less developed one), changed. The thinking type, then, would have to acquire the ability to use their feelings, which would have primitive connotations, while the feeling type would have to become familiar with the intellectual judgments, in itself very difficult for their ego to manage. The subsequent stages of therapy were similar for the different psychological types: first, there was the confrontation with the Shadow and then with the Anima, that is, with the increasingly deeply denied and repressed aspects of one's personality. In some cases, deeper and more archaic elements, linked to the chthonian world of the collective unconscious, could also emerge (Jung, 1928/1953b).

In the essay *Problems of Modern Psychotherapy* (Jung, 1929/1966d) the question of how the analysis proceeded was approached from a new and particular perspective: there would be a series of stages in the therapeutic process, which could be more or less appropriate with patients of different characteristics. These stages were defined as *confession, elucidation, education, transformation*. The first was linked to the religious tradition, although taken up by Freud; the second was unequivocally of Freudian derivation; the third was of the Adlerian brand; and the last was the specific contribution of Jungianism.

The effectiveness of both sacramental and psychotherapeutic confession, would have been due to the possibility of sharing a secret, the weight of which could crush a person who bears it alone. The effect of religious confession was cathartic, just as, according to Jung, the result of Freud's early therapeutic technique was an intense catharsis.

Confession and catharsis could in themselves be sufficient for the success of a therapy, but they could also be insufficient for two types of patients: those who could not really "perceive the shadows" (p. 60) despite the fact that analysis had put them in a position to do so; and the ones who enjoyed exploration and catharsis "at the expense of (. . .) adaptation to life" (p. 61). In this case, instead of healing, a new symptom was obtained, consisting of the creation of a dependence on the analysis and on the analyst. If the patient relived their relationship with their parents in the transference, then the existence of possibly incestuous desires never consciously understood in that relationship was an important obstacle to the solution of the transference. Having understood this dynamic, Freud realized the need to interpret the unconscious contents to bring them to consciousness (what Jung called elucidation). The result was "a minute elaboration of man's shadow-side unexampled in any previous age" (ibid., p. 63). However, Freud's most important contribution to psychotherapy would turn into the most dramatic limitation of psychoanalysis:

> Freud's interpretative method rests on "reductive" explanation which unfailingly leads backwards and downwards, and is essentially destructive, if overdone or handled one-sidedly. Nevertheless psychology has profited greatly from Freud's pioneer work: it has learned that human nature has its black side (. . .) Even our purest and holiest beliefs rest on very deep and dark foundations (. . .) The uproar over Freud's interpretations is entirely due to our barbarous or childish naïveté (. . .) Our mistake lies in supposing that the radiant things are done away with by being explained from the shadow-side. This is a regrettable error into which Freud himself has fallen.
>
> (p. 64)

Even the knowledge of one's personal unconscious and the solution of transference was not be enough for the symptomatic consequences of one's neurosis to be liquidated: "in many cases the most thorough elucidation leaves the patient an intelligent but still incapable child" (p. 66). The need for the third stage then arose, education, Adler's fundamental contribution to psychotherapy: "Whereas Freud is the investigator and the interpreter," writes Jung, "Adler is primarily the educator" (p. 67). The Adlerian technique pushed people to social adaptation that self-knowledge might not be sufficient to promote. If, however, it was not enough for the person analyzed to reach the normality of adaptation and they aspired to complete self-realization, the last stage, that of transformation, would be necessary. If one was faced with a case in which the early onset of neurosis was evident, however, it would have been problematic in any case to avoid resorting to a profound change of personality: it would therefore always have been necessary to achieve transformation.

Personality transformation implied the possibility of going through a large section of the individuation process. It was precisely the subjectivity of the possible outcomes, however, that made it more difficult to codify the theory of the technique. In this sense, the personal relationship between therapist and patient became decisive: analysis became a dialogue in which communication took place on both a conscious and an unconscious level. The interpretive attitude toward the symbolic contents coming from the unconscious then became much more open. It could no longer be assumed that the therapist knew and judged objectively what the patient brought to therapy. Interpretation consisted of a process that was not only dialogical, but even dialectical. There could be mutual influence, and the therapist had to always be ready to question their own ideas. Freud, as we have seen, had identified neutrality as one of the fundamental aspects of the analytic technique and had indicated in countertransference (the analyst's transference on the patient) an obstacle to therapy. Jung, on the other hand, considered countertransference inevitable, although he was well aware of its risks:

> Just as all doctors are exposed to infections and other occupational hazards, so the psychotherapist runs the risk of psychical infections which are no less menacing. On the one hand he is often in danger of getting entangled in the neuroses of his patients; on the other hand if he tries too hard to guard against their influences, he robs himself of his therapeutic efficacy. Between this Scylla and Carybdis lies the peril, but also the healing power.
>
> (Jung, 1935/1966a, p. 19)

Even the different concept of the unconscious had deep implications compared to the idea of psychotherapy advocated by Freud. If Freud considered analysis as a sort of reclamation and enlargement of the boundaries of the ego with respect to the unconscious, Jung believed that it could also provide illumination and suggestions:

> The unconscious is seen as a creative factor, even a bold innovator, and yet it is at the same time a stronghold of ancestral conservatism. A paradox, I admit, but it cannot be helped. It is no more paradoxical than man himself and that cannot be helped either.
>
> (Jung, 1930/1966c, p. 34)

In the analytic process, moreover, for Jung "the therapist is no longer the agent of treatment, but a fellow participant in a process of individual development (. . .). The therapist enters into relationship with another psychic system as questioner and answerer" (Jung, 1935/1966a, p. 12). This difference in attitude was also reflected in the face-to-face position assumed by the analyst/patient couple in the practice: Jung did not like the use of the couch, because it interfered with the potential for direct contact with the patient (Storr, 1973). In therapy, moreover, Jung focused much more on the possibility of tracing the causes of neurosis in the present, rather than in childhood, as did Freud.

From Jung's point of view, the confrontation with the unconscious and the process of individuation could, in several cases, be extended for a much longer duration than that of analysis. To this end Jung theorized a technique that he called *active imagination*, consisting of a sort of meditation to be conducted from symbolic contents emerging from one's unconscious (Innamorati, 1995, 2013). The *Red Book* is an interesting testimony of how Jung applied this technique, as are the *Black Books* published only recently (Jung, 2009, 2020) thanks to the work of Sonu Shamdasani.[15]

As will be seen in the following chapters, the psychoanalytic movement was bound to adopt many of Jung's ideas about psychotherapy, albeit in most cases without knowledge of (or at least without mention of) Jung's writings. One critic has appropriately called these psychoanalysts, "unknowing Jungians" (Samuels, 1985, p. 7). The idea that the relationship is the fundamental therapeutic factor has been one of the guiding principles of the Neo-Freudians as well as of Self Psychology, and has been developed through relational psychoanalysis. The principle of openness with respect to the interpretation of unconscious contents has been strongly confirmed by the whole group of hermeneuticists. The dialectical involvement of the analyst/patient couple has been advocated by the proponents of *bi-personal psychology* and especially by the *intersubjectivists*.[16]

In extreme synthesis, it can be said that most Jungian theoretical concepts had been introduced by 1921: very few new terms, which were not already included in the Lexicon that concludes *Psychological Types* (completed with the entry Self in 1928), would be found later. The main clinical writings were published by the beginning of the 1930s. All subsequent production by Jung was devoted to deepening his conceptions about the collective unconscious.

Behaviorism and psychotherapy

Psychoanalysis was the psychotherapeutic model best able to take root during the first part of the 20th century, the century of modernity, of electricity, of new productive systems, of liberal states in which new antagonistic political subjectivities were emerging (the fourth state, women) and new rights and duties of citizenship (vote, strike, wage labor, popular education). In this context, and with Freud's trip to America in 1909, psychoanalysis had become an object of interest for American psychologists since the first decade of the 20th century.

Meanwhile, beginning with the "manifesto" (1913) of John B. Watson (1878–1958), behaviorism made its appearance and gradually colonized American psychology, whose exponents were both proud opponents of psychoanalysis and diffusers of a model of psychological research that had enormous influence during the 20th century. Watson denied the idea that the study of mental content and internal states was the goal of scientific psychology: psychology as a natural science had to study and predict behavior.

Similarly, Burrhus Frederic Skinner (1909–1990), Watson's follower, thought that looking at a person's behavior was like looking at a physical or biological system (Skinner, 1956, p. 81). Behaviorism, then, was essentially an anti-mentalist

U.S. scholarly tradition, developed in opposition to both early experimental psychology, which primarily studied consciousness, and to psychoanalysis, whose primary object of interest was instead the unconscious. Behaviorism has influenced all the psychology of the 20th century in a direct and subterranean way, integrating and hybridizing social and cognitive instances over time. Behavioral epistemology continues, to this day, to influence research in the field of psychology and psychopathology (Millon, 2004; Mills, 1998).

In dealing with behaviorism, it is necessary to abandon the fairly widespread notion that behaviorists were originally uninterested in psychotherapy, and that the applications of this tradition of studies were merely the result of a late interest. On the contrary, from the very beginning, behaviorists also studied individuals from a clinical perspective, precisely in opposition to an alleged literariness and lack of scientificity of psychoanalysis. Moreover, from the very beginning, behaviorists dealt with pathology. From this point of view, behaviorists would have wanted, in their own way, to bring the pathological back to normality. The consequence was that the pathological manifestations empirically detectable through a whole series of psychophysiological correlates (sweat, redness, dizziness, etc.) became one of the targets of behavioral psychotherapy.[17] In this approach, conditioning was the keystone of treatment, and behavioral clinicians used, above all, theoretical models concerning learning. Edward Lee Thorndike (1874–1949) and Ivan Petrovič Pavlov (1849–1936) should be mentioned among those who paved the way for the behavioral theory of learning.

Thorndike, a student of William James and James McKeen Cattell (1860–1944), was an American psychologist influenced by functionalism and pragmatism. Although criticized by behaviorists because of his theory, still considered mentalistic and excessively focused on spontaneous modes of learning, he was also one of their theoretical-methodological references. Thorndike had studied the learning processes in particular, imagining very original experiments in which animals learned to solve problems according to feedback mechanisms based on trial and error, and on rewards and punishments. He developed the *law of effect*, according to which a behavior became more frequent (strong) if it was associated with a satisfaction, and remained less likely if it had unsatisfactory consequences. From this perspective, he had an incremental and automatic idea of learning, according to which the more a behavior was enacted, the more it was learned (*law of exercise*). Conversely, disused behaviors were forgotten. Thorndike was also convinced that the most recent response was also the one that would be most likely to be re-enacted (*principle of recency*). He then introduced the idea that behaviors learned in one condition were easily generalizable to situations that appeared similar. Thorndike was, therefore, among the first to show that certain behaviors could be reinforced by their positive consequences. This idea was later followed in behavioral psychotherapy.

The study of animal models of behavior and the eugenic approach also became predominant with Thorndike's work, which influenced American psychology in various ways in the years to follow (Thorndike, 1898; see Clifford, 1968).

The studies of animal learning by a very young Thorndike were even cited by Pavlov, a Russian physiologist and Nobel Prize winner, destined to leave an indelible mark on the history of psychology. As is well known, Pavlov's model of learning was very influential, especially because it showed how certain behaviors, once learned, could occur in situations seemingly unrelated to the original context. In Pavlov's classic experiment, food was presented to dogs after they had heard the ringing of a bell within a defined optimal time frame. First the amount of saliva produced by dogs after the presentation of food (unconditioned stimulus, because it is always able to produce salivation) was measured. Then, after a certain number of exposures, the amount of saliva produced after only hearing the sound of the bell was measured: the result was the same (demonstrating the possibility of learning a conditioned stimulus). Food was therefore associated in a consequential way to the sound of the bell, which assumed a symbolic meaning capable of evoking a behavior originally provoked by food alone, in an unconditioned way (Pavlov, 1927). A theory related to the extinction of learned behaviors through conditioned stimulation was also codified in the Pavlovian model. Pavlov showed that if the conditioned stimulus (ringing of the bell) was no longer followed by the unconditioned stimulus (food), the conditioned behavioral response (salivation after the bell) also died out. The disappearance of behavior was precisely the cornerstone of early behavioral psychotherapy. As Leon Trotsky creatively illustrated:

> Both Pavlov and Freud think that the bottom of the 'soul' is physiology. But Pavlov, like a diver, descends to the bottom and laboriously investigates the well from there upward; while Freud stands over the well and with penetrating gaze tries to pierce its ever-shifting and troubled water and to make out or guess the shape of things down below. Pavlov's method is experiment, Freud's method is conjecture, sometimes fantastic conjecture (Trotsky, 1927/1962, p. 105).

This comparison shows that Trotsky[18] grasped the clinical significance of the Pavlovian model of learning, which, although oriented mainly to the manifest behaviors and mechanisms of digestion, ended up reaching the symbolic meaning that stimulations of various kinds could have meant, if capable of soliciting behaviors in nature not associated with those same stimulations. The symbolic meaning was linked to the stimuli, and was continuously interpreted by the mind. This pushed Trotsky to assimilate the two models, the psychoanalytic and the psychophysiological, apparently and by all psy-scientists, considered very dissimilar.[19]

Pavlov in Russia had thus developed a theory and laboratory practice that would long influence experimental, clinical and personality psychology.[20] At the same time behaviorism was the psychological model that was integrating previous conceptions of learning into a successful and coherent model in the United States. Behaviorism was especially linked to the name of John B. Watson, who is usually remembered as one of the founding fathers of experimental psychology, whereas the role he played in clinical psychology is overlooked. A student of functionalist James Rowland Angell (1869–1949) in Chicago, he became a young and successful professor at Johns Hopkins University in Baltimore and editor of the *Psychological Review*. He was immediately concerned with giving psychology a solid biological foundation to encourage its classification within the natural sciences. In his famous article *Psychology as the Behaviorist Views It* (1913) he abandoned the idea, shared by both structuralist and functionalist psychology, that the main method of experimentation in psychology was through controlled introspection. Basic psychological research since the second half of the 19th century (especially in the German context) was in fact conducted using introspective analysis, more or less objectified by recording methods, of states of consciousness. For Watson the only way to make psychology a science was to put the study of manifest behavior at the center of the investigation.

Watson's psychology was aimed at investigating complex behavior, and not only single stimulus-response units, as is often suggested in the historiographical vulgate. Watson certainly derived from Pavlov the idea that complex behaviors were born from conditioned reflexes, but he rejected all those symbolic and physiological consequences to which the association between conditioned stimulus and conditioned response could have led. He was convinced that by means of specific learning techniques it would be possible to educate children to be exactly what one wished them to become in adulthood. This approach fascinated American culture, and Watson became a celebrated and recognized psychologist.

From a clinical point of view, Watson was able to produce experimental neuroses that he claimed to be able to extinguish. He famously experimented on little Albert, a child who had not yet turned one year of age, and associated a crying reaction originally produced with annoying noises, to the presence of a white rat. Albert then generalized the crying originally associated with the white rat – which before Watson's intervention did not frighten him – to other animals and situations.[21] He thus described the process of generalization of a behavior produced in the laboratory, which is similar to the emotional reactions described in the different forms of neurosis (Watson & Rayner, 1920). Watson and his collaborators affirmed they could deconstruct the emotional reactions they themselves created through a "reverse learning process" called desensitization, by which overlearned emotional reactions were reduced by a process of gradual and systematic exposure to the same stimulus that previously elicited disturbing emotional reactions.

The true extent of Watson's experiments is still a subject of heated historiographical debate, just as the actual induction of neurosis through conditioning techniques has been questioned by scholars who have specifically analyzed Watson's experiences (Harris, 1979). Although Albert's case is still obscure precisely because of the paucity of the initial account of Watson and his collaborator Rosalie Rayner (1898–1935), it is nevertheless certain that, as will be seen, it became the anchor point of behavioral psychotherapies which developed in the 1950s and 1960s,[22] especially with the passage from classical conditioning to operant conditioning by Skinner at the end of the 1930s (Skinner, 1938).[23] Indeed, it is possible to say that the case of Little Albert was then mythologized in the 1960s as a scientific and valid example to be contrasted with the "pseudoscientific" praxis of psychoanalysis and the fictional creation of cases by Freud, such as that of Little Hans.[24]

Being only forty-two years old, Watson had to abandon his academic career because of a scandal, arising from the fact that he left his wife to have an affair with his assistant Rosalie Rayner. Watson then embarked on a brilliant career as a psychologist in the world of advertising and marketing (Buckley, 1989). Watson's intellectual legacy bore fruit, especially in the work conducted by Skinner at the University of Minnesota in the latter half of the 1930s.

Behaviorism: therapies and cultures

Behaviorism, far from being a narrow laboratory practice, was actually a formidable lever for a whole series of applications of psychology: desensitization practices;[25] *aversive therapies*;[26] *biofeedback*;[27] techniques to treat phobias and some categories of psychosomatic disorders (muscle tension, psychosomatic hypertension, headache, etc.). On the other hand, by integrating internal mechanisms for the control of behavior (cognitive maps, motivations) and external mechanisms (environmental pressures, influence of the situation), behaviorism has changed greatly in the 20th century, turning into the cognitive behavioral theory and the social cognitivism that we will analyze in the next chapters.[28]

Skinner discovered that animals could be trained with food when placed in an enclosed area (a Skinner box), which would reinforce their behavior (operant conditioning). With a system of reinforcement, Skinner trained pigeons to undertake diverse activities (such as playing music or identifying a playing card). These experimental demonstrations led him to believe that it was even possible to build an ideal world in which the system of reinforcements or punishments would shape human behavior to create a society in which happiness was achieved by all through learning methodologies, and all undesirable behaviors were kept under control (on the political aspects of Skinner's behaviorism see Rutherford, 2009). This ideal community project was described into a novel, *Walden Two* (1948), which achieved much success in the United States during the so-called "counterculture" period of the 1960s and 1970s (Millon, 2004; Smith & Woodward, 1996).[29]

Behaviorism therefore exerted a long and strong fascination on Western culture, and the idea that psychology could modify behavior in ways that were useful to society greatly stimulated the imagination of politicians, artists, psychologists, and psychiatrists. At the same time, some questioned the extreme simplicity with which behavioral learning techniques would actually control complex phenomena related to mental functioning and society. The theories and experiments of behaviorists thus strongly and decisively influenced psychotherapy. All specific anxiety disorders could be treated through a desensitization plan and unlearning actions. Such psychotherapeutic techniques also showed great practical importance in some specific cases, such as phobias. For example, those who were afraid of flying in an airplane but at the same time needed to do so could benefit from desensitization techniques that proved to be effective. In particular, the effectiveness of these behavioral therapies was demonstrated across a broad spectrum of mental disorders (phobias, depression, anxiety, anger, stress, psychosomatic disorders) when hybridized with cognitivist techniques.[30] Skinner had promoted various behavioral reinforcement activities in psychological practice. He was convinced that precisely the most difficult cases (children, adolescents, the elderly, psychotics) could easily be mistreated in institutions if standardized techniques that could foster desired behaviors through reinforcement were not used. Skinner, for example, favored the *token economy* (symbolic economy or technique of reinforcement by means of objects of little value) as a mode of behavioral conditioning, which typically used plastic cards as a means of exchange to encourage desired behaviors and to oppose those deemed nonadaptive. This behavioral-derived technique was applied in psychiatric hospitals, as a reissue of moral treatment, with good results especially with chronic patients. It then spread and is also used to educate "difficult" children and teens.[31] The children obtain cards if they behave appropriately, or if they also took part in other therapies such as group therapy, and with the cards they bought free time and consumer goods provided by the institution itself (Ayllon & Azrin, 1968).[32]

The behavioral framework had consequences that went beyond the mere territory of psychotherapy. A significant example of the long-lasting influence of the behavioral culture throughout the 20th century is described in the film *A Clockwork Orange*, written and directed by Stanley Kubrick in 1971, and based on the novel of the same name (1962) by Anthony Burgess. The film and the novel are in fact a critique of the mechanicism inherent in the conception of humans proper to behaviorism. In an indeterminate future, the protagonist of the film uses violence in an eroticized manner, but is forced by behavioral techniques (the Ludovico Technique) to feel nauseous at the mere thought of being able to commit violence. A mechanical man who can be conditioned with scientific techniques was thus represented. This being, although emotionally flattened, finds a way to recover his ambivalent humanity, lost because of the Ludovico therapy, at the end of the film. Paradoxically, behaviorism is thus represented as a technique useful to all those conceptions of the state, progressive or conservative, which aim to control the behavior of citizens, even if the ultimate goal was the construction of a better society (such as in the society of Walden Two).

The utopian and simplistic idea of being able to manage behavior through an engineering system and some simple rules based on reinforcement or desensitization, on rewards and punishments, has managed to last until now even in the psychology inherent in the politics influenced by contemporary Monetarism and Ordoliberalism.[33] Freud, for his part, was the first to theorize the use of the analyst's fee as a reinforcement for the success of the treatment. Money was therefore considered an instrument with which to regulate behavior and to overcome resistance (Freud, 1915/1958f). On the other hand, money regulates not only the transactions between individuals, but also the behavior of citizens, in economic history. The measure of the use – or abuse – of money by states or citizens, starting from the German Ordo-liberal School and the Monetarism School of economic thought (the Chicago School), has today even become the yardstick by which we assess the need to modify the behavior of citizens of entire nations to bring them back to a virtuous normality, dictated by international agencies of governance that, in this case, also use technologies of the self with interventions for the individual, the group and the family (Arienzo, 2013; Miller & Rose, 2008).[34]

As we will see in later chapters, a certain naiveté of behaviorism led psychologists to revise its paradigm quite profoundly. Over the years, in fact, strong criticism developed against these practices of the self which, although showing elements of effectiveness, could be clearly marked by a paternalistic and authoritarian conception of intervention. This modality was also masterfully depicted by Milos Forman in the film *One Flew Over the Cuckoo's Nest* (1975), whose "therapeutic" scenes showed the cold implementation of dehumanizing reinforcement techniques in a hospital environment, which caused the protagonist of the film to revolt in the psychiatric hospital.

Paradoxically, some critics later attributed paternalism, authoritarianism and an instance of control of the masses to psychoanalysis alone,[35] which were actually present in a utilitarian and "anti-mentalist" conception of humans, such as organicist or behaviorist. On the contrary, dynamic psychology was instead based on the idea that therapy proceeded along a path of enlightenment, expansion of reason, mental enrichment, compensation and autonomy of the individual. The alternative psychodynamic models, more radical than the Freudian model, emphasized, on the one hand, the symbolic and cultural dimensions and, on the other hand, a critical conception of society. In practice, they led to the overturning of a traditional conception of the relationship between the state and the individual, no longer considered as a merely passive subject who must adapt to institutions, but also as the bearer of new needs, new freedoms and rights, claimed in various ways in the decades following World War II.

Notes

1 On Freud and De Sanctis, see Lombardo and Foschi (2008).
2 Ellenberger (1970) has shown that Freud reworked existing ideas far more than he cared to admit. According to Sonu Shamdasani (2003), the problem of the proper placement of the *Interpretation of Dreams* is due in part to the often uncritical acceptance by scholars of the review of previous literature proposed by Freud himself.

3   The mechanism of symbolization is also listed in order to simplify the exposition, which was actually introduced by Freud in 1909, mainly inspired by Stekel. The importance of the theoretical novelty, however, was such that both Jung (1909/1961a) and Ferenczi (1909/1994) immediately included it in their respective writings on dreams.

4   See infra, pp. 108–110.

5   The group that gathered around Freud highlighted an associative strategy that is often found in the history of the sciences. As we have seen, Mesmer had founded the Society of Harmony, a sort of brotherhood similar to Freemasonry. From 1897 Freud was a member of B'nai B'rith, a Jewish fraternity that at the time had initiation rites and simplified esoteric degrees, derived from Freemasonry, and the purpose of which was opposition to racism, the spread of Jewish culture and charitable activities. Freud had the opportunity to discuss his theories with the brothers of the B'nai B'rith on several occasions, and this affiliation, while enduring, is still little investigated, as is in general the relationship between secular fraternities and scientific-professional associations (see Cicciola, 2018; Meghnagi, 1992).

6   See infra, Ch. 5, pp. 206–213.

7   In 1907 Adler met Leon Trotsky (1879–1940) in Vienna who, as we shall see, was one of the few Marxist theorists and revolutionaries interested in psychoanalysis (Chemouni, 2004).

8   See supra, Ch. 2, p. 60 and p. 80, footnote 43.

9   See infra, Ch. 4, pp. 139–141.

10   See infra, Vol. 2 Ch. 8, pp. 147–149.

11   A note by Glover at the beginning of the text thanks a collaborator for collecting and collating quotes from Jung.

12   The introvert and extrovert types were probably the most widely used personality descriptions in 20th-century individual difference psychology. These traits were also studied from a psychophysiological and temperamental perspective (Lombardo & Foschi, 2002b).

13   See supra, Ch. 1, pp. 59–61.

14   This principle indeed received indirect confirmation when empirical research established that patient-therapist matching is a much more important predictor of therapeutic success than the theoretical model of reference (Dahl Kächele & Thomä, 1988).

15   The *Red Book* or *Liber Novus* was born from twelve fantasies that Jung had in the year that World War I would break out (in retrospect he considered them prophetic of the tragic impending war), and that he transcribed and elaborated in a series of notebooks known as *Black Books*. "He faithfully transcribed most of the fantasies from the *Black Books,* and to each of these added a section explaining the significance of each episode, combined with a lyrical elaboration" (Shamdasani, 2009, p. 202). This transcription (calligraphed like a medieval manuscript) was enriched with paintings by Jung himself.

16   See infra, Vol. 2, Ch. 8 and 9.

17   By extension, therefore, psychophysiological therapeutic approaches such as biofeedback or clinical sexology were also later rooted in the fertile soil of behaviorism.

18   On Trotsky and psychoanalysis see Chemouni (2004).

19   The juxtaposition of Pavlov and Freud must have been a topic that circulated in the Russian culture of the 1920s. Proof of this are the autobiographical short stories written in the 1930s by Michail Zoščenko (1894–1958), which, however, after their first publication in 1943, were immediately banned by the Soviets. His works were then published in full in Russia, with enormous success, only in 1987. These stories represent the author's attempt to self-analyze and make sense of his own existential state and his own discomforts based on the theories of Pavlov and Freud.

20   Pavlov's theory in fact also included a typology that differentiated the various nervous systems according to the different ease of conditioning of people with the idea that behavior depended on this natural psychophysiological component. The Pavlovian

tradition of studies on "temperament" was then hybridized with the English psychometric tradition and still promotes today, along the lines of a temperamental behaviorism, types of people (introvert/extrovert, sensation seekers, sensation avoiders, etc.) that are described as strongly influenced by their own typology in their adaptation to the environment (Lombardo & Foschi, 2002a, 2002b).

21 Watson and Rosalie Rayner (1898–1935) also presented the case of Little Albert through film. In the films (today easily available on YouTube) the psychologists showed a normal child who was not afraid of animals or other items (fire, monkey, dog, rabbit and finally a white rat), then the conditioning of the phobia of the white rat and finally the generalization of this phobia to all those stimuli that at the beginning of the film had not been found frightening. It was thus shown that Albert had learned a phobia, which could also have been deconstructed by a reverse process.

22 Mary Cover Jones (1897–1997) is remembered as the first true behavioral psychotherapist for having applied systematic desensitization in one of the famous clinical cases of children, very typical in the history of psychotherapy, the case of Little Peter. This case is only slightly later than Albert's but was rediscovered decades later (Rutherford, 2006).

23 See infra, Vol 2, Ch. 7, pp. 67–69.

24 Despite the importance of the case, even today there is no certainty about who Little Albert really was, and how much he was actually a "normal" child as shown by Watson and Rayner. A real science war has recently been unleashed regarding the identity of Albert between those who argue that Albert was a child with severe neuropsychiatric disorders, those who instead believe that he was a patient without obvious psychiatric problems and those who simply argue that Watson and Rayner's version of the facts was built for the purpose of justifying their thesis (see Powell et al., 2014; Harris, 2020). Paradoxically, in fact, it seems that Albert's case was, even at its inception, a constructed artifact with an anti-psychoanalytic function (Watson & Rayner, 1920; see Harris, 2011, p. 1; on the logic that led to the uncritical dissemination of Albert's case, see Digdon, 2020).

25 Systematic desensitization was the first successful therapeutic practice, an alternative to psychoanalysis. In practice, relaxation is associated with the anxious stimulus, which would replace the anxiogenic activation with a state of well-being. The patient then learns to generalize this well-being to all potentially anxiogenic situations.

26 Similar to desensitization, in aversive therapies an unwanted behavior (e.g., alcoholism, addiction, anger, aggression) is associated with an unpleasant stimulus with the idea of extinguishing the "pathological" behavior.

27 *Biofeedback*, unlike desensitization, is focused on learning the ability to manage the physiological activation that follows an anxiogenic stimulus. Derived from both behaviorism and meditative techniques, with the use of methods to monitor physiological activation (e.g., breath, heart rate, skin electrical conductivity, muscle relaxation), it promotes a patient's learning of states of relaxation and well-being, and also good physical and psychological functioning.

28 The psychotherapeutic ones were preeminent among these hybridizations, especially in the United States where behavioral therapy was integrated with other therapies (see infra, Vol. 2, Ch. 9, pp. 191–195). Even today, many academic psychologists who deal, for example, with infant research, conduct observational studies, in order to confirm their theories, which are based on the methods of behaviorists (see infra, Vol 2, Ch. 8).

29 See infra, Vol. 2, Ch. 7, pp. 62 ff.

30 See infra, Vol. 2, Ch. 8, pp. 154–157.

31 Today, behavioral techniques are also commonly used for the treatment of serious behavioral disorders, especially in the developmental years. For example, *applied behavior analysis* (ABA), in which various behavioral analysis methodologies are used in order to improve conduct from a functional perspective, is widely used for autism.

32 See the interview with Skinner contained in *Token Economy: Applied Behaviorism*, a 1972 documentary available at https://archive.org/details/tokeneconomybehaviorismapplied.

33 Ordoliberalism is a German liberal school, developed in Freiburg during the Cold War and established in Europe as a doctrine that, grafting meritocratic and regulatory criteria, intends to calm the wildest pushes of liberalism, making it more attentive to the needs of society and giving the state a control function. This socio-economic doctrine has gradually become hegemonic in the European Union, so much so as to represent a sort of democratic alternative to Neoliberalism and American Anarcho-capitalism, but also to the old collectivism of the Soviet Union (Foucault, 2015).

34 It must be stressed that this conception of the relationship between the state and the citizen does not take into account a whole series of internal dimensions and complex situational circumstances that determine behavior as the product of matrices of causes, which are difficult to control with mere programs of reinforcement or punishment, but which do prove useful in "controlling" behavior, albeit in a very limited way.

35 An example is the long documentary *The Century of the Self* by Adam Curtis, produced by the BBC. It is also an attempt to link Freud's fate to that of his nephew Edward Bernays (1891–1995), who in the first half of the 20th century was probably the "inventor," in the United States and in the Western world, of the modern idea of propaganda, with a function not only promotional but also aimed at controlling the masses through events, public relations, and mass media (Bernays, 1928). The author of this documentary, however, represents the various souls of psychoanalysis in a partial way, connecting it in one way to the relationship between Sigmund, his daughter Anna, and his grandson, thus reducing psychoanalysis itself to the version propagandized and used by Edward.

References

Abraham, K. (1955). Review of C.G. Jung "Attempt at a reresentation of psycho-analytic theory". In *Clinical paper and essays on psycho-analysis* (pp. 101–115). Brunner/Mazel. (Original work published 1914)

Adler, A. (2002). The neurotic character. In *The collected clinical works of Alfred Adler* (Vol. 1) Alfred Adler Institute. (Original work published 1912).

Adler, A. (2003a). Health manual for the tayloring trade. In *The collected clinical works of Alfred Adler* (Vol. 2, pp. 1–14). Alfred Adler Institute. (Original work published 1898)

Adler, A. (2003b). The penetration of social drives into medicine. In *The collected clinical works of Alfred Adler* (Vol. 2, pp. 15–18). Alfred Adler Institute. (Original work published 1902)

Adler, A. (2003c). City and country. In *The collected clinical works of Alfred Adler* (Vol. 2, pp. 22–27). Alfred Adler Institute. (Original work published 1903)

Adler, A. (2003d). State aid and self-help. In *The collected clinical works of Alfred Adler* (Vol. 2, pp. 28–31). Alfred Adler Institute. (Original work published 1903)

Adler, A. (2003e). The physician as educator. In *The collected clinical works of Alfred Adler* (Vol. 2, pp. 32–38). Alfred Adler Institute. (Original work published 1904)

Adler, A. (2003f). A study of organ inferiority and its physical compensation. In *The collected clinical works of Alfred Adler* (Vol. 2, pp. 15–18). Alfred Adler Institute. (Original work published 1907)

Adler, A. (2003g). The aggressive drive in life and in the neurosis. In *The collected clinical works of Alfred Adler* (Vol. 2, pp. 15–18). Alfred Adler Institute. (Original work published 1908)

Adler, A. (2003h). Psychological hermaphroditism in life and in the neurosis. In *The collected clinical works of Alfred Adler* (Vol. 3, pp. 1–8). Alfred Adler Institute. (Original work published. 1910)

Adler, A. (2003i). A declaration (Adler breaks with Freud). In *The collected clinical works of Alfred Adler* (Vol. 3, p. 74). Alfred Adler Institute. (Original work published 1911)

Adler, A. (2003j). Additional guiding principles for the practice of individual psychology. In *The collected clinical works of Alfred Adler* (Vol. 3, pp. 134–140). Alfred Adler Institute. (Original work published 1913)

Adler, A. (2003k). Individual psychological treatment of neuroses. In *The collected clinical works of Alfred Adler* (Vol. 3, pp. 115–129). Alfred Adler Institute. (Original work published 1913)

Adler, A. (2003l). On the role of the unconscious in neurosis. In *The collected clinical works of Alfred Adler* (Vol. 3, pp. 170–176). Alfred Adler Institute. (Original work published 1913)

Adler, A. (2003m). Dreams and dream interpretation. In *The collected clinical works of Alfred Adler* (Vol. 3, pp. 183–194). Alfred Adler Institute. (Original work published 1913)

Adler, A. (2003n). Individual psychology: Its presumptions and results. In *The collected clinical works of Alfred Adler* (Vol. 4, pp. 26–36). Alfred Adler Institute. (Original work published 1914)

Adler, A. (2003o). Child psychology and neurosis research. In *The collected clinical works of Alfred Adler* (Vol. 4, pp. 37–50). Alfred Adler Institute. (Original work published 1914)

Adler, A. (2003p). Individual psychology and upbringing. In *The collected clinical works of Alfred Adler* (Vol. 4, pp. 123–129). Alfred Adler Institute. (Original work published 1918)

Adler, A. (2015). *The education of children.* Routledge. (Original work published 1930)

Alexander, F. G., & Selesnick, S. T. (1966). *The history of psychiatry: An evaluation of psychiatric thought and practice from prehistoric times to the present.* Harper & Row.

Arienzo, A. (2013). *Governance.* Ediesse.

Arkin, A. M., Antrobus, J. S., & Ellman, S. J. (1978). *The mind in sleep: Psychology and psychophysiology.* Lawrence Erlbaum.

Aserinsky, E., & Kleitman, N. (1953). Regularly occurring periods of eye motility, and concomitant phenomena, during sleep. *Science, 118*(3062), 273–274.

Atwood, G. E., & Stolorow, R. D. (1979). *Faces in a cloud: Intersubjectivity in personality theory.* Jason Aronson.

Ayllon, T., & Azrin, N. H. (1968). *The token economy: A motivational system for therapy and rehabilitation.* Appleton-Century-Crofts.

Bernays, E. L. (1928). *Propaganda.* Liveright.

Bottome, P. (1939). *Alfred Adler: Apostle of freedom.* Faber & Faber.

Breuer, J., & Freud, S. (1955). Studies on hysteria. In *The standard edition of the complete psychological works of Sigmund Freud* (Vol. 2, pp. 1–307). Hogarth Press. (Original work published 1895)

Buckley, K. W. (1989). *Mechanical man: John Broadus Watson and the beginnings of behaviorism.* Guilford Press.

Burgess, A. (1962). *A clockwork orange.* Heinemann.

Chemouni, J. (2004). *Trotsky et la psychanalyse* [Trotsky and psychoanalysis]. In Press.

Cicciola, E. (2018). Scienza e Massoneria: Storia e storiografia [Science and freemasonry: History and historiography]. *Physis, 53*(1–2), 221–249.

Clifford, G. J. (1968). *Edward L. Thorndike: The sane positivist.* Wesleyan.

Cohen, E. D. (1974). *C. G. Jung and the scientific attitude.* Philosophical Library.

Dahl, H., Kächele, H., & Thomä, H. (Eds.). (1988). *Psychoanalytic process research strategies.* Springer.

De Sanctis, S. (1899). *I sogni. Studi clinici e psicologici di un alienista I sogni. Studi clinici e psicologici di un alienista* [Dreams. Clinical and Psychological Studies of an Alienist]. Bocca.

Digdon, N. (2020). The Little Albert controversy: Intuition, confirmation bias, and logic. *History of Psychology, 23*(2), 122–131.

Ellenberger, H. F. (1970). *The discovery of the unconscious: The history and evolution of dynamic psychiatry*. Basic Books.

Ferenczi, S. (1990). A proposito di "Contributo allo studio dei tipi psicologici" di C. G. Jung [Review of C. G. Jung, "A contribution to the study of psychological types"]. In *Opere* (Vol. 2, pp. 146–147). Raffaello Cortina. (Original work published 1914).

Ferenczi, S. (1994). The psychological analysis of dreams. In *First contributions to psycho-analysis* (pp. 94–131). Karnac. (Original work published 1909)

Ferenczi, S. (2005). Criticisms and review of C. G. Jung, transformations and symbols of the libido. *Psychoanalysis and History*, 7(1), 63–79. (Original work published 1913)

Fichtner, G. E., & Pomerans, A. J. (2003). *The Sigmund Freud-Ludwig Binswanger correspondence: 1908–1938*. Other Press.

Foucault, M. (2015). *Nascita della biopolitica. Corso al Collège de France (1978–1979)* [Birth of biopolitics. Course at the Collège de France (1978–1979)]. Feltrinelli. (Original work published 1978–1979)

Freud, S. (1953a). The interpretation of dreams. In *The standard edition of the complete psychological works of Sigmund Freud* (vols. 3–4). Hogarth. (Original work published 1900)

Freud, S. (1953b). Fragment of an analysis of a case of hysteria. In *The standard edition of the complete psychological works of Sigmund Freud* (Vol. 7, pp. 3–122). Hogarth. (Original work published 1905 [1901])

Freud, S. (1953c). Three essays on sexuality. In *The standard edition of the complete psychological works of Sigmund Freud* (Vol. 7, pp. 125–143). Hogarth. (Original work published 1905)

Freud, S. (1955). Beyond the pleasure principle. In *The standard edition of the complete psychological works of Sigmund Freud* (Vol. 18, pp. 7–61). Hogarth. (Original work published 1920)

Freud, S. (1957a). The future prospects of psycho-analytic therapy. In *The standard edition of the complete psychological works of Sigmund Freud* (Vol. 11, pp. 139–151). Hogarth. (Original work published 1910)

Freud, S. (1957b). 'Wild' psycho-analysis. In *The standard edition of the complete psychological works of Sigmund Freud* (Vol. 11, pp. 219–227). Hogarth. (Original work published 1910)

Freud, S. (1957c). On the history of the psycho-analytic movement. In *The standard edition of the complete psychological works of Sigmund Freud* (Vol. 14, pp. 7–66). Hogarth. (Original work published 1914)

Freud, S. (1957d). Instincts and their vicissitudes. In *The standard edition of the complete psychological works of Sigmund Freud* (Vol. 11, pp. 109–140). Hogarth. (Original work published 1915)

Freud, S. (1958a). Formulations on the two principles of mental functioning. In *The standard edition of the complete psychological works of Sigmund Freud* (Vol. 12, pp. 213–226). Hogarth. (Original work published 1911)

Freud, S. (1958b). Recommendations to physicians practising psycho-analysis. In *The standard edition of the complete psychological works of Sigmund Freud* (Vol. 12, pp. 109–120). Hogarth. (Original work published 1912)

Freud, S. (1958c). The dynamics of transference. In *The standard edition of the complete psychological works of Sigmund Freud* (Vol. 12, pp. 97–108). Hogarth. (Original work published 1912)

Freud, S. (1958d). On beginning the treatment. In *The standard edition of the complete psychological works of Sigmund Freud* (Vol. 12, pp. 121–144). Hogarth. (Original work published 1913)

Freud, S. (1958e). Remembering, repeating and working-through. In *The standard edition of the complete psychological works of Sigmund Freud* (Vol. 12, pp. 123–144). Hogarth. (Original work published 1913)

Freud, S. (1958f). On beginning the treatment (technique of psycho-analysis, I). In *The standard edition of the complete psychological works of Sigmund Freud* (Vol. 12, pp. 157–171). Hogarth. (Original work published 1915)

Freud, S. (1959). Some general remarks on hysterical attacks. In *The standard edition of the complete psychological works of Sigmund Freud* (Vol. 9, pp. 227–234). Hogarth. (Original work published 1908)

Freud, S. (1960a). The psychopathology of everyday life. In *The standard edition of the complete psychological works of Sigmund Freud* (Vol. 6). Hogarth. (Original work published 1901)

Freud, S. (1960b). Jokes and their relations to the unconscious. In *The standard edition of the complete psychological works of Sigmund Freud* (Vol. 8). Hogarth. (Original work published 1905)

Freud, S. (1964a). Analysis terminable and interminable. In *The standard edition of the complete psychological works of Sigmund Freud Freud* (Vol. 23, pp. 216–253). Hogarth. (Original work published 1937)

Freud, S. (1966). Project for a scientific psychology. In *The standard edition of the complete psychological works of Sigmund Freud* (Vol. 12, pp. 281–397). Hogarth Press. (Original work written 1895)

Freud, S. (1987). Einleitungspassagen zu› Über einige Übereinstimmungen im Seelenleben der Wilden und der Neurotiker [Introductory passages to' On some similarities in the soul life of savages and neurotics.]. In *Gesammelte Werke: Texte aus den Jahren 1885 bis 1938* [Complete Works – Texts 1885–1938) (pp. 740–742). (Original work published 1912).

Glover, E. (1950). *Freud or Jung*. W. W. Norton.

Greenberg, J. R., & Mitchell, S. A. (1983). *Object relations in psychoanalytic theory*. Harvard University Press.

Harris, B. (1979). Whatever happened to little Albert? *American Psychologist, 34*, 151–160.

Harris, B. (2011). Letting go of Little Albert: Disciplinary memory, history, and the uses of myth. *Journal of the History of the Behavioral Sciences, 47*(1), 1–17.

Harris, B. (2020). Journals, referees, and gatekeepers in the dispute over Little Albert, 2009–2014. *History of Psychology, 23*(2), 103–121.

Haynal, E. (Ed.). (1992) *The correspondence of Sigmund Freud and Sándor Ferenczi Volume 1, 1908–1914*. Harvard University Press.

Innamorati, M. (1995). *La relazione analitica: Oltre la terapia* [The analytical relationship: Beyond therapy]. In L. Aversa (a cura di), *Psicologia analitica* [Analytical psychology] (pp. 285–312). Laterza.

Innamorati, M. (2013). *Jung*. Carocci.

Jaffé, A. (Ed.). (1989) *Memories, dreams, reflections by CG Jung*. Vintage Books. (Original work issued 1961)

Janet, P. (2004). *La psychanalyse de Freud* [Freud's psychoanalysis]. L'Harmattan. (Original edition published 1913)

Jones, E. (1953–1957). *The life and work of Sigmund Freud* (3 vols). Hogarth.

Jung, C. G. (1920a). The psychology of dreams. In *Collected papers on analytical psychology* (pp. 299–311). Baillière, Tindall & Cox. (Original work published 1914)

Jung, C. G. (1920b). The psychology of unconscious processes. In *Collected papers on analytical psychology* (pp. 354–444). Baillière, Tindall & Cox. (Original work published 1917)

Jung, C. G. (1953a). The psychology of the unconscious. In *The collected works of C. G. Jung* (Vol. 7, pp. 3–117). Routledge & Kegan Paul. (Original work published 1943)

Jung, C. G. (1953b). The relations between the ego and the unconscious. In *The collected works of C. G. Jung* (Vol. 7, pp. 121–239). Routledge & Kegan Paul. (Original work published 1928)

Jung, C. G. (1953c). The structure of the unconscious. In *The collected works of C. G. Jung* (Vol. 7, pp. 263–292). Routledge & Kegan Paul. (Original work published 1916)

Jung, C. G. (1953d). Psychology and alchemy. In *The collected works of C. G. Jung* (Vol. 12). Routledge & Kegan Paul. (Original work published 1944)

Jung, C. G. (1957). On the psychology and pathology of so-called occult phenomena. In *The collected works of C. G. Jung* (Vol. 1, pp. 3–88). Routledge & Kegan Paul. (Original work published 1902).

Jung, C. G. (1960a). The psychology of dementia praecox. In *The collected works of C. G. Jung* (Vol. 3, pp. 1–151). Routledge & Kegan Paul. (Original work published 1907)

Jung, C. G. (1960b). The transcendent function. In *The collected works of C. G. Jung* (Vol. 8, pp. 67–91). Routledge & Kegan Paul. (Original work published 1916–1958)

Jung, C. G. (1960c). Instinct and the unconscious. In *The collected works of C. G. Jung* (Vol. 8, pp. 129–138). Routledge & Kegan Paul. (Original work published 1919–1948)

Jung, C. G. (1960d). General aspects of dream psychology. In *The collected works of C. G. Jung* (Vol. 8, pp. 237–280). Routledge & Kegan Paul. (Original work published 1916–1948)

Jung, C. G. (1960e). On the nature of dreams. In *The collected works of C. G. Jung* (Vol. 8, pp. 281–297). Routledge & Kegan Paul. (Original work published 1945–1948)

Jung, C. G. (1961a). Freud's theory of hysteria: A reply to Aschaffenburg. In *The collected works of C. G. Jung* (Vol. 4, pp. 3–9). Routledge & Kegan Paul. (Original work published 1906)

Jung, C. G. (1961b). The analysis of dreams. In *The collected works of C. G. Jung* (Vol. 4, pp. 25–34). Routledge & Kegan Paul. (Original work published 1909)

Jung, C. G. (1966a). Principles of practical psychotherapy. In *The collected works of C. G. Jung* (Vol. 16, pp. 3–20). Routledge & Kegan Paul. (Original work published 1935)

Jung, C. G. (1966b). What is psychotherapy? In *The collected works of C. G. Jung* (Vol. 16, pp. pp. 21–28). Routledge & Kegan Paul. (Original work published 1935)

Jung, C. G. (1966c). Some aspects of modern psychotherapy. In *The collected works of C. G. Jung* (Vol. 16, pp. 29–35). Routledge & Kegan Paul. (Original work published 1930)

Jung, C. G. (1966d). Problems of modern psychotherapy. In *The collected works of C. G. Jung* (Vol. 16, pp. 53–75). Routledge & Kegan Paul. (Original work published 1929)

Jung, C. G. (1966e). Medicine and psychotherapy. In *The collected works of C. G. Jung* (Vol. 16, pp. 84–93). Routledge & Kegan Paul. (Original work published 1945)

Jung, C. G. (1966f). The psychology of the transference. In *The collected works of C. G. Jung* (Vol. 16, pp. 163–323). Routledge & Kegan Paul. (Original work published 1946)

Jung, C. G. (1971a). Psychological types. In *The collected works of C. G. Jung* (Vol. 6, pp. 1–495). Routledge & Kegan Paul. (Original work published 1921)

Jung, C. G. (1971b). A contribution to the study of psychological types. In *The collected works of C. G. Jung* (Vol. 6, pp. 499–509). Routledge & Kegan Paul. (Original work published 1913)

Jung, C. G. (1971c). Psychological typology. In *The collected works of C. G. Jung* (Vol. 6, pp. 542–555). Routledge & Kegan Paul. (Original work published 1936)

Jung, C. G. (1973a). Psychoanalysis and the association experiment. In *The collected works of C. G. Jung* (Vol. 2, pp. 88–317). Routledge & Kegan Paul. (Original work published 1906)

Jung, C. G. (1973b). The association method. In *The collected works of C. G. Jung* (Vol. 2, pp. 439–465). Routledge & Kegan Paul. (Original work published 1910)

Jung, C. G. (1977a). Symbols and the interpretations of dreams. In *The collected works of C. G. Jung* (Vol. 18, pp. 185–264). Routledge & Kegan Paul. (Original work published 1961)

Jung, C. G. (1977b). Adaptation, individuation, collectivity. In *The collected works of C. G. Jung* (Vol. 18, pp. 449–454). Routledge & Kegan Paul. (Original work written 1916)

Jung, C. G. (1983). *The Zofingia lectures*. Routledge & Kegan Paul.

Jung, C. G. (1984). *Dream analysis: Notes of the seminar given in 1928–30*. Routledge & Kegan Paul.

Jung, C. G. (2009). *The red book. Liber novus*. W. W. Norton.

Jung, C. G. (2012a). *Jung contra Freud: The 1912 New York lectures on the theory of psychoanalysis*. Princeton University Press.

Jung, C. G. (2012b). *Children's dreams: Notes on the seminar given in 1936–1941*. Princeton University Press.

Jung, C. G. (2019). *Psychology of the unconscious: A study of the transformations and symbolisms of the Libido* [Transformations and symbols of the libido]. Routledge. (Original work published 1912)

Jung, C. G. (2020). *The black books*. W. W. Norton.

Jung, C. G., & Riklin, F. (1973). The associations of normal subjects. In *The collected works of C. G. Jung* (Vol. 2, pp. 3–196). Routledge & Kegan Paul. (Original work published 1904).

Lombardo, G. P., & Foschi, R. (2002a). The European origins of 'personality psychology'. *European Psychologist, 7*(2), 134–145.

Lombardo, G. P., & Foschi, R. (2002b). *La costruzione scientifica della personalità* [The scientific construction of personality]. Bollati Boringhieri.

Lombardo, G. P., & Foschi, R. (2008). Escape from the dark forest: The experimentalist standpoint of Sante De Sanctis' psychology of dreams. *History of the Human Sciences, 21*(3), 45–69.

Mahony, P. (1996). *Freud's Dora: A psychoanalytic, historical, and textual study*. Yale University Press.

Masson, J. M. (1985). *The complete letters of Sigmund Freud to Wilhelm Fliess 1887–1904*. Belknap Press.

McGuire, W. (Ed.). (1974) *The Freud/Jung letters*. Princeton University Press.

Meghnagi, D. (1992). *Il padre e la legge: Freud e l'ebraismo* [The father and the law: Freud and Judaism]. Marsilio.

Miller, P., & Rose, N. (2008). *Governing the present: Administering economic, social and personal life*. Polity Press.

Millon, T. (2004). *Masters of the mind: Exploring the story of mental illness from ancient times to the new millennium*. Wiley.

Mills, J. A. (1998). *Control: A history of behavioral psychology*. New York University Press.

Nunberg, H., & Federn, E. (Eds.). (1962). *Minutes of the Vienna psychoanalytic society, Vol. 1. 1906–1908*. International Universities Press.

Parenti, F. (1987). *Alfred Adler*. Laterza.

Paskauskas, A. (Ed.). (1993). *The complete correspondence of Sigmund Freud and Ernest Jones*. Harvard University Press.

Pavlov, I. P. (1927). *Conditioned reflexes. An investigation of the physiological activity of the cerebral cortex*. Oxford University Press.

Powell, R. A., Digdon, N., Harris, B., & Smithson, C. (2014). Correcting the record on Watson, Rayner, and Little Albert: Albert Barger as "Psychology's lost boy". *American Psychologist, 69*(6), 600–611.

Rutherford, A. (2006). Mother of behavior therapy and beyond: Mary Cover Jones and the study of the "Whole Child". In D. A. Dewsbury, L. T. Benjamin, & M. Wertheimer (Eds.), *Portraits of pioneers in psychology* (pp. 189–204). American Psychological Association; Lawrence Erlbaum Associates Publishers.

Rutherford, A. (2009). *Beyond the box: BF Skinner's technology of behavior from laboratory to life, 1950s–1970s*. University of Toronto Press.

Samuels, A. (1985). *Jung and the post-Jungians*. Routledge.

Shamdasani, S. (2003). *Jung and the making of modern psychology: The dream of a science*. Cambridge University Press.

Shamdasani, S. (2009). Introduzione [Introduction]. In C. G. Jung (Ed.), *Il libro rosso* [The red book] (pp. 193–221). Bollati Boringhieri.

Skinner, B. F. (1938). *The behavior of organisms: An experimental analysis*. Appleton-Century.

Skinner, B. F. (1948). *Walden two*. Macmillan.

Skinner, B. F. (1956). What is psychotic behavior? In F. Gildea (Ed.), *Theory and treatment of the psychoses: Some newer aspects* (pp. 77–99). Washington University Press.

Smith, L. D., & Woodward, W. R. (1996). *B. F. Skinner and behaviorism in American culture*. Lehigh University Press.

Storr, A. (1973). *Jung*. Routledge.

Thorndike, E. L. (1898). *The animal intelligence: An experimental study of the associative processes in animals*. Macmillan.

Trotsky, L. (1962). Culture and socialism. *Labour Review*, 7(3), 101–113. (Original work published 1927)

Vaihinger, H. (2021). *The philosophy of 'as if'*. Routledge. (Original work published 1911)

Watson, J. B. (1913). Psychology as the behaviorist views it. *Psychological Review, 20*, 158–177.

Watson, J. B., & Rayner, R. (1920). Conditioned emotional reactions. *Journal of Experimental Psychology, 3*, 1–14.

4

Depth psychology between the World Wars

World War I

The year 1914 found Freud, Jung, and Adler seeking to strengthen their identity. Freud was in the strongest and most visible position: Freudian doctrine had already begun to spread in many countries. In Hungary, Ferenczi had obtained the first university chair specifically for psychoanalysis. Nevertheless, Freud felt the need to publish a paper in which he claimed his role as the sole creator of psychoanalysis, accusing Jung and Adler of compromising its purity by abandoning the libido theory (Freud, 1914/1957a). At the same time, Freud was attempting to resolve the most significant difficulty that libido theory had encountered, that of explaining the origin of psychosis. Jung, in fact, had repeatedly stressed the impossibility of linking the symptoms of psychosis, and of schizophrenia in particular, to sexual themes (Jung, 1907/1960, 1912/2019). In *On Narcissism: An Introduction* (Freud, 1914/1957b), an integration of the theory of psychosexual development was proposed to overcome this difficulty. The human beings would go through an initial phase of existence in which they would invest all their libido in themselves (primary narcissism): it would have been a phase of autoeroticism. The individual would feel a sense of omnipotence, which would have been overcome when the first object investments began. Part of the libido was then invested in objects, that is, in significant others. In psychosis there would be a withdrawal of libido from object investments, to return to a condition similar to the initial one (and for this reason called secondary narcissism). However, this was a theoretical adjustment that did not change Freud's assessment of the treatment of psychosis, which in his eyes remained impossible through psychoanalysis, because a transference would have been impossible when people had completely invested libido in themselves.

Surprisingly, Freud went through a (brief) period of near euphoria at the outbreak of World War I, marked by the conviction that Austria-Hungary would quickly emerge victorious from the conflict. The subsequent disillusionment led to a radical rethinking of the meaning of existence and human nature, which was already evident in Freud's *Thoughts for the Time on War and Death* (Freud, 1915/1957d) and *On Transience* (Freud, 1915/1957e), and which

DOI: 10.4324/9781003252405-4

would lead to a profound revision of the theory a few years later. Important writings of theoretical systematization, namely *Papers on Metapsychology* (Freud, 1915/1957c) and *Introductory Lectures on Psychoanalysis* (Freud, 1915–1916/1961k, 1917/1963), belong to the war years.

After leaving the psychoanalytic movement, Jung went through a period of relative isolation, which was also sanctioned by his abandonment of the Zurich psychiatric hospital. The war years corresponded with the distillation of analytical psychology as an autonomous discipline with respect to psychoanalysis: some of Jung's decisive writings were written during this period. Although a citizen of neutral Switzerland, Jung abandoned his private clinical practice several times in order to run an internment camp at Château d'Oex between 1917 and 1919, with the rank of medical captain.

Adler, who had left the Freudian group before Jung, was engaged in organizing his own movement at the outbreak of the conflict, certainly in a more informal way than the now hierarchical Psychoanalytic Society. Such a circumstance also reflected more progressive political convictions than Freud's. It seems that the Adlerian group used to meet in Viennese cafés rather than in institutional venues, which did not fail to attract criticism from medical circles (Ellenberger, 1970). Having applied for a professorship at the University of Vienna as early as 1912, Adler received a (negative) response only after the war broke out in 1915. The doors of the academy remained closed to him, nor would they open before he emigrated to the United States, several years later. Like Jung, Adler was employed as a military doctor, from 1916. He initially worked close to the front, in the neuropsychiatric department of the military hospital in Semmering (where Stekel was later sent), until he was transferred to Krakow and finally to Grinzing.

The war, experienced more directly by Adler and Jung but not less intensely by Freud (whose sons Ernst and Martin took part in the conflict), certainly exerted a fundamental influence on the ideas of the three main protagonists of depth psychology. Not only, moreover, could the nature of human conduct be interpreted differently, in a general sense, after having ascertained its destructive capacity. Specifically, the war neuroses, determined by the extreme experiences on the battlefield, constituted an unprecedented form of psychopathology, involving a very significant number of soldiers. In fact, the last conflict had introduced strong elements of discontinuity compared to the previous ones, both in terms of the weapons used (more effective artillery, heavy machine guns, chemical aggression, aircraft) and from the point of view of the soldiers' condition (life in the trenches and the need for constant vigilance due to the threat posed by snipers). The consequences of all this will be examined in the following paragraphs.

In the meantime, a young psychiatrist on the Russian front observed the consequences of the war on the soldiers' minds: Aleksandr R. Lurija (1902–1977). Lurija was one of the first to introduce psychoanalysis in the Soviet Union, but he soon had to abandon it because of the regime's highly critical attitude toward the new discipline. This forced choice, however, had a paradoxically positive outcome: Lurija was to become the founder of modern neuropsychology.

The death drive

Interest in psychoanalytic theory within the German and Austro-Hungarian bloc was revived at the beginning of 1918 by the publication of a book on the treatment of war neuroses by Ernst Simmel (1882–1947), who was not part of the Freudian movement. Simmel illustrated positive therapeutic results obtained through the use of the cathartic method. The topicality of the subject and Simmel's success stimulated the convening of a psychoanalytic congress in Budapest the same year, specifically devoted to war neuroses. The congress, of course, was not attended by analysts from the other side of the front. Both Ferenczi and Abraham, two of Freud's closest collaborators, presented papers in which they tried to demonstrate that war neurosis was a phenomenon perfectly compatible with psychoanalytic theory. Ferenczi believed that war neuroses were typically assimilated to conversion hysterias and anxiety hysterias triggered by trauma. In particular, it seemed clear to Ferenczi that the shock had easily provoked neurotic regression: a return to a stage of development long since passed. Abraham, for his part, endeavored to show that war neuroses are not understandable if sexuality is not taken into account. By the time the papers presented at the congress were brought together for publication in a book, the war was over and Jones was also able to add his own point of view, which raised some doubts about the relationship between sexuality and war neurosis. Freud, for the time being, dismissed these doubts as follows: "If the investigation of the war neuroses (and a very superficial one at that) has *not shown* that the sexual theory of the neuroses is *correct*, that is something very different from its *showing* that that theory is *incorrect*" (Freud, 1920/1955d, p. 208; emphasis in the original; all other papers cited here in: Ferenczi et al., 1921).

The caution was, however, provisional. A shocking observation had caught Freud's attention in his *Thoughts for the Time on War and Death*: "Indeed, our unconscious will murder even for trifles" (Freud, 1915/1957d, p. 297): in dreams and fantasies the human being shows a death wish for anyone who causes even the slightest offence. The massacres of 1914–1918 induced in Freud the decisive doubt: how was it possible that millions of people went to war, certain that they would kill other human beings or be killed by them, just because they had been ordered to do so? It was more likely that their unconscious drove them to the front with even greater force. Finally came the painful theoretical breakthrough represented by *Beyond the Pleasure Principle* (Freud, 1920/1955f), which consisted in the theorization of the *death drive* alongside the sexual drive as a basic motivating factor of psychical life.

It was precisely the war neurosis that offered one of the starting points for the reflections contained in Freud's essay, and in particular the apparently inexplicable alteration of the dream life of the soldier traumatized by the fighting, which seemed to bring him back continually to the situation of the trauma. In other words, the war neurosis showed a patient "fixated to his trauma" (p. 13). But war neurosis was not the only situation in which human beings tended to repeat previous experiences, in a way that seemed entirely independent of the search for pleasure. Children could repeat games inspired by deeply distressing experiences: the famous wooden reel game by one of Freud's nephews was a striking example. The child accompanied the throwing of a spool of thread across his bed (out of his field of vision) with an enthusiastic "fort!" ("go!"), the spool was then withdrawn with the exclamation "da!" ("there!"). The meaning of the game was related "to the child's great cultural achievement – the instinctual renunciation (that is, the renunciation of instinctual satisfaction) which he had made in allowing his mother to go away without protesting." The child, then, "compensated himself for this, as it were, by himself staging the disappearance and return of the objects within his reach" (p. 15). The child performed the first part of the game independently of the second. The possible interpretation that the disappearance was only the necessary premise for the symbolic pleasure induced by the reappearance of the mother reel evidently was not possible. Moreover, Freud observed, if on the one hand the child passively suffered the mother's absence, "he took an active part" in the game (p. 16). The most logical explanation, from Freud's point of view, was based on the hypothesis of a revenge impulse toward the object, evidently repressed in real life. The mother had left and the child had taken revenge (by displacement). This hypothesis was corroborated by Freud's further observation of the same child who, a year later, vented his anger on a toy by throwing it and saying "Go to the *fwont!*" (when his father was actually "at the front"). It should be remembered, on the one hand, that Freud had already observed that children could throw and break objects in order to give vent to an impulse concerning people (Freud, 1918/1955c); and, on the other hand, that the father of the child in question was away from home, in the war, and the child did not seem to miss him at all.

A further doubt Freud felt about the hegemony of the pleasure principle concerned the circumstance of how tragedy and other forms of art could provoke the highest enjoyment while being accompanied by painful impressions. Freud had already observed how widespread was the insuppressible tendency to repeat past experiences in the present and called it *repetition-compulsion* (Freud, 1914/1958a, 1915/1958b). In the transference, in particular, the patients repeated, within the relationship with the analyst, experiences already lived in the relationship with the significant figures of their past life, largely unpleasant experiences. Expectations of exclusive love from the parent of the opposite sex were frustrated; infantile sexuality had to be repressed; education suppressed drives. Too many phenomena, then, seemed to Freud to remain unexplained unless he postulated that compulsion to repeat "overrides the pleasure principle" (Freud, 1920/1955f, p. 22). Freud therefore believed that it was possible to suppose the existence of drives of organic origin, but acquired in the course of phylogeny. They tended toward regression, in the attempt to restore a previous state. Freud called them *death drives*. A second class of drives would have operated against the death drives (among which the sexual drives were to be counted), which would have driven organisms to survival and would therefore have been defined overall as *life drives*. The possible (reversible) mixing of drives could explain the aggressive component of the libido (present even when sadism does not turn into a real perversion) (Freud, 1922/1955h). The existence of the death drive, moreover, seemed to throw a new light on the fact that "the dominating tendency of mental life" is "the effort to reduce, to keep constant or to remove internal tension due to stimuli" (Freud, 1920/1955f, p. 4). The principle of constance could in this sense legitimately be renamed the nirvana principle (Freud, 1920/1955f).

Ego, id, and superego: the structural model of Freud

Already in *Beyond the Pleasure Principle*, Freud had changed his conception of the ego, which he no longer considered to be identified with the conscious or even with the conscious/preconscious system. The rethinking was linked to a reflection on resistance: it could not be the "repressed" that offered resistance to interpretation, since its drive was rather to emerge. The resistance therefore had to come from the patient's ego. Therefore, only the hypothesis of an unconscious part of the ego made it possible to explain the phenomenon (Freud, 1920/1955f).

In *Group Psychology and the Analysis of the Ego*, the idea of a psychic instance, the ego ideal, liable to differentiate itself from the rest of the ego and come into conflict with it, was also assumed (or revived):

> (The ego ideal was) the heir to the original narcissism in which the childish ego enjoyed self-sufficiency; it gradually gathers up from the influences of the environment, the demands which that environment makes upon the ego and which the ego cannot always rise to; so that a man, when he cannot be satisfied with his ego itself, may nevertheless be able to find satisfaction in the ego ideal which has been differentiated out of the ego.
>
> (Freud, 1921/1955g, p. 110)

In the meantime, Freud had made it increasingly clear that the unconscious could not be identified solely as the site of the repressed (even apart from the unconscious part of the ego and the ego ideal). Evidently, the time was ripe for a profound revision of the theory of mind, which indeed came, with *The Ego and the Id* and a series of fundamental writings in the years immediately following, such as *Neurosis and Psychosis* and *Inhibitions, Symptoms and Anxiety*.

From *The Ego and the Id*, Freud developed the *structural model* or *second topic*. At the heart of the new model was the tripartition of the psyche into ego, id, and superego (a term that came to sit alongside and eventually replaced the term ego ideal in Freud's language). Two attributes seemed to be character-istic of the ego in Freud's new theory: organization and control. On the one hand, the ego was entrusted with the task of self-observation and the control of perception and movement. On the other hand, it would depend on the ego itself whether a representation or a tendency was allowed to cross the thresh-old of consciousness. This implied that oneiric censorship and repression were the responsibility of the ego. Elaborating further on this conclusion, Freud attributed to the ego all the *defenses* or *defense mechanisms*, that is, the strategies used to manage drives (Freud, 1925/1959a). In this perspective, he recovered a concept, that of defense, first conceived in 1894 and subsequently aban-doned in the conviction that all defenses were tied to repression. In fact, Freud reflected, the thesis was tenable only in certain cases. The use of *isolation* meant that only the memory of the affect was lost from a traumatic event and not the memory of the historical circumstances. In the case of *undoing*, on the other hand, nothing would be forgotten about a first act, but a second act would be performed (ritualistic, corresponding to the archaic conviction of being able to work magic) in order to "blow away" the first, so as to render it in the eyes of the subject as not occurring. Both of these mechanisms, incidentally, had long been described by Freud (1909/1955a).

Defenses were, according to Freud, triggered by a signal of anxiety, emit-ted by the ego when faced with unpleasant situations (Freud, 1925/1959a). In childhood traumatic episodes, there was a feeling of helplessness. In later life, anxiety would arise in two ways: when actual dangerous situations occurred or when a threat seemed to be looming. The ego would then generate anxiety precisely in order to avoid the feared unpleasant situation. Freud also empha-sized that, on the one hand, there was a link between neurosis and anxiety and, on the other, that anxiety reactions were not always to be considered neurotic. From this point of view, the distinction between *realistic anxiety* and *neurotic anxiety* was born: the first would have originated from a real danger (p. 162ff), to which one would have reacted in a natural way both on an affective level (precisely with anxiety) and on a motor level (with protective action). Faced with the drive danger, anxiety would have been the *signal* to start an action to avoid it. It could happen, however, that confronted with a real danger, an exag-gerated and therefore neurotic reaction was produced: the known real danger had to be linked to an unknown drive danger.

However, according to Freud, the main characteristic of neurotic anxiety was the expectation of the possible repetition of a traumatic situation and the related feeling of helplessness: this would lead to an anticipation of the possi-ble trauma and to avoidance behavior. In short, in Freud's conception the ego would elaborate a "fantasy of the traumatic situation" (Brenner, 1955, p. 76) and would react to this fantasy with *signal anxiety*.

The superego, like the ego, was described as partly conscious and partly unconscious. In the context of the new model, Freud stated that "the differenti-ation of the superego from the ego is no matter of chance" (Freud, 1923/1961a,

p. 25): the process leading to the formation of the superego was thus no longer described as a (possible) split but as a (necessary) differentiation. The superego would be formed from the ego through identification with the parents. The child would form an ideal on the model of its parents to which it would want to conform. As Roy Schafer summarizes:

> In practice and in fantasy the boy begins to become his own parent; in this development he uses his representations of his parents as his models (merging his self-representations and the representation of his parents).
>
> (Schafer, 1968, p. 196)

The child would then begin to perceive the presence of norms above him, with which he would have to comply: these norms were those imposed from outside (i.e., by the parents) and began to come from within (from the mind). Moral consciousness was described as conscious and would be expressed through a *categorical imperative* (an expression taken from Kant, 1785/2002) to which the ego had to conform (Freud, 1923/1961a, p. 48): if one did not act in accordance with the categorical imperative, the resulting guilt would be perfectly conscious and would not need analytical interpretation to be ascertained and explained. But guilt could also be unconscious: its presence would be inferred from a phenomenon typical of analysis, the *negative therapeutic reaction*. With this expression Freud identified those situations characterized by a worsening of symptoms that followed a progress in the analysis of certain neurotics: "There is no doubt that there is something in these people that sets itself against their recovery, and its approach is dreaded as though it were a danger" (p. 49).

If the superego was formed from the ego, the latter in turn developed and differentiated from the entirely drive-oriented and unconscious part of the personality, which at the beginning of the human being's life would constitute the totality of the psyche. Freud called Es (id) the third psychic instance (first in order of formation), using the suggestion of the writer Georg Groddeck (1866–1934), who in turn had been inspired by Nietzsche (Groddeck, 1923/2015, 1977). "Es" corresponds to the third-person neuter personal pronoun in the German language: its use in this sense suggested the principle that "our ego behaves essentially passively in life (...) we are 'lived' by unknown and uncontrollable forces" (Freud, 1923/1961a, p. 23). The Es/id would also be the reservoir of psychical energy. In summary:

> The id is the part of psychical life furthest removed from consciousness, from rational logic, from a sense of reality, from the rules of civilized life. The id is in fact the matrix of the mind: it is the deepest part of the unconscious, the "primary" set of instinctual energies in their magmatic and prestructured aspects, and of the most archaic, contradictory, unrealistic and primitive fantasies and desires.
>
> (Jervis & Bartolomei, 1996, p. 63)

The perceptual system is said to have influenced the formation of the ego both as a source of information about the external world and as a carrier of bodily and proprioceptive sensations.

The resolution of Oedipus' complex

The process of identification with the parents that generated the superego was not described as linear, because of both the "triangular character of the Oedipus situation" and the "constitutional bisexuality of each individual" (Freud, 1923/1961a, p. 31) of the human being. The male child developed above all love (*object cathexis*) for the mother and identification with the father. When the child began to realize that his desire for his mother was hindered by the presence of his father, the Oedipal complex arose: the identification was tinged with hostility and the behavior toward the father took on the character of ambivalence. Ambivalence toward the father and affection toward the mother would thus be the content of the Oedipal complex in its simplest (positive) form. When the Oedipal complex waned, opening the *latency period*, the investment in the mother could be replaced by an identification with the mother herself or by strengthening the identification with the father. The latter possibility would have been the most common, making it possible both to partially preserve the positive affection for the mother and to consolidate the boy's masculinity. In *The Ego and the Id*, Freud declared himself convinced that the story of the girl was a mirror image: there would be the twilight of the Oedipus and identification with the mother which would reinforce the feminine character or identification with the father, the lost object, which would amplify the masculine tendencies.

If human bisexuality was already the basis of a possible crossroads in character determination from a simple Oedipal complex, it was even more influential in the case Freud considered most frequent (especially for neurotics): that of the complete positive and negative Oedipal complex. In this case the male child, in addition to expressing ambivalence toward the father and affection toward the mother, behaved like a girl, revealing a feminine tenderness toward the father and his corresponding jealous-hostile attitude toward the mother. From this perspective, every human being would therefore have manifested object identification and choice, affection and ambivalence toward both parents. The formation of the superego would then be the result of this complicated interweaving of relational tendencies. Later, Freud began to place more and more emphasis on the likelihood that a fundamental role in the Oedipal affair would be played by the castration complex, the nature of which would necessarily assume different traits for the two sexes:

> At the height of the course of development of infantile sexuality, interest in the genitals and in their activity acquires a dominating significance which falls little short of that reached in maturity. At the same time, the main characteristic of this "infantile genital organization" is its *difference* from

the final general organization of the adult. This consists in the fact that, for both sexes, only one genital, namely the male one, comes into account. What is present, therefore, is not a primacy of the genitals, but a primacy of the *phallus*.

(Freud, 1923/1961b, p. 142; emphasis in the original)

Thus, the situation was not to be described as an attitude toward the possession of "genitals," but toward the presence or absence of the male genitals. The question of its perishing, then, would also have taken on different connotations for the two sexes.

Freud drew attention to the fact that the male child was exposed first to the trauma of separation from the mother at birth, then to the trauma of separation from the mother's breast at the end of breast-feeding, then to a series of daily separations from his intestinal contents. The adults' disapproval of the child's own interest in his own genitalia during the phallic phase would have been expressed in an anxiety of castration that he still would not have taken seriously if, in addition to his past traumas, he had not discovered that there were beings (girls) without a phallus. The child's hypothesis must have been that the girls had been castrated and were therefore living testimony that castration was a real danger. On the other hand, the girl, having also been confronted with the male genitals, would have been in a state of lack, although she would probably have hoped to be put in a position to possess a similar genitalia herself in the future. Ultimately, according to Freud, "the girl accepts castration as an accomplished fact, whereas the boy fears the possibility of its occurrence" (Freud, 1924/1961d, p. 178). As the actual anxiety of castration and hence the attendant anxiety disappeared, the reasons for the formation of a strong superego in the girl became, in Freud's eyes, much less pressing. The only plausible threat would be that of losing the love of her parents. Another rethink with respect to *The Ego and the Id* was the conviction that the female Oedipus complex was much simpler, that is, much more characterized by love for the father alone. On these premises was grafted the impression that the Oedipus complex is never abandoned as well as the idea that the desires to possess a penis and to possess a child remain strongly invested in the unconscious, thus helping the female to prepare for her future sexual function. In other words, an unresolved Oedipus and a never fully structured superego would be inevitable features of female identity. In a further paper, Freud assumed that in women the desire for a child replaced the desire for a penis, but he confirmed and even enhanced the difference between male development and its consequences for the formation of the superego and female morality (Freud, 1925/1961g). The idea of a difference between male and female moral consciousness would never leave Freud, who would, if anything, tend to accentuate it (e.g. Freud, 1933/1964a). Even the idea that women were intellectually inferior to men was called a fact in *The Future of an Illusion*, even if it was considered the result of a wrong upbringing, aimed at distancing them from what would interest them most, namely sexuality (Freud,

1927/1961i). Freud was aware of possible criticism from the female side early on and sought refuge in the partially similar ideas of two female analysts, Helene Deutsch (1884–1982) and Karen Horney (1885–1952), about the psychosexual development of women (Freud, 1925/1961g). Both Deutsch and Horney took up critically the Freudian idea that women were characterized by a natural masochism, due to the receptivity and passivity that seemed inherent in female sexuality. Both attributed female masochism to factors that were not innate but educational and cultural. Deutsch, however, remained an orthodox Freudian, while Horney later became a leading exponent of the culturalist movement in psychoanalysis, criticizing Freudian thought for its link to a masculine and ethnocentric perspective.[1]

If in *The Ego and the Id* it might have seemed that there was a direct relationship between parental suppression and the severity of the superego, in *Civilization and Its Discontents* it was made clear that things were in fact different. Actually, Freud argued that the severity of the superego was not correspondent to the severity expected from the father but was as strong as the aggressive feelings against the father (Freud, 1930/1961j). Finally, in the second series of *Introductory Lectures on Psychoanalysis*, Freud proposed that the superego is modeled not so much on the (perceived or real) attitude of the father to the son as on the superego of the father himself (Freud, 1933/1964a).

The introduction of the structural model also changed the general conception of psychopathology. In the light of the structural model, neurosis would be the effect of a conflict between the ego and the id, while psychosis was the analogous outcome of a similar disturbance in the relations between the ego and the external world (Freud, 1924/1961c). Clarifying the formula, with regard to neurosis, Freud stated:

> The transference neuroses originate from the ego's refusing to accept a powerful instinctual impulse in the id or to help it to find a motor outlet (...). The ego defends itself the instinctual impulse by the mechanism of repression. The repressed material struggles against this fate. It creates for itself, along paths over which the ego has no power, a substitutive representation (which forces itself upon the ego by way of a compromise) – the symptom.
>
> (pp. 149–150)

In turn, the ego would undertake a new struggle against the symptom, attempting a new repression. This dialectical framework would determine the neurosis. The ego, in undertaking the repression, would put itself at the service of the demands coming from the superego, which in turn were the result of internalized external influences. It could therefore be said that the ego, in carrying out the defense, had placed itself at the service of the superego and of reality, against the drives' demands.

The ego would normally be influenced by the external world in two ways: through current perceptions and through memory. In psychosis, this influence would be altered in several possible ways. In amnesia, according to Freud, the external world was no longer perceived (or the perception had no effect), while the internal world in its characteristic (mnestic) reproduction of the external world also lost its significance. The resulting state was comparable to a perpetual dreamlike condition, the result of the severe and unbearable frustration of desire by reality. In schizophrenia, there was also a loss of interest in external reality in favor of an internal world that replaced it. In this sense, the delusional formations constituted an unsuccessful "attempt at a cure or a reconstruction" (p. 151).

There was also the possibility that some mental illnesses were the result of conflict between the ego and the superego, as in the case of melancholia. In any case, both neurosis and psychosis would have been the result of a failure in the functioning of the ego, whose efforts are clearly intended to make compatible the demands that come to it from various sides. It should be emphasized that in both neurosis and psychosis the relationship with reality would be altered, although to different degrees:

> Neurosis does not disavow the reality, it only ignores it; psychosis disavows it and tries to replace it. We call behavior "normal" or "healthy," if it combines certain features of both reactions – if it disavows the reality as little as does a neurosis, but if it then exerts itself, as does a psychosis, to effect an alteration of that reality.
>
> (Freud, 1924/1961e, p. 185)

The alternative to the use of defenses against the demands of the id was perversions, "through the acceptance of which (people) spare themselves repressions" (Freud, 1924/1961c, p. 153). The conception of the original perverse-polymorphous condition of the child, outlined in the *Three Essays on the Theory of Sexuality* (Freud, 1905/1953), remained firm.

Reorganization of the psychoanalytic movement

The reorganization of the Freudian movement after World War I was rather slow, so that the first congress that brought together analysts from the nations in conflict between 1914 and 1918 was held in The Hague only in 1920. A mere 62 members of the IPA participated, of which only two were American. The American branch, led by Abraham A. Brill (1874–1948), had even considered disbanding (Fine, 1979): no one could have foreseen the leadership role (theoretical and organizational) that this group was destined to acquire after 20 years and to maintain to this day.

Once they resumed contact with each other, the psychoanalysts began a capillary penetration of the European continent, through the foundation of new national societies (in Switzerland in 1919 and in Italy in 1925), new local groups (Dresden, Leipzig, and Munich in 1921; Kazan in 1923), the first specific clinics (the Psychoanalytic Institute of Berlin in 1920 and that of Vienna in 1922). The foundation of the Berlin Institute was the occasion to institutionalize psychoanalytic training according to standards that would be made universally mandatory from the Bad Homburg Congress of 1926. The delegation of this demanding task was entrusted by Freud to Max Eitingon, a choice that could certainly appear surprising given that several analysts seemed much more qualified than him for such a purpose. However, Eitingon represented, in Freud's eyes, a character of rare fidelity and very little ambition for originality (he never wrote anything, considering superfluous any theoretical proposal that transcended the Freudian dictate). Freud therefore supported Eitingon unconditionally, sending Hanns Sachs (1881–1947) to Berlin to become the Institute's first training analyst (Fine, 1979).

The model of the training organized by Eitingon was tripartite. First of all, there was the obligation of a personal analysis of the future therapist, following a proposal that originally came from Jung, although no one seemed to remember it (so much so that many still believe it was formulated by Nunberg). The duration of the training analysis was originally rather short, but it was destined to increase progressively (from a few months to eventually spanning several years after World War II). Second, the future analyst had to follow theoretical courses which, following Freud's wish, should include not only psychoanalysis but also related fields: "elements from the mental sciences, from psychology, the history of civilization and sociology, as well as from anatomy, biology and the study of evolution." On the contrary, Freud stated that medical education seemed to him "to be an arduous and circuitous way of approaching the profession of analysis" and "a convoluted and heavy way to reach analytical professionalism" (Freud, 1927/1959b, p. 252). Finally, analysts would have to begin their practice under specific supervision by a more experienced colleague. Which analysts could take on the task of analyzing other analysts in training and could act as supervisors was determined by the Institute and could not be the result of personal initiative.

The functionality of the tripartite education system with formalized and centralized organization quickly became an accepted standard in all psychoanalytic institutions (not only within the IPA but also in external analytic societies, such as the Jungian). Eitingon took on the chairmanship of an international commission to standardize analytical training and had to deal with American dissent from Freud's position that *lay* people (non-doctors) could train as analysts. The Commission broke the deadlock by stipulating that each national society could determine whether or not the candidate should have a medical degree. "In practice, this meant that the training of lay analysts was officially outlawed in the United States but permitted in all other countries" (Fine, 1979, p. 97).

Analytic therapy: further evolution of Freud's ideas

After defining the structural model, Freud profoundly rethought some fundamental questions within the theory of technique (in particular the related questions of resistance and negation) and even the very meaning and possibilities of analytic treatment.

The concept of resistance was a very complex theoretical knot. Freud was aware of the risk that what the analyst asserted could not be rejected by the patient, because "if the patient agrees with us, the interpretation is right, but if he contradicts us, that is only a sign of his resistance, which again shows that we are right." It was therefore a matter of demonstrating that the analyst was not using the technique of "heads I win, tails you lose" (Freud, 1937/1964c, p. 257). In reality, Freud stressed, it is not assent or refusal as such that constitutes the criterion of confirmation of an interpretation. The refusal could constitute the manifestation of resistance. On the other hand, assent could be hypocritical or condescending; or even functional in its turn to resistance, masking a deeper unconscious content not detected by interpretation. The value of the patient's response to interpretation should have been assessed on three basic criteria: (a) the amount of *affect* that accompanied the response; (b) the immediate presence of concomitant confirmatory data; (c) the consistency of the response to the interpretation (positive or negative) with further confirmatory data that emerged later in the course of the analysis (Freud, 1937/1964c).

With regard to point (a), the patients' sense of deep insight was of course proof of a correct interpretation: the emotional recognition that the interpretation grasped something essential of their inner world. Rejection accompanied by intense negative emotions (feelings of indignation, horror, and the like) was also to be regarded as confirmation: it would be the typical sign of resistance, and therefore in any case proof of the correctness of the analytic interpretation. On the contrary, the patient's impassivity and indifference to the interpretation were to be considered as evidence against it (as long as it was not merely a momentary postponement of the emotional explosion). Freud believed, however, that errors on the part of the analyst were always possible and not particularly detrimental to the therapy, except for the bad impression that could be given by the analyst who made a long sequence of interpretative mistakes.

Point (b) occurred in special and fortunate circumstances. The clearest case was the interpretation rejected before the analyst had a chance to formulate it:

"Now you'll think I mean to say something insulting, but really I have no such intention." We realize that this is a rejection, by projection, of an idea that has just come up. Or: "You ask who this person in this dream can be. It's *not* my mother." We emend this so: "So it *is* my mother." In our interpretation, we take the liberty of disregarding the negation and picking out the subject matter alone of the association. It is as though the patient had said: "It's true that my mother came into my mind as I thought of this person, but I don't feel inclined to let the association count."

(Freud, 1925/1961f, p. 235)

Similar was the meaning of dissent from the content of an interpretation accompanied by characteristic verbal reactions:

> One of these is a form of words that is used (as though by general agree-ment) with very little variation by the most different people: "I didn't ever think" (or "I shouldn't ever have thought") "that" (or "of that"). This can be translated without any hesitation into: "Yes, you're right this time – about my unconscious." Unfortunately this formula, which is so welcome to the analyst, reaches his ears more often after single interpretations than after he has produced an extensive construction.
>
> (Freud, 1937/1964c, p. 253)

A "particularly striking" mode of confirmation would be observed when assent to the interpretation insinuates itself into the explicit formulation of a dissent "by means of a parapraxis" (Freud, 1937/1964c). A clinical example of this kind had already been published by Freud in a 1907 addition to *The Psy-chopathology of Everyday Life*:

> I once had to interpret a patient's dream in which the name "Jauner" occurred. The dreamer knew someone of that name, but it was impos-sible to discover the reason for his appearing in the context of the dream; I therefore ventured to suggest that it might be merely because of his name, which sounds like the term of abuse "*Gauner*" (swindler). My patient hast-ily and vigorously contested this; but in doing so he made a slip of the tongue which confirmed my guess, since he confused the same letters once more. His answer was "That seems to me too 'jewagt'" [instead of "gewagt" (far-fetched)]. When I had drawn his attention to his slip, he accepted my interpretation.
>
> (Freud, 1901/1960, p. 94)

Criterion (c), however, was the most important one, the one in which Freud relied most for the confirmation of the validity of the clinical data accumu-lated by psychoanalysis. In fact, Freud maintained that only the continuation of the analysis would allow the validity of an interpretation to be judged. Ideally, the confirmation would come from the emergence of a previously repressed memory (Freud, 1937/1964c).

However, other associative contents could also have a confirmatory value (it could happen, for example, that an analyst's interpretation was followed by the narration of another situation experienced by the patient to which the inter-pretation just given fitted and gave meaning). A very particular criterion was the worsening of the symptoms (*negative therapeutic reaction*) which, in Freud's opinion, inevitably followed the listening to significant interpretations by that category of patients to whom one could ascribe "sense of guilt, a masochistic need for suffering or repugnance to receiving help from the analyst" (Freud,

1937/1964c, p. 265). It has also been rightly observed that the analyst should anticipate this type of reaction before it occurs, in order for it to be considered a confirmation of the interpretation (Wisdom, 1967).

Freud never used a triumphalist tone in boasting about the successes of psychoanalysis. We have already remembered that, at the beginning of his own path, he supposed he could transform "hysterical misery into common unhappiness" (Breuer & Freud, 1895/1955, p. 304). However, he had claimed that psychoanalysis was the only truly effective form of psychotherapy. Only analysis, according to Freud, could offer the neurotic a true and complete knowledge of his inner world, and only this could lead to results: the conflicts of a patient "will only be successfully solved and his resistance overcome if the anticipatory ideas he is given tally with what is real in him" (Freud, 1917/1963, p. 452). Positive results were to be considered linked to the dissolution of the transference and could be considered definitively acquired.

Later, Freud referred to analysis no longer as the only effective method but as the "most powerful," and as such not to be applied in minor cases, being "also the most laborious and time consuming." On the contrary, "In suitable cases it is possible by its means to get rid of disturbances, bring about changes for which in pre-analytic times one would not have ventured to hope" (Freud, 1933/1964a, p. 153). In his later writings, Freud seemed to take an even more cautious attitude. The analytic process was not only a long and tiring work: one also had to admit that an apparently finished therapeutic path did not always preserve the analysand from later psychical problems. Freud (1937/1964b) recalled, in this regard, the case of the Wolf Man who, after an apparent success (Freud, 1918/1955b), reopened less than ten years later with a new treatment by Freud, followed by further periods of analysis with another therapist (see Gardiner, 1971; Mahony, 1984). We now know, moreover, that the patient in question never considered himself completely cured and even had serious doubts about the efficacy of psychoanalysis from the beginning, and finally gave an interview, which appeared posthumously, in which he denied ever having derived any benefit from his analyses (Borch-Jacobsen & Shamdasani, 2011; Obholzer, 1982). While Freud was certainly far from an admission of failure, there is no doubt that such a case (not unique) was a reason to reflect on the meaning and possibilities of psychoanalytic therapy.

Eventually, Freud made it clear that the concept of the end of analysis could be interpreted in different ways. Ideally, the therapy would end when "no further change can be expected to take place" from a continuation of the analysis, in the sense of having reached "absolute psychical normality" (Freud, 1937/1964b, pp. 219–220). Less ambitiously, an analysis could be considered terminated when patient and analyst agreed on two circumstances:

> First, that the patient shall no longer be suffering from his symptoms and shall have overcome his anxieties and his inhibitions; and secondly, that the analyst shall judge that so much repressed material has been made

conscious, so much that was unintelligible has been explained, and so much internal resistance conquered, that there is no need to fear a repetition of the pathological processes concerned.

(p. 219)

Even such an outcome would not necessarily occur but was conditioned by the nature of the neurosis. Assuming that all psychopathology depended on both constitutional and experiential factors, it was only when the latter prevailed that analysis could achieve the best results. This was because analytic work could be carried out starting from an *alliance* of the analyst with the ego of the patient – an alliance that can be made only with a normal ego. Evidently, however, even the therapeutic alliance with the patient's ego had a relative and unstable value, because "defense mechanisms directed against former danger recur in the treatment as resistance against recovery": in practice "the ego treats recovery as a new danger." Therapy therefore had to proceed "between a piece of id-analysis and a piece of ego-analysis" (p. 238). The work on the emergence of new content from the id and the correction of something in the ego proceeded in parallel: taking up the Freudian metaphor, it was as if the alliance had to be continually renewed so that the ego would avoid surrendering after each battle. The paradox was that surrender might seem all the more attractive the clearer the previous victory seemed. On the other hand, "the power of the instruments with which analysis operates is not unlimited but restricted, and the final upshot always depends on the relative strength of the psychical agencies which are struggling with one another" (p. 230).

Freud pointed out that further obstacles to treatment could come from "the individuality of the analyst" (p. 246). The normal training analysis could prove insufficient. Each analyst would then have to undergo a new period of analysis every five years: even the therapist's analysis could be *interminable*. Other forms of resistance already described in the past now appeared to Freud as almost insurmountable obstacles. The *adhesiveness of the libido* (i.e., the difficulty of abandoning old investments) and *psychical inertia* could slow down any kind of psychotherapy in an unpredictable way (pp. 241–242). The unconscious sense of guilt already recognized as being "localized by us in the ego's relation to the super-ego" was thus only one component of the resistance, which was now described as "a force which is defending itself by every possible means against recovery" (p. 242). All of this meant that only a less disturbed personality could really benefit from analytic psychotherapy, although, in the end, the difference between an unanalyzed person and the analyzed one could be not so radical as one would like or expect. It could be so intangible that the analyst could consider a therapy concluded without the patient having felt any real advantages. The opposite (but sometimes complementary) risk was that the analysis could be considered finished only in a very limited number of cases (thus justifying treatment courses lasting more than ten years). To complete the overall picture, there was also the idea, now more than overshadowed, that the unconscious could only be known in a partial and distorted way.

In particular, in the conclusions of *Analysis Terminable and Interminable*, Freud called the masculine defense against feminine aspects (passivity) and the feminine defense against masculine aspects (envy) of the personality a *bedrock*, which might not even have allowed any change in a patient's mind. To transform the id into a province of the ego would have been anything but easy. The conviction (which had never failed Freud before) that it was possible to know the historical truth about the patient's past was therefore shaken. That this possibility was not always realized was, however, clear from the emergence of the concept of *construction*, as opposed to mere *interpretation*. Construction constituted a larger fresco, a narrative of the patient's past that started from the elements that had already emerged in order to paint a broad and coherent picture of events that had not yet emerged from repression:

> "Interpretation" applies to something that one does to some single-element of the material, such as an association or a parapraxis. But it is a "construction" when one lays before the subject of the analysis a piece of his early history that he has forgotten, in some such way as this: "Up to your *n*th year you regarded yourself as the sole and unlimited possessor of your mother; then came another baby and brought you grave disillusionment. Your mother left you for some time, and even after her reappearance she was never devoted to you exclusively. Your feelings towards your mother became ambivalent, your father gained a new importance for you," . . . and so on.
>
> (p. 261)

Initially Freud attributed an anticipatory value to the construction, which did not replace insight. Still at the beginning of *Constructions in Analysis*, Freud seemed to keep the point: "It depends only upon analytic technique whether we shall succeed in bringing what is concealed completely to light" (p. 260). In the end, however, he felt forced to admit:

> The path that starts from the analyst's construction ought to end in the patient's recollection; but it does not always lead so far. Quite often we do not succeed in bringing the patient to recollect what has been repressed. Instead of that, if the analysis is carried out correctly, we produce in him an assured conviction of the truth of the construction which achieves the same therapeutic result as a recaptured memory.
>
> (pp. 265–266)

This position implicitly opens up the possibility of a hermeneutic outcome of psychoanalytic theory.[2] If the historical evidence of the recovery of the repressed memory was not decisive for the purposes of therapy, if conviction had the same therapeutic value as memory, then the analyst's real objectives could become narrative coherence and the rhetorical persuasiveness of the analyst's narration. This was far from Freud's original intentions, but it was consistent with his later statements.

Otto Rank and the trauma of birth

Otto Rank, Sándor Ferenczi, and Wilhelm Reich (1897–1957), who will be discussed in this and the following paragraphs, shared a singular destiny: for a long time they were considered leading elements of the Freudian psychoanalytic movement, but all three were marginalized during the 1920s and 1930s. The intention to reform psychoanalysis was in fact matched by a hostile attitude on the part of psychoanalytic institutions and even a posthumous ostracism that bordered on historical falsification.

In this respect, the fates of Rank and Ferenczi are particularly similar: for a long time they remained in Freud's inner circle of collaborators and were even members of the Secret Committee[3] since its creation, yet were destined to live out their final years outside the Freudian circle. Both were guilty of introducing a theoretical novelty, which was initially greeted with mere perplexity by Freud and later violently abhorred by him. The historiography of psychoanalysis, based on the testimony of Ernest Jones, has long regarded the two as traitors, as has been the case with all those whom Freud dismissed for reasons of theoretical disagreement. Both have more recently been re-evaluated. Ferenczi is in fact now considered a fundamental theoretical reference point by relational psychoanalysis (Aron & Harris, 1993).[4] Reich, on the other hand, despite the obvious historical relevance of *Character Analysis* and *The Mass Psychology of Fascism*, both of 1933, continues to be a little-read author, probably because of the peculiar drift of his later writings.

These are certainly not isolated cases. The fact that the psychoanalytic movement tended to exalt the figure of Freud as heroic and to devalue all those who questioned his ideas, while he was alive, has long been pointed out by independent historians (Ellenberger, 1970; Sulloway, 1979). However, reconsidering the cases of these three figures, so unfairly treated by their contemporaries, offers interesting food for thought. Rank, Ferenczi, and Reich were marginalized for daring to propose reforms, which in many ways appeared too precocious.

When Otto Rank's *The Trauma of Birth* was published in December 1923, the author had already played, and was still playing, an exceptionally important role in the psychoanalytic movement. He had even written essays that were included in the 1914 and 1922 editions of Freud's *The Interpretation of Dreams*. Moreover, he had published *The Double* (Rank, 1914/2012), a psychoanalytic interpretation of the literary theme of the double which had strongly impressed Freud himself, who drew inspiration from it in *The Uncanny* (Freud, 1919/1955e); he had promoted a collected work which has gone down in history: *The Myth of the Birth of the Hero* (Rank, 1909/2015).

In *The Trauma of Birth*, however, Rank expounded the peculiar idea that the primary origin of psychical pathologies was fundamentally to be found in the human being's experience of coming into the world (though without denying the importance of subsequent psychosexual development, and of the Oedipal complex in particular). Initially Freud was not particularly shocked by this, not least because he himself had assumed that the distress experienced at birth was prototypical for all subsequent forms of anxiety (Freud, 1909/1955a, 1923/1961a). Rank's view, however, radicalized such a hypothesis, when he wrote:

> (The aim of analysis is) the correct severance of the primal libido from its fixation, by the removal or the lessening of the primal repression, and this ultimately means going back to a repetition of the birth trauma, with the help of an experienced midwife.
>
> (Rank, 1923/2010, p. 204)

In 1924, Rank published a coauthored paper with Ferenczi: *The Development of Psychoanalysis* (Ferenczi & Rank, 1924/1980). This too was of no particular concern to Freud, although it contained potentially radical theoretical innovations. Here Rank and Ferenczi "challenged the prevailing notion that remembering was the chief aim of analytic work, whereas repetition was a sign of resistance." In their view, for treatment to work, "a 'phase of experience' had to precede the customary 'phase of understanding'" (Ragen & Aron, 1993, p. 218). Thus, the analyst's aim would be to enable the patient to relive the traumatic experiences in some way. Rank had also provisionally convinced Ferenczi that setting an end to each analysis was an almost infallible way to shorten it. Rank, however, later withdrew his adherence to the universal applicability of such a stratagem, without denying its possible appropriateness in certain cases (Ferenczi, 1926/1994c). Freud, too, had – quite occasionally – used such a tactic to overcome moments of stalemate in the analysis.

The book on psychoanalytic technique, published later (Rank, 1926), argued that the real therapeutic factor of analysis was specifically to relive, under the analyst's guidance, the affective experience of birth. This singular innovation was fiercely criticized by Abraham and Jones (Gay, 1988). Even Ferenczi (1927) disassociated himself, going so far as to write that Rank's ideas had become more unilateral than Adler's and Jung's. Ferenczi seemed to suggest anathema and excommunication, which finally came officially from Freud's work *Inhibitions, Symptom, Anxiety*. Freud conceded: "(Rank) remains on psychoanalytic ground and pursues a psychoanalytic line of thought" (Freud, 1925/1959a, p. 150). However, the sentence that Rank's theory "floats in the air instead of being based upon ascertained observations" (ibid., p. 299) seemed quite a final condemnation.

In fact, the process of estrangement had already begun when Rank found a very favorable reception in both France and the United States and finally decided to move to New York, where he could appear for the moment as Freud's most distinguished disciple on American soil. Moving away from Vienna led first, in 1924, to his replacement by Sándor Radó (1890–1972) as editor of the *Zeitschrift*, announced in a laconic communiqué (Freud, 1924/1961h), and then, in 1925, to his replacement by Anna Freud (1895–1982) in the Committee. On April 12, 1926, Sigmund Freud and Otto Rank met for the last time, and the latter presented Freud with a complete edition of Nietzsche's works, which Freud took with him to London in 1938. In his later years, Rank, by now permanently based in New York (where he died in 1939), continued to practice as an analyst but as an outsider. Just as Jung had drawn closer to Adler's work in his estrangement from Freud, so Rank, after his forced secession, incorporated Jungian ideas, such as archetype, self, individuation, extroversion/introversion, into his theoretical model (Marchioro, 2016). For the same reasons, Jung's rapprochements with Adler, and Rank's rapprochements with Jung, went unnoticed in the psychoanalytic movement. The path of theoretical integration was thus ignored for decades.

Active analysis and its results

Ferenczi, for his part, had also played an extraordinarily important role in the development of the psychoanalytic movement until his relationship with Freud began to deteriorate. Ferenczi's estrangement from the Freudian circle was linked to the development of what the Hungarian called *active technique*, which at first did not raise negative reactions from Freud, and in part even seemed to have been suggested by him (Ferenczi, 1921/1994b). The expression "active technique" implied a more interventionist behavior on the part of the therapist, compared to the well-established psychoanalytic attitude. Usually the analyst waited for the patient to walk the path leading to the understanding of the symptoms, through free association. As Ferenczi observed, after all, the history of psychoanalytic psychotherapy had gone through an initial phase in which the therapist used a *very active* approach: he hypnotized the patients in order to influence them or to favor abreaction. Only later did Freud adopt a passive stance, employing the principle of free association. In a certain sense, then, the use of interpretation could be classified as an active moment on the part of the analyst, because it gave the patient's thoughts "a given direction," facilitating "the appearance of ideas that otherwise would have been prevented by the resistance from becoming conscious" (Ferenczi, 1921/1994b, pp. 200–201). Also specifically active were psycho-educational interventions (Ferenczi called them *education of the ego*): such interventions can even be qualified as suggestion, even if a kind of suggestion completely different from the non-psychoanalytic one (Ferenczi, 1921/1994b, pp. 200–201).

What characterized the active technique in Ferenczi's sense was the assignment of tasks to the patient in order to overcome impasse situations. In the cases of anxiety hysteria, the first to which Ferenczi applied the technique, the patients "could not get beyond 'dead points' in the analysis until they were compelled to venture out from the retreat of their phobia, and to expose themselves experimentally to the situation they have avoided because of their painfulness" (Ferenczi, 1921/1994b, p. 201). According to Ferenczi, exposure involved a temporary increase in anxiety, but also the overcoming of resistance to the recovery of unconscious material that became available for analysis. In other cases, patients were asked to forgo acts that were pleasurable to them (such as masturbation): the aim was still to unlock unconscious material. Ferenczi warned that the use of orders and prohibitions should never be implemented before the transference was established, or else there would be the typical failure of *wild analysis*, when uninformed therapists tried to force patients into a rapid resolution of symptoms. Instead, "Active technique desires nothing more and nothing less than to lay bare latent tendencies to repetition and by this means to assist the therapy to these triumphs a little oftener than hitherto" (Ferenczi, 1921/1994b, p. 217).

Ferenczi later enumerated other possible applications of the activity principle, which in his view could also be used to interrupt the verbal flow of the patient who was apparently continuing in his free associations, overlooking some important aspect that had emerged but was buried under the logorrhea. In this sense the task of unmasking resistance was not to be neglected even in those cases where resistance tended "to employ the fundamental rule of association to frustrate the objects of the treatment" (Ferenczi, 1924/1994a, p. 69). In the case of patients with particularly poor phantasmatic activity, the active technique found new fields of application. When, for example, someone did not seem to react to situations or interpretations that would arouse intense feelings, Ferenczi intervened "forcing the patient to recover the adequate reactions." If he insisted that nothing came to mind, he would allow him "to discover such reactions in phantasy" (Ferenczi, 1926/1994c, p. 219). These inventions would later be transformed into cues for the full emergence of deeply repressed unconscious content. Progressively Ferenczi began to believe that after an initial phase of study and a subsequent phase in which the analytic interventions were only of an interpretative nature, one could begin to prescribe rules of behavior that would advance the analytic work (Ferenczi, 1925/1994d), thus influencing important interpersonal relationships, habits, and behavior. The experiments were not without risk, and Ferenczi had the intellectual honesty to admit this, suggesting that the provocative measures should not be imposed as in a repetition of the parent-child relationship: the therapist should obtain rational consent from the patient (Ferenczi, 1926/1994c). After the introduction, in certain cases, of tasks to increase urethral and sphincter tension (Ferenczi, 1925/1994d), Ferenczi also began to experiment with relaxation techniques during the session (Ferenczi, 1926/1994c).

The evolution toward ever more radical technical experiments was decisively influenced by Elizabeth Severn (1875–1959), a patient who entered Ferenczi's life in 1924 and remained in analysis with him, albeit with seasonal interruptions, practically until the Hungarian psychoanalyst's death in 1933. Severn was the patient whom Ferenczi's *Clinical Diary* (1995) identified as RN. She was a severely disturbed person, repeatedly on the verge of suicide, who came to a self-diagnosis of schizophrenia even though she started her own practice as a psychotherapist. Ferenczi made superhuman therapeutic efforts with her, holding multiple sessions on the same day for up to five hours in total (even overnight), continuing the analysis at weekends or even during holidays abroad (Fortune, 1993). Finally, the experiment of *mutual analysis* also arrived, which is extensively documented in the *Clinical Diary*. Although the manuscript remained unpublished until 30 years after Ferenczi's death, many aspects of his new technical elasticity filtered into his later writings (Ferenczi, 1928/1994e). Through his analysis with Severn, Ferenczi also became convinced of the need to re-evaluate the theory of childhood sexual trauma, which caused Freud's consternation (Rachman, 2018). In the case of Ferenczi, Freud's estrangement in his later years was not made official (although Ferenczi's disappointment was no less painful). Indeed, Freud wrote an impassioned obituary of Ferenczi. When, in *Analysis Terminable and Interminable* (1937/1964b), Freud described the problems that followed the analysis of a pupil that had not been sufficiently thorough, he alluded to Ferenczi, although he did not mention him. Jones's condemnation, however, would weigh heavily on the evaluation of Ferenczi's work for a long time, despite his obvious influence on the likes of Clara Thompson (1893–1958) (Shapiro, 1993) or Erich Fromm (1900–1980) (Bacciagalluppi, 1993), and despite Michael Balint's (1896–1970) tenacious efforts to enhance his contribution (Balint, 1968/2013).

The encounter of psychoanalysis and Marxism

As has been mentioned, a very fortunate historical interpretation sees Karl Marx, Friedrich Nietzsche, and Sigmund Freud as *philosophers of suspicion*. Starting with these three thinkers, in fact, it would finally have become possible to *suspect* that commonly accepted morality, established order, and consciousness are not what they appear to be, and that their current manifestation is not the only possible one (Ricoeur, 1965/1972). A relative value can be attributed to this formula, as in the case of all historical formulas and simplifications. There is no doubt, however, that when psychoanalysis has been confronted with philosophy, Marx and Nietzsche have been privileged references. The encounter between depth psychology and Nietzsche was very early: Freud, Adler, and Jung were directly influenced by him (although, as has been shown, admitting the influence in different ways). The encounter between Marxism and psychoanalysis came later (Freud and Jung were not politically committed to the left, while Adler was oriented toward social democratic thought) and can be dated to the 1920s. His parallel sources were the birth of the Frankfurt School and the conversion to communism of Wilhelm Reich, active as a psychoanalyst first in Vienna and then in Berlin (and later a much discussed outsider). The encounter was 'in the air' at that particular historical moment. On the one hand, psychoanalysis was experiencing an extraordinary affirmation. On the other hand, the victory and consolidation of a communist regime in Russia had been witnessed with the birth of the Soviet Union. So the idea of a Marxist social revolution in Western Europe seemed a real possibility. The possibility, however, did not materialize. On the contrary, the West saw rather a progressive advance of fascism, a scenario certainly not foreseen by Marx.

The so-called Freudo-Marxism was developed in different ways but started from a common root: the conviction that it was not enough to cure the individuals in order to heal their neurosis. Society itself was sick and necessarily neuroticized individuals. Without changing the system, therefore, it would not have been possible at all to restore sanity to the human being. The Marxist anthropology on which this approach was based drew on the writings of the young Marx, in particular the *Economic and Philosophic Manuscripts of 1844* (Marx, 2012), *The Holy Family* (Engels & Marx, 1845/2013), and *The German Ideology* (Marx & Engels, 1845/1976), which historicized human needs and desire.

The psychological insights in these early writings of Marx produced a long echo and influence in the Freudo-Marxist camp, contaminating psychology and psychoanalysis with *historical materialism*. In these writings, there was an anthropology in which natural needs interacted with their possibility of satisfaction; needs (Marxian) were identified with desires (Freudian), changing dynamically when confronted with reality. For example, hunger is different if it is satisfied with a simple food or with a culturally reworked food. Hunger in humans thus changes as the material conditions of satisfaction change: the nature of hunger changes when it turns from a need into a desire for sophisticated food. This psychological use of Marx led to a conception of psychology and psychoanalysis that took into account the limits placed on human evolution by the historical and material conditions in which people were (Fromm, 1961).

As we will see in the following paragraphs, both Reich (1933/2013a) and the Frankfurt School (Horkheimer et al., 1936) convinced themselves that the social framing of the individual started from the family experience, through which the repressive instances conveyed by society were absorbed very early. Reich, however, resolved to propose a strategy of action based on sexual liberation. The Frankfurt theorists, as a whole, conceived Freudian thought rather as a diagnostic tool than as a lever of change (the revolution should have been economic–political). Moreover, Erich Fromm, the most prominent element of the Frankfurt School for the history of psychotherapy, was destined to soon abandon his Marxist faith and to place himself in an eccentric position even with respect to the psychoanalytic movement. As will be seen, together with Karen Horney, Frieda (Fromm) Reichmann (1889–1957), Harry Stack Sullivan (1892–1949), and Clara Thompson, Erich Fromm will generally be classified as a *neo-Freudian*.

Wilhelm Reich and character analysis

Wilhelm Reich trained as a doctor and psychiatrist in Vienna after fighting on the Italian front in World War I between 1915 and 1918. His studies were swift and brilliant, and he graduated in medicine in 1922 and later specialized in neuropsychiatry. By 1920, however, he had already joined the Vienna Psychoanalytic Society and only two years later began his private practice as a psychoanalyst. His meeting with Freud was facilitated by his interest in sexology. Reich had become the leader of a group of Viennese students who complained about the lack of teaching in this field at the university and decided to organize seminars on their behalf. The invitation to Freud was a predictable step, but the meeting resulted in love at first sight. Both Freud's personality and ideas made an immediate and indelible impression on Reich. In particular, he found himself drawn to Freud's conception of the libido as energy (a conception that was later to receive a particular elaboration in his hands).

Like Adler, Reich showed a keen interest in social problems from the outset and promoted (even at his own expense) the establishment of sexual advice centers for the lower classes. It was precisely his contact with the "sexual misery of the working masses" (Reich, 1945) that led him to doubt the classical psychoanalytic approach, based on practice with upper-middle-class patients (who could above all cope with the time and cost of therapy). In his eyes, sexual restraint, rather than a means of preserving civilization, as Freud saw it, was a tool of implementing political oppression, especially on the poor.

A sympathizer and member of the Austrian Socialist Party, he left it in 1927, shaken by the socialists' inaction in the face of the deaths of innocent people during demonstrations at the hands of right-wing provocateurs and the police (De Marchi, 1970). He then joined the Communist Party and immersed himself in the reading of Marx and Friedrich Engels (1820–1895), the first fruit of which was *Dialectical Materialism and Psychoanalysis* (Reich, 1929), a text in which he attempted to show the intimately dialectical nature of psychoanalysis and to contest its tendency (to which Freud himself had not been immune) to lose its original *revolutionary* characteristics and become an instrument of domination of the bourgeoisie over the proletariat. Taking up the research of the anthropologist Bronislaw Malinowski (1884–1942), who questioned the alleged universality of the Oedipus complex (Malinowski, 1924), Reich (1931) came to overturn Freud's assumption that civilization was based on the suppression of drives. Instead, in his view, civilization generated suppression in order to control the subordinate classes. Rather than being a factor in social order, suppression degraded love life. Naturally, after Hitler's rise to power, Reich, Fromm, and all the Frankfurt theorists were forced to flee abroad. Even before the exodus, however, Reich was thrown out of the IPA, not so much for his almost heretical positions as for his open communist militancy. Fellow analysts feared that Reich's presence in their ranks might attract less than benevolent attention from the Nazis. Reich incredulously accepted the invitation to retire *sine ira* from the IPA at the 1934 Lucerne Psychoanalytic Congress. However, he was a good prophet in predicting that it would not be his exit that would prevent psychoanalysis from being banned from German territory (Reich, 2013b).

Wilhelm Reich's theoretical-clinical activity, since the 1920s and even immediately after his nonconsensual divorce from the IPA, attracted considerable attention within the psychoanalytic movement and exerted an influence greater than that actually acknowledged by official psychoanalysis later on. It could be said that his contribution constituted a sort of bridge between Rank and Ferenczi's ideas and those of the later Ego psychology: in fact, his most important book, *Character Analysis* (Reich, 1980/1933), was based on Rank and Ferenczi's proposals of active technique and was later mentioned by Anna Freud in *The Ego and the Defense Mechanisms* (A. Freud, 1936/1993) for the importance of its clinical proposals. Anna Freud's recognition was all the more significant because she herself had in the meantime influenced the dismissal of Reich (Reich, 2013b). Even more remarkable is the circumstance, if one considers that the expulsion order followed the cowardly decision to deny the publication of precisely *Character Analysis* by the official publishing house of psychoanalysis in Germany. And this despite the fact that Reich was still, in 1933, within his rights to request it, as a full member of both the German and the International psychoanalytic societies.

Reich's contribution was based on a fundamental problematic issue in Freudian psychoanalysis. Freud had initially believed that the emergence of unconscious contents in consciousness should necessarily lead to healing. He later realized that the analysis of the unconscious could only be a prerequisite for healing, but that this prerequisite was not always sufficient. Reich wondered, therefore, why some patients remained resistant to any improvement despite a long and thorough analysis, while others, who had sometimes gone through a less complete analytic process, recovered completely from their neurosis. Comparing what differentiated the patients in the first group from those in the second, Reich concluded that the key was sexual activity. Patients improved if they were able to initiate a satisfactory sexual life with the help of analysis and did not improve if they remained abstinent. Moreover, the likelihood of recovery was higher the more "the genital primacy was established" during the developmental age, whereas "the prognosis was poorer the less the libido had been attached to the genital in childhood" (Reich, 1980/1933, p. 13).

A remarkable feature of Reich's clinical texts is the courage he showed in recounting therapeutic failures, a courage he had in common with the best moments of Freud's work, such as the case of Dora. And just as with Freud, the impasse situations were a cue to illustrate new technical suggestions. Just as Dora's escape offered a reason to stress the importance of transference management, Reich's reflection on unfinished cases suggested a new attitude to the progress of analysis. Reich went so far as to say: "Every unresolved stoppage in an analysis is the fault of the analyst" (p. 22). The polemical target, for Reich, was first and foremost the

> misconception of the Freud's rule that the course of the analysis should be left to the patient. This rule can only mean that one should not disturb the work of the patient as long as it proceeds according to the patient's wish to get well and our therapeutic intentions.
>
> (p. 28)

However, Reich observed, it would never be the patients who would speak first about their resistance. It would therefore be the analyst who would have to direct the course of the associations and look for a red thread to follow in the progressive unraveling offered on the analytic path. From this point of view, the closeness with Ferenczi's and Rank's theses on active analysis was evident. Of the two colleagues, however, he found erroneous the conviction that fixing a term for the analysis in advance could break through the wall of resistance. Just as he was convinced that simply telling the patient that resistance was being put in place was a wrong and unnecessarily guilt-ridden approach. Only an understanding of the nature of resistance could dismantle its strength.

Reich also assumed with the utmost clarity that the analysis of resistance should always precede the explication of the deeper contents: "Our principle is: no interpretation of meaning when a resistance interpretation is needed" (p. 27). Just as it was necessary to continue "avoiding any deep-reaching interpretations of the unconscious as long as the wall of conventional politeness between patient and analyst continues to exist" (p. 31). As a general rule, "one cannot act too early in analyzing resistances, and one cannot be too reserved in the interpretation of the unconscious, apart from resistances" (p. 38). In this sense, indeed, interpretation "may be likened to a valuable drug which has to be used sparingly, if it is not to lose its efficacy" (p. 37).

The issue of resistance analysis led Reich to propose other technical innovations of great interest, first, by emphasizing an often underestimated aspect of patient communication, namely the nonverbal. One of the fundamental problems of the prevailing analytic practice was, in his view, the overvaluation of content at the expense of form. Instead, it was not only what the patients said that was important but also how they said it, or even how much they did not say, and the very apparent absence of material: "There is hardly any situation in which the patient brings 'no material'; it is our fault if we are unable to utilize the patient's behavior as 'material'" (p. 45). Conversely, it was also possible that the overabundance of dreams and associations constituted a paradoxical form of resistance: the patient displayed a positive transference which the analyst enjoyed, while the negative transference remained hidden and the analysis inexplicably stalled after years of seemingly endless work.

It was better to begin with character analysis, that is, on a "thorough working through of the conflicts assimilated by the ego" (p. 62) rather than concentrating on the material usually taken into consideration first, that is, childhood memories. According to Reich, in fact, the most important thing was "to see the present-day meaning of the character resistance: this is usually possible without the infantile material" (p. 51). Moreover, the neurotics would have tended to bring relatively less of this material to the analysis, if the therapeutic process had not first led them to dismantle the strongest resistances, instrumental in maintaining the unstable equilibrium they had achieved:

> The totality of the neurotic character traits makes itself felt in the analysis as a compact defense mechanism against our therapeutic endeavor. (. . .) Since the neurotic character, in its economic function, has established a certain equilibrium, albeit a neurotic one, the analysis presents a danger to this equilibrium.
>
> (p. 44)

According to Reich, neurosis therefore tended to forge the character in such a way as to behave similarly both in analysis and in everyday life, so that one could speak of *character armor* against the outside world and against the id.

Character Analysis was a milestone in the history of the development of analytic therapy because it proposed, for the first time in a clear way, a precise strategy on the due time of interpretation. Reich's general principles were later assimilated by Ego psychology, but this was not adequately recognized, not least because of Reich's theoretical twists and turns, which would take him further and further away from the psychoanalytic orbit, when finally, in advocating a utopia of complete sexual liberation of humanity, he began to develop singular theories about a vital (or *orgone*) energy that would permeate the Universe.

After *Character Analysis* and *The Mass Psychology of Fascism* (1933/2013a), Reich developed his concept of the character armor, assuming that emotional blocks corresponded to muscular or physical blocks. He therefore began to introduce techniques designed to induce relaxation or, on the contrary to provoke in the patient real crises of weeping and laughter, fury and anxiety. The aim of these techniques was to unearth those energies buried in the individual and often used precisely to feed the repressive force of the character armor. This approach paved the way for what later, with Alexander Lowen (1910–2008), became known as *bioenergetic therapy*. Lowen (1958/1971, 1975/1994), moreover, explicitly attributed to Reich the theoretical origin of the psychotherapeutic technique he developed.[5]

Eventually, however, Reich turned to almost delusional ideas. The same critic, who calls his *Character Analysis* "a significant contribution to the understanding of character structure" (Fine, 1979, p. 128), describes his *orgonomy* as "a connection of blatant absurdities for which he nonetheless found some followers" (p. 129). His bizarre therapeutic experiments attracted the attention of the judiciary rather than the scientific world. When Reich began to lock his patients in metal containers, in which he irradiated them with *orgone energy*, he was arrested by the American police. His life ended in prison, where he died of a heart attack in 1957. The imprint of the early Reich is, however, recognizable in several authors that we will discuss later, from Deleuze and Guattari of *Anti-Oedipus*, to Marcuse of *Eros and Civilisation*, from the anti-psychiatrists Laing and Cooper to the already mentioned Anna Freud (De Marchi, 1970; Vegetti Finzi, 1987).

The Frankfurt School

One of the most successful combinations of psychoanalysis and Marxism was promoted by the so-called Frankfurt School. Thanks to the financial support of the billionaire Hermann Weil (1868–1927), the Institute for Social Research was founded in Frankfurt in 1922 with the intention of introducing Marxism into the German Academy. The Institute was accepted at the University of Frankfurt thanks to the considerable funding it was guaranteed and immediately began to bring together philosophers, sociologists, and later psychologists of the highest caliber. The group was consolidated around the charismatic figure of Max Horkheimer (1895–1973), director of the Institute from 1929. He was committed to building Critical Theory: an attempt to take up and update Marx's thinking, adapting it to the new historical and cultural climate. In addition to Horkheimer, the Frankfurt School is linked to such important names as Theodor W. Adorno (1903–1969), Herbert Marcuse (1898–1979), Walter Benjamin (1892–1940), Karl Wittfogel (1896–1988), and, more recently, Jürgen Habermas. For the history of psychotherapy, the most prominent name has undoubtedly been that of Erich Fromm.[6]

A characteristic feature of the movement became the use of psychoanalysis as an instrument for the investigation of contemporary society, an instrument that stood alongside the philosophy of history and the economic theory of Marx. Erich Fromm, in this sense, was a decisive element. He was not the first to stimulate his colleagues to read Freud (to whom Adorno had dedicated his doctoral thesis), but he was indeed the first psychoanalyst to join the Frankfurt School.

For the Frankfurt School, the whole of the Western world lived under the assertion of capitalism at the expense of the subordinate classes. In this sense, there was no real qualitative difference between the democratic-liberal states (such as Weimar Germany or the United States) and the Nazi regime: liberalism was, in their eyes, nothing more than fascism in disguise. The present situation was seen as the outcome of a historical process, the origin of which could be traced back to the Enlightenment, and whose "dialectic" led in any case to the alienation of man proper to "bourgeois" society. It was with the Enlightenment, in fact, in the eyes of the Frankfurt theorists, that instrumental reason, or apparent rationality, was established in the West, bent to control the physical world and, once applied to the production of goods, destined to accentuate more and more the domination of the capitalists over the working class. The Enlightenment, therefore, could not be interpreted as a movement for the liberation of the human beings but as the source of their increasing alienation (Horkheimer & Adorno, 1947/1972). The rationalization of the productive system coincided in fact with an exasperated division of labor, which in turn increasingly alienated the workers, who were dedicated to simpler tasks with a tighter rhythm. Marx saw well, according to the Frankfurt theorists, how this historical process led to a concentration of economic power in the hands of a few and the increasing subjugation of the working class. Marx failed, however, to see the aspect of repression linked to sexuality, as was only possible since Freud: society would in fact also stand on the sublimation of sexual instincts, as argued in *Civilisation and Its Discontents* (Freud, 1930/1961j). Furthermore, Marx had made a mistake in predicting that bourgeois society, founded on the *exploitation of man by man*, would be overthrown by the rebellion of the proletariat. On the contrary, neither the German nor the American workers had shown any particular impetus for political change in society. In itself, the use of propaganda, however new and extraordinarily effective an instrument of consensus, could not be a sufficient explanation for the stalemate of the historical dialectic and conflict that was supposed to lead to revolution in purely Marxian terms.

The understanding of individual and group psychological reasons became a fundamental hermeneutic tool for understanding the recent evolution of Western societies. It was Fromm (1932/1971) who coined the expression *analytical social psychology*, which would indicate, in the language common to the Frankfurt theorists, the application of psychoanalysis to the study of society. Fromm had, in particular, an insight of great depth: since the individuals had no direct contact with society in the first stages of his existence, so until their personality was already formed, it was the family that was the principal psychological agency of society (Fromm, 1932/1971). This insight constitutes the germ of the later *Studies on Authority and the Family* (Horkheimer et al., 1936), probably the most important testimony to Erich Fromm's collaboration with Horkheimer's group. Here Fromm – who was entrusted with the psychological contribution – argued extensively on how the family was the foundation of political authority, since the relationship established by the children with their father was the model of the attitude toward constituted authority. In the same way, however, it was the social model that founded the family structure, namely the type of relationship established between parents and children.

Fromm's collaboration with the Frankfurt group, however, did not survive long after he moved to the United States in 1934 because of the Nazis. This was partly due to economic divergencies (Fromm was asked somewhat brutally to give up the lifetime salary provided for in his contract with the Institute), partly due to Adorno's personal hostility, and partly due to a different position with respect to Freud: the naturalistic and materialistic view of psychoanalysis, which Fromm increasingly tended to criticize, while constituting a reason of specific interest for Adorno and Horkheimer. Fromm later also distanced himself from Marxism, making the rift completely irremediable.

Even after Fromm's departure, however, the Frankfurt School continued to make extensive use of Freud in the development of Critical Theory. Here it is worth mentioning at least two texts that can be traced back to exponents of the School who have exerted a particular historical influence: the first is *The Authoritarian Personality*, which constituted a powerful attempt to study the latent tendency to accept fascist regimes. Theodor W. Adorno and his collaborators carried out a wide-ranging empirical study, based on the construction of ad hoc psychological scales and their application to large samples, in order to understand the personality characteristics of those who tend to integrate easily into an authoritarian society (Adorno et al., 1950/2019). Although widely criticized on a methodological level, Adorno's attempt remains an indispensable reference in studies on authoritarianism (see, e.g., Altemeyer, 2006; Lauriola et al., 2015; Montuori, 2005). The second is *Eros and Civilisation*, a book in which Marcuse (1955) proposed a socialist utopia based on economic and sexual liberation and which turned out, for better or worse, to be one of the manifestos of 1968.[7]

While in the 1960s, Fromm and Marcuse, as we will discuss analytically, represented two different ways of understanding Freudo-Marxism, in Europe Jürgen Habermas, the illustrious heir of the Frankfurt theorists, was one of the first proponents, with Paul Ricoeur (1913–2005), of the hermeneutic interpretation of psychoanalysis (Habermas, 1971), later transposed on the clinical level by Roy Schafer and Donald Spence.[8]

Notes

1 See infra, Ch. 5, pp. 215–217.
2 See infra, Vol. 2., Ch. 8, pp. 144–147.
3 See supra, Ch. 3, p. 97.
4 See infra, Vol. 2, Ch. 9, pp. 180–186.
5 See infra, Vol. 2, Ch. 7, p. 98.
6 See infra, p. 165, ch. 5, pp. 213–215, and Vol. 2, Ch. 7, pp. 76–78.
7 See infra, Vol. 2, Ch. 7, pp. 76–78.
8 See infra, Vol. 2, Ch. 8, pp. 144–147.

References

Adorno, T., Frenkel-Brenswik, E., Levinson, D. J., & Sanford, R. N. (2019). *The authoritarian personality*. Verso. (Original work published 1950)
Altemeyer, B. (2006). *The authoritarian specter*. Harvard University Press.
Aron, L., & Harris, A. (Eds.). (1993). *The legacy of Sándor Ferenczi*. Analytic Press.
Bacciagalluppi, M. (1993). Ferenczi's influence on Fromm. In L. Aron & A. Harris (Eds.), *The legacy of Sándor Ferenczi* (pp. 185–198). Analytic Press.
Balint, M. (2013). *The basic fault*. Routledge. (Original work published 1968)
Borch-Jacobsen, M., & Shamdasani, S. (2011). *The Freud files: An inquiry into the history of psychoanalysis*. Cambridge University Press.
Brenner, C. (1955). *An elementary textbook of psychoanalysis*. Doubleday.

Breuer, J., & Freud, S. (1955). Studies on hysteria. In *The standard edition of the complete psychological works of Sigmund Freud* (Vol. 2, pp. 1–307). Hogarth. (Original work published 1895)

De Marchi, L. (1970). *Wilhelm Reich.* Sugar.

Ellenberger, H. F. (1970). *The discovery of the unconscious: The history and evolution of dynamic psychiatry.* Basic Books.

Engels, F., & Marx, K. (2013). *The holy family.* Windham. (Original work published 1845)

Ferenczi, S. (1927). Review of *Technik Der Psychoanalyse*: by Otto Rank. *International Journal of Psycho-Analysis, 8,* 93–100.

Ferenczi, S. (1994a). On forced phantasies. In *Further contributions to the theory and technique of psycho-analysis* (pp. 68–77). Karnac. (Original work published 1924)

Ferenczi, S. (1994b). The further development of an active therapy in psycho-analysis. In *Further contributions to the theory and technique of psycho-analysis* (pp. 198–217). Karnac. (Original work published 1921)

Ferenczi, S. (1994c). Contra-indications to the 'active' psycho-analytic technique. In *Further contributions to the problems and methods of psycho-analysis* (pp. 217–230). Karnac. (Original work published 1926)

Ferenczi, S. (1994d). Psycho-analysis of sexual habits. In *Further contributions to the theory and technique of psycho-analysis* (pp. 259–297). Karnac. (Original work published 1925)

Ferenczi, S. (1994e). The elasticity of psycho-analytic technique. In *Final contributions to the theory and technique of psycho-analysis* (pp. 87–101). Karnac. (Original work published 1928)

Ferenczi, S. (1995). *The clinical diary of Sándor Ferenczi.* Harvard University Press.

Ferenczi, S., Abraham, K., Simmel, E., & Jones, E. (1921). *Psychoanalysis and the war neuroses.* International Psycho-Analytical Library.

Ferenczi, S., & Rank, O. (1986). *The development of psychoanalysis.* JUP. (Original work published 1924)

Fine, R. (1979). *A history of psychoanalysis.* Columbia University Press.

Fortune, C. (1993). The case of 'RN': Sándor Ferenczi's radical experiment in psychoanalysis. In L. Aron & A. Harris (Eds.), *The legacy of Sándor Ferenczi* (pp. 101–120). Analytic Press.

Freud, A. (1993). *The ego and the defense mechanisms.* Karnac Books. (Original work published 1936)

Freud, S. (1953). Three essays on sexuality. In *The standard edition of the complete psychological works of Sigmund Freud* (Vol. 7, pp. 125–143). Hogarth. (Original work published 1905)

Freud, S. (1955a). Notes upon a case of obsessional neurosis. In *The standard edition of the complete psychological works of Sigmund Freud* (Vol. 10, pp. 155–249). Hogarth. (Original work published 1909)

Freud, S. (1955b). From the history of an infantile neurosis. In *The standard edition of the complete psychological works of Sigmund Freud* (Vol. 17, pp. 7–122). Hogarth. (Original work published 1918)

Freud, S. (1955c). A childhood recollection from "Dichtung und Wahrheit". In *The standard edition of the complete psychological works of Sigmund Freud* (Vol. 17, pp. 145–156). Hogarth. (Original work published 1918)

Freud, S. (1955d). Introduction to "Psychoanalysis of the war neuroses". In *The standard edition of the complete psychological works of Sigmund Freud* (Vol. 17, pp. 205–210). Hogarth. (Original work published 1920)

Freud, S. (1955e). The 'Uncanny'. In *The standard edition of the complete psychological works of Sigmund Freud* (Vol. 17, pp. 217–252). Hogarth. (Original work published 1919)

Freud, S. (1955f). Beyond the pleasure principle. In *The standard edition of the complete psychological works of Sigmund Freud* (Vol. 18, pp. 3–61). Hogarth. (Original work published 1920)

Freud, S. (1955g). Group psychology and the analysis of the ego. In *The standard edition of the complete psychological works of Sigmund Freud* (Vol. 18, pp. 79–143). Hogarth. (Original work published 1921)

Freud, S. (1955h). The libido theory. In *The standard edition of the complete psychological works of Sigmund Freud* (Vol. 18, pp. 255–259). Hogarth. (Original work published 1922)

Freud, S. (1957a). On the history of the psycho-analytic movement. In *The standard edition of the complete psychological works of Sigmund Freud* (Vol. 14, pp. 7–66). Hogarth. (Original work published 1914)

Freud, S. (1957b). On narcissism: An introduction. In *The standard edition of the complete psychological works of Sigmund Freud* (Vol. 14, pp. 73–102). Hogarth. (Original work published 1914)

Freud, S. (1957c). Papers on metapsychology. In *The standard edition of the complete psychological works of Sigmund Freud* (Vol. 14, pp. 109–258). Hogarth. (Original work published 1915).

Freud, S. (1957d). Thoughts for the time on war and death. In *The standard edition of the complete psychological works of Sigmund Freud* (Vol. 14, pp. 275–300). Hogarth. (Original work published 1915)

Freud, S. (1957e). On transience. In *The standard edition of the complete psychological works of Sigmund Freud* (Vol. 14, pp. 303–307). Hogarth. (Original work published 1915)

Freud, S. (1958a). Remembering, repeating and working-through. In *The standard edition of the complete psychological works of Sigmund Freud* (Vol. 12, pp. 145–156). Hogarth. (Original work published 1914)

Freud, S. (1958b). Observations on transference-love. In *The standard edition of the complete psychological works of Sigmund Freud* (Vol. 12, pp. 157–171). Hogarth. (Original work published 1915)

Freud, S. (1959a). Inhibitions, symptoms, anxiety. In *The standard edition of the complete psychological works of Sigmund Freud* (Vol. 20, pp. 87–172). Hogarth. (Original work published 1925)

Freud, S. (1959b). The question of lay analysis: Postscript. In *The standard edition of the complete psychological works of Sigmund Freud* (pp. 251–258). Hogarth. (Original work published 1927)

Freud, S. (1960). The psychopathology of everyday life. In *The standard edition of the complete psychological works of Sigmund Freud* (Vol. 6). Hogarth Press. (Original work published 1901)

Freud, S. (1961a). The ego and the id. In *The standard edition of the complete psychological works of Sigmund Freud* (Vol. 19, pp. 12–66). Hogarth. (Original work published 1923)

Freud, S. (1961b). The infantile genital organization. In *The standard edition of the complete psychological works of Sigmund Freud* (Vol. 19, pp. 141–148). Hogarth. (Original work published 1923)

Freud, S. (1961c). Neurosis and psychosis. In *The standard edition of the complete psychological works of Sigmund Freud* (Vol. 19, pp. 149–156). Hogarth. (Original work published 1924)

Freud, S. (1961d). The dissolution of the Oedipus complex. In *The standard edition of the complete psychological works of Sigmund Freud* (Vol. 19, pp. 173–182). Hogarth. (Original work published 1924)

Freud, S. (1961e). The loss of reality in neurosis and psychosis. In *The standard edition of the complete psychological works of Sigmund Freud* (Vol. 19, pp. 183–190). Hogarth. (Original work published 1924)

Freud, S. (1961f). Negation. In *The standard edition of the complete psychological works of Sigmund Freud* (Vol. 19, pp. 235–242). Hogarth. (Original work published 1925)

Freud, S. (1961g). Some psychical consequences of the anatomical distinction between the sexes. In *The standard edition of the complete psychological works of Sigmund Freud* (Vol. 19, pp. 243–250). Hogarth. (Original work published 1925)

Freud, S. (1961h). Editorial changes in the "Zeitschrift". In *The standard edition of the complete psychological works of Sigmund Freud* (Vol. 19, p. 293). Hogarth. (Original work published 1924)

Freud, S. (1961i). The future of an illusion. In *The standard edition of the complete psychological works of Sigmund Freud* (Vol. 21, pp. 5–56). Hogarth. (Original work published 1927)

Freud, S. (1961j). Civilization and its discontents. In *The standard edition of the complete psychological works of Sigmund Freud* (Vol. 21, pp. 64–145). Hogarth. (Original work published 1930)

Freud, S. (1961k). Introductory lectures on psycho-analysis (parts I-II). In *The standard edition of the complete psychological works of Sigmund Freud* (Vol. 15). Hogarth. (Original work published 1915–1916)

Freud, S. (1963). Introductory lectures on psycho-analysis (part III). In *The standard edition of the complete psychological works of Sigmund Freud* (Vol. 16). Hogarth. (Original work published 1917)

Freud, S. (1964a). New introductory lectures on psycho-analysis. In *The standard edition of the complete psychological works of Sigmund Freud* (Vol. 22, pp. 5–182). Hogarth. (Original work published 1933)

Freud, S. (1964b). Analysis terminable and interminable. In *The standard edition of the complete psychological works of Sigmund Freud* (Vol. 23, pp. 216–2534). Hogarth. (Original work published 1937)

Freud, S. (1964c). Constructions in analysis. In *The standard edition of the complete psychological works of Sigmund Freud* (Vol. 23, pp. 255–269). Hogarth. (Original work published 1937)

Fromm, E. (1961). *Marx's concept of man*. Ungar.

Fromm, E. (1971). The method and function of an analytic social psychology. In *The crisis of psychoanalysis* (pp. 135–162). Cape. (Original work published 1932)

Gardiner, M. (Ed.). (1971). *The wolf-man and Sigmund Freud*. Penguin.

Gay, P. (1998). *Freud: A life for our time*. W. W. Norton.

Groddeck, G. (1977). *The meaning of illness: Selected psychoanalytic writings including his correspondence with Sigmund Freud*. Hogarth.

Groddeck, G. (2015). *The book of the it*. Ravenio. (Original work published 1923)

Habermas, J. (1971). *Knowledge and human interests*. Beacon.

Horkheimer, M., & Adorno, T. W. (1972). *Dialectic of enlightenment*. Seabury. (Original work published 1947)

Horkheimer, M., Fromm, E., & Marcuse, H. (1936). *Studien über Autorität und Familie* [Studies on authority and family]. Alcan.

Jervis, G., & Bartolomei, G. (1996). *Freud*. La Nuova Italia Scientifica.

Jung, C. G. (1960). The psychology of dementia praecox. In *The collected works of C. G. Jung* (Vol. 3, pp. 1–151). Routledge & Kegan Paul. (Original work published 1907)

Jung, C. G. (2019). *Psychology of the unconscious: A study of the transformations and symbolisms of the Libido* [Transformations and symbols of the libido]. Routledge. (Original work published 1912)

Kant, I. (2002). *Critique of practical reason*. Hackett. (Original work published 1785)

Lauriola, M., Foschi, R., & Marchegiani, L. (2015). Integrating values and cognitive style in a model of right-wing radicalism. *Personality and Individual Differences, 75*, 147–153.

Lowen, A. (1971). *The language of the body*. Collier. (Original work published 1958)

Lowen, A. (1994). *Bioenergetics*. Penguin. (Original work published 1975)

Mahony, P. J. (1984). *Cries of the Wolf Man*. International Universities Press.

Malinowski, B. (1924). Psychoanalysis and anthropology. *Psyche, 4*, 293–332.

Marchioro, F. (2016). Prefazione [Foreword]. In O. Rank (Ed.), *Essere felici* [Being happy] (pp. 5–12). Castelvecchi.

Marcuse, H. (1955). *Eros and civilization*. Beacon.

Marx, K. (2012). *Economic and philosophic manuscripts of 1844*. Start.

Marx, K., & Engels, F. (1976). *The German ideology*. Progress. (Original work published 1845)

Montuori, A. (2005). How to make enemies and influence people: Anatomy of the anti-pluralist, totalitarian mindset. *Futures, 37*, 18–38.

Obholzer, K. (1982). *The Wolf-Man: Conversations with Freud's Patient – sixty years later*. Burns & Oates.

Rachman, A. W. (2018), *Elizabeth Severn: The "Evil Genius" of psychoanalysis*. Routledge.

Ragen, T., & Aron, L. (1993). Abandoned workings: Ferenczi's mutual analysis. In L. Aron & A. Harris (Eds.), *The legacy of Sándor Ferenczi* (pp. 217–226). Analytic Press.

Rank, O. (1926). *Technik der Psychoanalyse* [Technique of psychoanalysis]. Deuticke.

Rank, O. (2010). *The trauma of birth*. Martino. (Original work published 1923)

Rank, O. (2012). *The double: A psychoanalytic study*. UNC. (Original work published 1914)

Rank, O. (2015). *The myth of the birth of the hero*. JHU. (Original work published 1909)

Reich, W. (1929). *Dialektischer Materialismus und Psychoanalyse* [Dialectical materialism and psychoanalysis]. Unter dem Banner des Marxismus.

Reich, W. (1931). Die charakterologische Überwindung des Ödipus-Komplexes [The characterological overcoming of the Oedipus complex]. *Internationale Zeitschrift für Psychoanalyse, 17*, 55–71.

Reich, W. (1945). *The sexual revolution*. Vision.

Reich, W. (1980). *Character analysis*. Macmillan. (Original work published 1933)

Reich, W. (2013a). *The mass psychology of fascism*. Farrar, Straus & Giroux. (Original work published 1933)

Reich, W. (2013b). *Sex-pol: Essays 1929–1934*. Verso.

Ricoeur, P. (1972). *Freud and philosophy: An essay on interpretation*. Yale University Press. (Original work published 1965)

Schafer, R. (1968). *Aspects of internalization*. International Universities Press.

Shapiro, S. (1993). Clara Thompson: Ferenczi's messenger with half a message. In L. Aron & A. Harris (Eds.), *The legacy of Sándor Ferenczi* (pp. 159–174). Analytic Press.

Sulloway, F. J. (1979). *Freud, biologist of the mind: Beyond the psychoanalytic legend*. Harvard University Press.

Vegetti Finzi, S. (1987). *Storia della psicoanalisi* [History of psychoanalysis]. Mondadori.

Wisdom, J. (1967). Testing an interpretation within a session. *International Review of Psychoanalysis, 48*, 44–52.

5

New approaches to psychotherapy before and after World War II

The various origins of group psychotherapy

What has been observed with regard to the origin of psychotherapy in a general sense can be repeated, and perhaps with greater emphasis, with regard to group psychotherapy specifically. Depending, in fact, on which element is considered decisive in defining the expression "group psychotherapy," it will be possible to identify very different dates of birth. Treatments involving groups can be considered as ancient as the shamanic magic tradition, since typically the shaman performed his rites involving the whole tribe (Alexander & Selesnick, 1966). As above mentioned, in classical Greece, the theater assumed a therapeutic role through catharsis, according to a perspective already clearly theorized by Aristotle. Both Mesmer and Emile Coué (1857–1926), a hypnotist of the Nancy School, held group sessions for their proto-psychotherapeutic treatments, but without considering groupality as a curative factor in itself.

It should be noted, however, that throughout the course of the 19th century, in psychology, the small group was not considered an object of research, as was the crowd. Different theories about the crowd spread, based on different interpretations of evolutionism. A primitive, regressed, and passionate mentality was considered typical of the crowd, and this psychology of the crowd did not concern the influence that the small group had on the individual, but rather the effect that the mass had in regressing individual behavior, dissolving many selves in the mass. In this sense, in France, the relationship that binds people to each other or to a leader had been investigated, and suggestion for the psychologists of the crowd was the main mechanism creating bonds. Similarly, Gabriel Tarde (1843–1904) had used the notion of conscious or unconscious imitation to explain the collective mind and describe how the members of a mass are interconnected (Van Ginneken, 1992). In this scientific tradition, for all psy-scientists, the crowd had regressive and incurable pathological characteristics. Only an almost forgotten Italian social psychologist, Pasquale Rossi (1867–1905), argued that the crowd could be educated (Rossi, 1898).

Only when the small group replaced the crowd as the object of study, during the 20th century and especially in Anglo-American countries, did psy-scientists

DOI: 10.4324/9781003252405-5

begin to consider the group as a key to new types of psychotherapy. Pioneering initiatives of the therapeutic use of the group with the aim of encouraging self-help among patients suffering from the same medical condition (tisics, psychotics, alcoholics, neurotics), led by doctors and mental health workers, are often reported in the literature. Generally, however, these techniques were paternalistic, sometimes authoritarian, and merely aimed at ensuring the smooth running of hospital departments.

The development of a working group for psychological help is usually traced back to the initiative of Joseph Hersey Pratt (1872–1956). Pratt was a doctor who organized sessions or classes for tuberculosis patients of 20 to 25 participants who met weekly (Pratt, 1907). The aim of the meetings was to raise morale by exchanging information on the physical improvements of each of the patients (Badolato & Di Iullo, 1979).

Freud was probably also the first psychotherapist to take an interest in group phenomena and to provide an interpretative and theoretical scheme that started from the observation of a common awareness of the influence of unconscious factors on group behavior (Freud, 1921/1955c). He pointed out that the less rational and more emotional behavior of human beings in a larger social context, previously explained through the phenomenon of suggestion, was precisely what needed to be explained. According to Freud, the key to interpreting group phenomena was to be found in the link between leader and group members, which consisted of love drives that, without operating less energetically, were diverted from their original goals. The basic mechanism that created group bonds was *identification*. In this sense, the members of the group put a single object (the leader) in place of the ego ideal, identifying with each other.

Freud never derived a therapeutic application for groups from his ideas. Several psychoanalysts tried to do so, however. Edward W. Lazell (1921), at Washington Hospital, assuming that schizophrenic patients were inaccessible to individual therapy, decided to give them a series of lectures on psychoanalysis. Finding significant participation by even the most apathetic patients, Lazell identified the socialization of issues such as sexuality and death as an important therapeutic factor. A similar approach was proposed a decade later in New York by L. Cody Marsh (1931), a doctor and priest. He did not use psychoanalysis but a kind of psychological equivalent of religious awakening. It was instead the psychoanalyst Nicholas Trigant Burrow (1875–1950) who developed the idea of *group analysis* from the Freudian theoretical framework. Burrow (1927) believed that intra-individual conflicts were in fact the reflection of interpersonal conflicts and that the group situation was the best way to highlight their dynamics and thus treat them. While Trigant Burrow shared Freud's view that society as such was neurotic, he believed that this fact was not unchangeable and was merely the result of adopting a code of behavior that excluded spontaneity and creativity from interpersonal relationships. This approach led him to conceive a group setting in which the therapist's personality was also brought into play, according to a vision that was widely developed later by the so-called

Encounter movement. Trigant Burrow wanted to place patient and doctor on the same horizontal and symmetrical plane, in the belief that the mutual analysis of the defense mechanisms among the members of the small circle was possible. In this way each participant, with the function of both analysand and analyst, would have helped to make emotions more tolerable and to heal from neurotic disorders all the members of the small group (Pertegato & Pertegato, 2013).

From the 1930s onward, a series of American psychoanalysts used the group setting but focused their treatment on the individual. Along these lines, Louis Wender (1889–1966) conceived of the group as a reenactment of the patient's family, in which the therapist was the parent and the group members represented siblings (Wender, 1936). In this case, group treatment typically alternated with individual treatment. Paul Schilder (1886–1940) brought together patients who were already being treated individually in groups to discuss specific issues, resulting in a decrease in the sense of personal isolation (Schilder, 1939). Samuel R. Slavson (1890–1981), who began his experiments around 1934, used the group for essentially practical reasons, linked to the unfavorable ratio between the number of therapists and the number of patients. He also highlighted an interesting effect of group therapy, which consisted in multilateral transference, that is, the possibility of projecting onto the group members the characters of other family members, such as brothers and sisters (Slavson, 1943).

A real diffusion of a psychoanalytically oriented psychotherapy focused on the group did not take place, however, until after World War II. Its forerunners were the works of Siegmund Heinrich Fuchs (1898–1976), known as Michael Foulkes, and Wilfred Ruprecht Bion (1897–1979). In the meantime, Alfred Adler (1930/2015) had already experimented with educational-therapeutic interventions on children in the presence of other children and their parents. A disciple of Adler, Rudolph Dreikurs (1897–1972), had in turn started to work with groups of adults in the 1920s, claiming that in reality he had done no more than apply principles that were implicit in the Adlerian approach (Dreikurs, 1956).

The true pioneer in this field, however, was probably Jacob Levi Moreno (1889–1974), unanimously recognized as the inventor of psychodrama. Moreno's experiences, which began in Freud's Vienna, were destined to influence the birth of group psychotherapy, co-therapy, couple therapy, self-help groups, family psychotherapy, and the therapeutic community (Blatner, 1995). Moreno, moreover, claimed the *invention* of the expression *group psychotherapy*, feeling the need to stress that he performed therapy and not simply a sociological or psychological analysis (Moreno, 1964).

Moreno and the "cradle of psychodrama"

An anecdote told by Moreno himself describes his alleged meeting with Sigmund Freud. Although it is impossible to assess its authenticity, the story clearly illustrates Moreno's histrionic personality and how his attitude was alternative to psychoanalysis:

> I met Dr. Freud only on one occasion. It occurred in 1912 when, while working at the Psychiatric Clinic in Vienna University, I attended one of his lectures. Dr. Freud had just ended his analysis of a telepathic dream. As the students filed out, he asked me what I was doing. "Well, Dr. Freud, I start where you leave off. You meet people in the artificial setting of your office. I meet them on the street and in their home, in their natural surroundings. You analyze their dreams. I try to give them the courage to dream again. I teach the people here to play God." Dr. Freud looked at me as if puzzled. But psychoanalysis had developed an atmosphere of fear among young people. Fear of neurosis was the measure of the day. A heroic gesture, a noble aspiration made its bearer immediately suspect.
>
> (Moreno, 1946, pp. 5–6)

Freud, moreover, constituted the main polemical target of Moreno, who formulated his theoretical proposals presenting himself as the counterbalance of psychoanalysis. Moreover, in pointing out the fundamental limits of Freudian thought, namely the rejection of religion and indifference to social movements (Moreno, 1946), Moreno simply neglected to note that in the first case Freud had already found an explicit alternative in Jung, and in the second, in Adler.

Among his sources of inspiration, Moreno mentioned Henri Bergson (1859–1941) and Charles Sanders Peirce (1839–1914), one of the founders of American pragmatism. They introduced the reflection on spontaneity into philosophical thought, although they remained spectators rather than actors. In his view, they "did not try to change the universe, merely to understand it" (Moreno, 1946, p. 9). Moreno's statement also clearly echoed the famous passage from *Theses on Feuerbach*, according to which "[t]he philosophers have only interpreted the world in various ways; the point is to change it" (Marx, 1845/1998, p. 101). But perhaps a mention of Marx in the United States, where he wrote *Psychodrama*, might have seemed politically inappropriate to him.

The beginnings of Moreno's activity, what he himself called the "cradle of psychodrama" (Moreno, 1946), can be traced back to his time at the University of Vienna, where he studied philosophy and medicine. It was here that Moreno used to take a stroll through the city's gardens between 1908 and 1911 and gather groups of children together to put on impromptu plays. In 1913, he took steps to bring Vienna's prostitutes together in a self-managed mutual aid organization. In 1914, he published *Invitation to an Encounter*, a "poetic piece of writing centered on the importance of being in contact and experiencing the relationship with the other with one's whole being" (Badolato & Di Iullo, 1979, p. 70). Between 1915 and 1917 (the year in which he finished his medical studies), Moreno became interested in the Tyrolean refugees in the Mittendorf camp, working to understand and facilitate their group relations.

According to Moreno, however, psychodrama as such had a real date of birth: April 1, 1921, between 7 and 10 p.m. (Moreno, 1946), at the Komödienhaus in Vienna. On this occasion, an experiment in theater was staged for the first time, in which neither a script nor actors were planned in advance. When the curtain rose, there was only a throne and a crown on the stage.

Moreno's proposal to the astonished spectators was that they themselves should represent the drama the world was experiencing by finding a person among them to act as ruler. Moreno's basic aspiration was in fact to "help society as a whole develop more effective forms of practical democracy, interpersonal freedom, and interactive creativity" (Blatner, 1995, p. 415). Neither this nor other attempts by Moreno to reintroduce improvisation theater in other contexts, in Austria and in the rest of Europe, were particularly successful and even attracted open criticism (which Moreno, moreover, dismissed with the words *nemo propheta in patria*). The situation changed when Moreno decided to emigrate to the United States in 1925 and to limit the application of his ideas to the treatment of mental disorders.

In the United States, Moreno found a mentality more open than the European one to accepting the use of action (fundamental in psychodrama) in a psychotherapeutic setting. Psychoanalysis classified the so-called *acting out* – a process in which the patient in psychotherapy *acts* the impulses and desires rather than *verbalizing* them – as being in itself symptomatic and dangerous to the integrity of the setting. Psychiatry only considered acting possible when carrying out precise instructions from the doctor, for example in *occupational therapy*. The development of psychodrama techniques was matched by an increasingly significant response, which led Moreno to open a sanatorium in Beacon in 1936, then a theater-institute in New York, and later to found the first professional organization oriented toward the use of group psychotherapy, the American Society for Group Therapy and Psychodrama. Until his death in 1974, Moreno remained the undisputed leader and theoretical-clinical reference point for psychodramatists.

Therapeutic elements of psychodrama

Moreno claimed to have "picked up the trend of thought from where Aristotle had left off" (Moreno, 1946, p. 14), paying attention to the therapeutic effect of the theater in order to change its mode of action. Aristotle, in fact, in *Poetics*, argues that the purpose of drama is to purify the spectators through the artistic excitement of certain emotions that function as a kind of relief from their personal passions (Moreno, 1940/1987b). On the contrary, psychodrama would have produced a therapeutic effect not in the spectator (this was a *secondary catharsis*) but in the people themselves who performed the drama and, at the same time, got rid of it (Moreno, 1923). This effect would have been determined by the fact that the action was based not on invented written texts but on real events, on the experience of the members of the group. Each of them shared with the others the story of autobiographical episodes of their lives and with their help re-enacted them. The therapeutic effect would be promoted not only by the action itself but also by the possibility of improvising new solutions, new possibilities of interaction in recalling the old problems. Moreno defined these two procedures as *catharsis of abreaction* and *catharsis of integration*, without the latter, the former had only a provisional value.

Among the key concepts of psychodrama theory, fundamental was *role theory* (Moreno, 1961/1987c), which had become central, one might say, in the social sciences in general (Mead, 1934; Merton, 1957). According to Moreno, the individual personality, the self, would be formed through the integration of a series of roles that each person was called upon to play, including the expectations of the interactive context in which they found themselves. When a person assumed a defined social role, like being, married, and chose a certain job, he would tend to identify with his role and behave as such (as Jung had illustrated it with the concept of the *persona*). Role-driven behavior tended to be static and lacking in spontaneity. Conflicts would become inevitable basically because, by avoiding spontaneity, a person would not be able to see alternative possibilities of conduct. Staging one's own life made it possible, according to Moreno, to assume the distance from the role that was a necessary condition for change.

As the relational modality within the therapeutic setting changed, so did the conception of transference in psychodrama theory, or rather, it was integrated. Moreno recognized the existence of transference as a projection onto the therapist of the patient's inner world. In his view, however, another process also took place "in that part of his ego which is not carried away by autosuggestion" (Moreno, 1946, p. 230): it was the *tele* (which in Greek means far), developed from the feelings individuals had toward others, estimating and assessing what kind of people they were. The tele was the result of affinity toward others, and the preference "has no neurotic motivations but is due to certain realities which this other person embodies and represents" (p. 229). According to Moreno, the tele was the cement that holds groups together: it phenomenologically anticipates transference and remains even when this is resolved; it stimulates stable association and permanent relationships. Ultimately, it constituted the decisive factor in therapeutic progress (Moreno, 1937/1987a). However much the therapist might have been trained to prevent countertransference (Moreno also expressed doubts about this), he could never have been in a position to prevent different tele relationships with different patients. What Moreno jokingly called *tele limitations* would be the reason why therapists could perform better with some patients and worse with others, regardless of their training.

Moreno, therefore, developed techniques that would allow the participants to act their dysfunctional conflicts and, through catharsis, to unblock themselves and improve their psychological state. In order for psychodrama to take place, several people had to be present. First of all, there had to be a *director*, corresponding to the therapist, who had to facilitate the staging and implement all the techniques aimed at achieving role distance and empathy. The *protagonist* occupied the center of attention (especially of the director) and usually played himself or a key person in his life. At least one *auxiliary ego* helped the protagonist, playing a role in interaction with him. The *audience* consisted of the other members of the therapeutic group, who could sometimes take on an active role individually or collectively (as a chorus). In order for psychodrama to take place, it was also necessary to use a *stage*. Moreno built real stages in the institutions he created; he emphasized the need to use at least a specific area prepared for theatrical action.

Each psychodrama-based psychotherapy session consisted of three phases. In the *warming up*, the therapist-director had to facilitate the interaction between the members of the group and make possible the participation of all the members. The choice of the protagonist of the actual *action* (the second phase) would be made by the group on the basis of maximum sharing in the *here and now* of the collective interest in the problem brought by an individual. During the action – that is, the psychodramatic representation of what was proposed by the protagonist – the therapist used a series of techniques to facilitate the acquisition of awareness by the protagonist, the mutual empathy of the group members, and ultimately catharsis. The most classic techniques invented by Moreno were the *double*, the *mirror*, the *soliloquy*, and the *role reversal*. The double and the mirror allowed the protagonist to understand how others saw him or imagined he was feeling (in the first case, an auxiliary verbalized what he thought the protagonist was thinking or should say, in the second case, the protagonist momentarily left the scene, and his role was taken by an auxiliary). The possibility of soliloquy was suggested by the director to a protagonist in difficulty to explore and verbalize his emotions. Role reversal, on the other hand, allowed the protagonist to explore what he thought the internal world of the person momentarily played by the auxiliary ego expressed. The *cooling-off* phase involved sharing with the group what had been experienced, by both the protagonist and the auxiliaries, and by those who had not participated on stage (group echoes). This was followed by a final discussion. Thus, in classical Morenian psychodrama, the therapist-director was not expected to make use of interpretation.

Similar to psychodrama was *sociodrama*, where collective roles (parent, employer, etc.) were enacted and not specific to personal experience. Only after many years, with the contamination between psychodrama and psychoanalysis and the birth of the so-called *analytical psychodrama*, would the therapist introduce interpretive interventions in the last phase of the session.[1]

Kurt Lewin: a hidden source

Among the sources of group psychotherapy we must remember Kurt Lewin (1890–1947), one of the most influential psychologists of the first half of the 20th century, a unique scholar because, although he was not a psychotherapist, he developed a series of epistemological concepts that profoundly influenced various psychotherapeutic applications, both group and individual. His name will recur several times in the following pages.

Paradoxically, Moreno accused Lewin of plagiarizing his sociometric movement (1953). Actually, Lewin did not have a psychotherapeutic background and came to his own elaborations in an independent way. He studied in Berlin at the Institute of Psychology directed by Carl Stumpf (1848–1936) and was therefore influenced by Gestalt psychology, but also by the philosophy of symbolic forms of Ernst Cassirer (1874–1945), by the logical neo-positivism of Hans Reichenbach (1891–1953), and by the critical Western Marxism of Karl Korsch (1886–1961). During World War I, he volunteered in the army and wrote an essay entitled *The War Landscape* in which his concept of living space was already sketched. In a later period, Lewin theoretically investigated the scientific organization of work, and in 1920 he wrote *Socializing the Taylor System*. In this work he presented a critical analysis of applied psychology, seen as an expression of the entrepreneurial culture of the 20th century, from a socialist point of view. The *internal* or psychological value of work was distinct from the *external* value of classical economics. The concrete objective of psychology was therefore to intervene positively in the working condition, to achieve worker satisfaction and the humanization of the factory, not productivity or added value (see Ash, 1998; Mecacci, 1992). In the 1930s, Lewin published some important contributions on personality that in the United States were collected in the volumes *A Dynamic Theory of Personality* (1935) and *Principles of Topological Psychology* (1936). Close to Frankfurt scholars, during Nazism he was one of the psychologists forced to leave Germany and emigrate to America. In 1939, Lewin and Korsch presented a communication to the Fifth International Congress for the Unity of Science held in Cambridge (MA), *Mathematical Constructs in Psychology and Sociology*. It stated that psychology and sociology had made only embryonic use of the mathematics underlying their research. In psychology, as in sociology, a transition from the descriptive to the dynamic stage was desirable, resulting in the development of new mathematical constructs. Lewin criticized the "Aristotelian" use of measurement in psychology, which primarily used the correlational method. The analysis of correlations between psychological variables was considered merely descriptive and juxtapositional. It said nothing about interdependence and the transformative dynamics that such interdependence exerted on phenomena. It was necessary to move from data collection to the study of dynamic functions and pragmatic transformations. For Lewin (1931), psychology needed to move from an "Aristotelian" to a "Galilean" level of inquiry. A starting point for mathematization would be provided by *field theory* (which considered individual action to be always a function of context) and the materialistic conception of history in the social sciences. Development, personality, economy, society, and politics would be interdependent phenomena (Lewin & Korsch, 1939). In fact, the very idea of a psychology of individual character or personality was not appropriate, because the object of investigation was not to be the isolated individual but the person in a situation. Lewin distinguished between a "being-thus" (*Sosein*) and a "being-there" (*Dasein*). The research proceeded from the being-thus of the individual empirical case and led to the causes represented by the being-there (Danziger, 1990).

For Danziger (1990), in the Lewinian perspective, personality or character as reified static entities were replaced by types of psychological contexts considered real objects of psychological inquiry. In *A Dynamic Theory of Personality*, the theme of the evolution of the dynamic structures of personality was included in a conceptualization that considered the individual to be the product of the interaction between motivational dimensions and his context or, precisely, the psychological field, within a temporal dimension characterized above all by the *principle of contemporaneity*. In Lewin's elaboration, therefore, the analysis of the space in which the motivational processes that qualify the person in relation to the goals that this sets itself assumed particular importance (Lewin, 1935). In *A Dynamic Theory of Personality* were therefore contained the methodological orientations of Lewin on the scientific understanding of the individual and also the fundamental notions concerning the psychological field and the principle of contemporaneity that would be codified in the following paper, *Principles of Topological Psychology* (1936).

In these writings Lewin elaborated the so-called universal equation of behavior:

$$B = f(P, E)$$

Behavior (B) was a function (f) of the person (P) and the environment (E). In Lewin's theory of personality, the environment retained a fundamental value and specific determinant of behavior. It was not to be understood as a generic set of elements surrounding the individual but as a context perceived by him. In *Field Theory of Learning*, Lewin (1942) listed instead some distinctive foundations of field theory: the method, which should be genetic, never classificatory, and as such gives an account of how a people construct themselves in a concrete environment; the dynamic setting, directed at identifying the forces that determine actions in specific contexts; the psychological setting, whereby the field concretely resulted as the space perceived by the individual in contemporaneity; and the analysis of the situation as a starting point, whereby the researcher assumed the totality of a situation as the initial moment and then analyzed and deepened the elements of the totality. Behavior was to be interpreted as a function of the field that presented itself from time to time, so the past was only one of the determinations of action in the present. The psychologist should have primarily had as his goal the knowledge of the determinants of behavior, seen in its contemporaneity. The final result should have been the mathematical representation of the psychological situation, since for Lewin the person in a situation needed to be rigorously described, by means of topological notions and vector qualities.

As mentioned above, Lewin emigrated to the United States because of the racial persecution of the Nazis. In 1945 he founded at the Massachusetts Institute of Technology the first research center on small group dynamics (Lewin, 1945). The Gestaltist approach pushed him to study groups as entities whose nature is different from the sum of individuals and to observe how the group influences the behavior of individuals more than any other individual learning condition. Lewin thus inaugurated a long season of training groups (or T-groups) to promote cohesion and the solution of problems related to discrimination and prejudice (but also to the modification of habits, increased productivity, etc.) between members belonging to institutional or social groups (work, school, university). In training groups he employed practices that facilitated communication, expression of emotions and mirroring between members of groups, consisting of up to fifteen people. In addition to role playing and problem solving, feedback was used in T-groups, or the sharing of impressions aroused by other group members in the sessions. These expressive techniques were thus originally used in non-therapeutic contexts: the T-groups were always directed by a guide or facilitator who promoted spontaneity but did not try to *cure*. However, T-groups were later integrated into the group psychotherapy of various theoretical orientations. In particular, they became the backbone of the Rogersian groups, which in the Sixties were spread by the so-called "Encounter" movement, and were aimed at the development of the human potential of the participants (Rogers, Mintz, Schutz) (Rogers, 1970; see also Back, 1987; Badolato & Di Iullo, 1979).

Ludwig Binswanger and the birth of *Daseinsanalyse*

As mentioned above, Ludwig Binswanger had met Freud in 1907 together with Jung. A positive human relationship was immediately established between Freud and Binswanger, documented in an exchange of letters that lasted until Freud's death (Fichtner & Pomerans, 2003) and recalled in Binswanger's moving testimony (1936). Although Binswanger was the only member of the Swiss group who did not follow Jung in his secession from the psychoanalytic movement, his position with regard to psychoanalytic doctrine was destined to become very eccentric. In 1917, Freud, on receiving a (lost) piece of writing by Binswanger, addressed him with some alarm: "What are you proposing to do about the unconscious, or rather, how will you manage without the unconscious? Does the philosophical devil finally got you in his clutches?" (Freud to Binswanger, 8/20/2017, in Fichtner & Pomerans, 2003 p. 139).

In fact, it was the "devil of philosophy" that influenced Binswanger in his progressive march away from orthodox psychoanalysis toward the creation of an original theory, namely "existential analysis" (*Daseinsanalyse*). The reading of authors such as Søren A. Kierkegaard (1813–1855), Edmund Husserl (1859–1938), and Martin Heidegger (1889–1976), who determined the birth of phenomenology and existentialism, was decisive in Binswanger's path, alongside Freudian texts.

Kierkegaard was the first to enucleate the philosophical value of the concepts of anxiety and despair, which lost their marginal and pathological connotations to assume a fundamental feature within existence (Innamorati, 1993). The depth of a human being's spirit would be a function of the capacity to feel anxiety in the face of the meaninglessness of existence. Despair was merely the logical consequence of the impossibility of finding satisfaction in both the aesthetic stage (the search for pleasure in a single moment of enjoyment) and the ethical stage (the search for pleasure in the repetition of the same experience) of life. Kierkegaard was also a key thinker in overcoming the objective conception of truth (as expressed at its peak in Hegel). Truth, for Kierkegaard, made sense only for its subjective value, as Binswanger (1930/1963a) fully recognized.

Husserl was (like Freud!) a pupil of Franz Brentano, from whom he borrowed the concept of intentionality as a characteristic of all psychic processes. From this point of view, what distinguished an intentional process was its being necessarily in reference to something else. Human consciousness would therefore always be expressible as consciousness-of or reference-to. The foundation of knowledge was therefore to be based on phenomenology, that is, on the analysis of the immanent perception of experience (Husserl, 1913/2012). The phenomenological method, by means of the suspension of judgment (*epoché*), made it possible to overcome the naive realism of the sciences and to understand the true nature of their data, which would claim to be objective, as an expression of human consciousness. In this sense, phenomenology constituted the study of the conditions of possibility of consciousness and therefore preceded psychology. Husserl's phenomenology was also the product of a reworking of Brentano's phenomenological psychology, a very important source for the origins of psy-sciences. In fact, the historiography of psychology tends to underestimate Brentano's work. On the other hand, Mecacci (1992) has rightly reconstructed how the different introspections, Wundt's experimental and Brentano's phenomenological, promoted different methodological points of view in 20th-century psychology. Apart from Husserl, many of his pupils were Gestaltists and phenomenologists. As we have seen, even Freud followed his lessons, and it is not clear how much he was influenced by the Austrian psychologist. Certainly, the theory of intentional relation seems to provide a theoretical context on which then relational theories were described. Even the theory of transference may have been a creative reworking of the notion of intentionality.

Husserl and Kierkegaard were also the main sources for Heidegger, especially in *Being and Time* (Heidegger, 1927/2010), in his analytics of human existence. This is understood as *being-there* (*Dasein*), that is, being in the world in a situation, the premises of which it was necessary to understand as the foundation of any knowledge. The human being was in a condition of "thrownness": it was a kind of project that was precisely "thrown" into the world, in an inevitable relationship with others. The being-there was therefore also a *being-with* (*Mitsein*). But the being-there also had another fundamental characteristic, that of *being-toward-death*.

Anguish, despair, consciousness as a reference to another, subjective truth, and existence as thrownness were therefore not existential data that belonged to pathology, but constituted the ontological foundation of the human being as such, the foundation of man's spiritual being, which for Binswanger was the premise for understanding the humanity of his patients. As Eugenio Borgna wrote:

> *Daseinsanalyse* has shown how psychological illness can no longer be considered a "natural event" but must be recognized as an original possibility of the human condition: marked, that is, by the same fundamental structures, albeit in their metamorphosis, of corporality, temporality, spatiality, and being-in-the-world with others-from-self in an inexhaustible circularity of experiences and perceptions.
>
> (Borgna, 2006, p. 9)

Through Binswanger, then, spirit re-enters psychotherapy but, his "notion of spirit (. . .) could only have emerged after Freud" (Needleman, 1963, p. 4). The psychiatry of the world in which Freud began his work was marked, according to Binswanger, by full adherence to the creed of Wilhelm Griesinger (1817–1868), for whom mental illnesses were brain diseases and psychological phenomena could be described in a naturalistic way, as organic phenomena (Griesinger, 1845). Psychoanalysis presented itself, for the early Binswanger (1909, 1911), as a completely different clinical approach, open to the humanity of the patient, although the Swiss never seemed fully convinced of Freud's theoretical viewpoint (Molaro, 2016). Binswanger's perplexities were already quite evident in the speech presented at the Psychoanalytic Congress of The Hague (Binswanger, 1920) and were certainly not dispelled in the subsequent *Introduction to the Problems of General Psychology* (Binswanger, 1922), rather lukewarmly received by Freud (Freud to Binswanger, 2/7/1923, in Fichtner & Pomerans, 2003, pp. 162–162). Certainly, it is significant that the *Introduction* was to be the first part of a two-volume work, the second of which was specifically to deal with psychoanalytic theory, but was never written. The initial intention to "do justice to basic psychoanalytic ideas in an historical sense as well," expressed in a letter from Binswanger to Freud dated 7 January 1920 (Fichtner & Pomerans, 2003, p. 148), was no longer of interest to Binswanger.

That Binswanger wanted to take a completely personal path is already evident from that sort of fundamental *ballon d'essai* constituted by the work *Dream and Existence* (Binswanger, 1930/1963a). Here Binswanger proposed a theory of dream interpretation that differed both from the Freudian one (based on the idea of unconscious desire) and from the Jungian one, in which Binswanger found contradictions, especially in the reference to the collective unconscious. Rather than from the drive world or the common inheritance of primordial experiences, Binswanger assumed that the dream originated "out of language itself" (p. 222). The dream, then (following a much more Jungian procedure than Binswanger admits), was interpreted with an emphasis on the manifest content, rather than the presumed latent content. With attention to the possible correspondence between the characters and the possible opposing tendencies of the dreamer. Its spiritual dimension could in no way be reduced to pure instinct. Binswanger, instead of preventing the possible criticism of excessive accentuation of the philosophical aspects in his thought, tended to turn them into a sort of manifesto:

> It would be rather unfortunate if our patients had to understand Heraclitus or Hegel in order to get well, but none can attain genuine health unless the physician succeeds in awakening in him that spark of mind that must be awake in order for the person to feel the slightest breath of koinòs cosmós (common universe).
>
> (Binswanger, 1930/1963a, p. 244)

In this sense there was a real reversal of Freudian positions on spiritual life, understood as a sublimation of drives: "interpretations that are either one-sidedly biological or that misguidedly view the spirit as an enemy of life" can be considered "a fraud and a self-conceit" (p. 243).

Freud's thought was then gradually identified by Binswanger both as the turning point toward the overcoming of the "depersonalization of man" (Binswanger, 1936/1963c p. 189), typical of classical psychiatry, and as a burden to be discarded in order to overcome the conception of man as a purely instinctual being. Freud was thus transformed into the most consistent theorist of man as *homo natura*:

> One might even formally express Freud's whole life by stating that the idea of *homo natura* can lead to the possibility of expressing psychic processes in a mathematical functional equation. Freud succeeded in demonstrating a mechanism at work in what was apparently the freest reaches of the human mind, thereby creating the possibility of mechanically "repairing" the mind (with the psychoanalytic techniques of unmasking and annulling repression and regression by means of the transference mechanism).
>
> (Binswanger, 1936/1963b, pp. 163–164)

In this light, even desire becomes a physical, material thing: "Wishing is not constitutive of mankind as such, however constitutive it may in fact be for the psychic apparatus built into *homo natura*" (p. 164).

If, however, through psychoanalysis one could arrive at a coherently scientific knowledge of man, as Binswanger believed, such knowledge did not exhaust what reason could discover. And on the other hand, even a philosophical knowledge, by itself, would have been as one-sided as a purely scientific knowledge:

> Certainly science, and particularly natural science, is not and ought not to be prohibited from illuminating all regions of being, including human

being. It must, however, realize that all modes of human existence and experience are autonomous (. . .). Every form that reason takes may be exposed to criticism (. . .). Each of these modes of apprehending being represents an essential form of human existence.

(Binswanger, 1936/1963b, pp. 172–173)

Binswanger, however, always continued to recognize the momentous role of Freud's thought. Before his advent, man lived in a world of consciousness with secure boundaries, but he showed how limited this world was by how little we could influence it. Moreover, the fact that he had not only thought, but also experienced and represented in detail, the subject as a natural process related to other natural processes was responsible for the transformation of our knowledge of the human being and our idea of scientificity (Binswanger, 1957).

Little Hans and the birth of child psychoanalysis

Children represented a new category of people at whom psychological and educational sciences had begun to look with interest in the late nineteenth and early twentieth centuries. The target was partly solving social problems, such as illiteracy, in the context of the modernization of educational institutions in the new liberal states. The first signs of this renewed interest were the pedagogical models inspired by positivism and, in psychology, the mental tests that had been perfected for the first time in the first decade of the new century (Cicciola, 2019; Foschi & Cicciola, 2006).

In most cases, the child continued to be seen, as in the past, as an adult in a state of development. In the positivist environment, children, women, southerners, ethnic groups different from the European one, and, finally, the insane shared the same fate. They were all considered inferior individuals, closer to the animal world than the white man of the north, and therefore presented the need for orthopedic interventions that would favor a socially desirable path of development. In this sense, Freud's perverse-polymorphic children were no exception: they represented an immature being, lacking a value system and at the mercy of drives, which only with growth would be placed under the control of the ego (see Guarnieri, 2006).

Sigmund Freud, however, despite the ample space devoted in his writings to theories of child development, never directly applied the analysis to children and indeed almost never devoted himself to their observation. The episodes of childhood life reported in Freud's works refer mainly to memories and associations of adult patients: in two cases to childhood memories of two illustrious figures from the past, namely Leonardo (Freud, 1910/1957a) and Goethe (Freud, 1917/1955b); or to his own family members. The only true Freudian clinical case relating to a child is that of little Hans (Freud, 1909/1955a). Little Hans was the son of one of Freud's pupils, Max Graf (1873–1958), and it was the latter who observed the course of his son's phobia toward horses. Freud met little Hans only once during his childhood neurosis, when he saw him with his father. When Hans returned to meet him, he was already nineteen years old and apparently no longer retained any memory of his former fears. Hans's phobia was considered to be the result of the displacement onto horses of the fear toward his father, linked to the castration anxiety, characteristic of the Oedipus complex in full bloom.

The treatment of Hans consisted in the progressive facilitation by his father of "confessing" his thoughts, under Freud's supervision. Also, the case of little Árpád, recounted by Ferenczi, was the result of observation rather than of an actual treatment. Árpád showed a phobia of roosters and in turn implemented a behavior of imitation of the same animals, coinciding with Oedipal concerns. In fact, after being pecked by a rooster on his penis around the age of two and a half, the child had not shown any abnormal behavior, according to his parents, until he had shown a certain interest in manipulating his own genitals, followed by the threat of possible castration if he did not cease his unacceptable behavior – a threat that was not uncommon in the education of the time (Ferenczi, 1913). Ferenczi himself, on the other hand, far from foreseeing the possibility of actual child analysis, had simply defined as "not impossible" an educational science that would aim to prevent neurosis by exerting some influence on infants (Ferenczi, 1908/1994a). This was certainly not the manifestation of an optimistic attitude.

In publishing the account of Hans's story, Freud was far from thinking that child analysis could become a universally applicable procedure. He seemed convinced of the contrary when he affirmed:

> It was only because the authority of a father and of a physician were united in a single person, and because in him both affectionate care and scientific interest were combined, that it was possible in this one instance to apply the method to a use to which it would not otherwise have lent itself.
>
> (Freud, 1909/1955a, p. 5)

A few years later, he was no less skeptical about the cognitive results that the analysis of the child could present:

> An analysis which is conducted upon a neurotic child itself must, as a matter of course, appear to be more trustworthy, but it cannot be very rich in material; too many words and thoughts have to be lent to the child, and even so the deepest strata may turn out to be impenetrable to consciousness.
>
> (Freud, 1914/1957b, pp. 8–9)

Freud, however, hoped instead for the possible role of some specifically female figure in supporting psychoanalytically oriented children. In fact, he wrote to Binswanger on 5 January 1909:

> This letter carries what is still a hypothetical question but one that may soon become of practical importance: would your clinic be able to take

children (from about eight years onwards) who need psychic treatment of our kind, i.e., do you have nurses whom you feel you can trust yourself to train for this, as the physician himself will not have an easy time with this kind of treatment?

(Fichtner & Pomerans, 2003, p. 3)

This orientation of Freud's could be the reason why the first protagonists of the use of psychoanalysis with children were all women: Hermine Hug-Hellmuth (1871–1924), Melanie Klein (1882–1960), and Sigmund's daughter, Anna Freud. In any case, the father of psychoanalysis had in mind to try treatments on children who had already reached the age of latency and considered possible the use of paramedical or "para-psychoanalytical" staff. He could not foresee the enormous development that child psychoanalysis was destined to experience in a few years' time.

The real pioneer in this field was Hug-Hellmuth, a character unjustly, albeit understandably, neglected by historians, especially psychoanalysts. Despite her undoubted merits, in fact, Hug-Hellmuth was hit by two different scandals and her name became a source of embarrassment for the psychoanalytic movement. Her beginnings were marked by an interesting paradox: the individual who initiated her into psychoanalytic studies was Isidor Sadger (1867–1942), one of the first members of the Vienna Society and the very person who had initially fought against the possibility of women being admitted. Hug-Hellmuth began her work with children along the lines that had been imagined by Sigmund Freud and that would later be followed by his daughter Anna: help for children in difficulty was based on an intervention of a primarily educational nature, in which transference was not even considered possible. Having started her own clinical experience, Hug-Hellmuth wrote a text that obtained immediate success, the so-called *A Young Girl's Diary*. The booklet, however, was published anonymously and pretended to have been written by a young girl who witnessed the awakening of her sexuality according to a path that seemed to resoundingly confirm Freudian theories (Hug-Hellmuth, 1919/1971). The forgery was discovered, however, because the style in which the text was written betrayed a control of concepts and language that could only belong to an adult.[2]

Despite the misstep, she continued her own work, which found historically significant fruit in the first paper (Hug-Hellmuth, 1921) and the first book (Hug-Hellmuth, 1924) devoted to the application of psychoanalysis to children. Unfortunately, the author did not survive long: in 1924 she died, strangled by her nephew Rolf, a young thug who wanted to extort money from her. Hug-Hellmuth probably feared that such a circumstance would occur, because in her last will was found the explicit request that no one would write an obituary after her death (so that the psychoanalytic environment would not be placed in difficulty). So she was recalled for what happened to her rather than for what she wrote, at least until relatively recent times (Appignanesi & Forrester, 1992).

Melanie Klein (1882–1960) is therefore usually remembered as the first analyst of childhood: she herself, after all, tried to accredit herself as such by devaluing the real importance of her colleague's contribution (see Klein, 1955). About Hug-Hellmuth, however, Klein wrote:

> She makes it very clear that she deprecated the idea of analyzing very young children, that she considered it necessary to content oneself with "partial success" and not to penetrate too deep in analysis with children, for fear of stirring up too powerfully the repressed tendencies and impulses or of making demands which their power of assimilation are unable to meet.
>
> (Klein, 1927/1948c, p. 153)

These are, in fact, the same criticisms that Klein believed she could make to Anna Freud, with whom she had a heated disagreement, which led to the first major theoretical conflict within the International Psychoanalytic Association not to end with the exodus of one of the two parties involved. In any case, for the history of the psychoanalytic movement, Klein's contribution represented an enormously significant turning point, whatever evaluation one might propose of her work.

Melanie Klein: play and therapy

Melanie Klein was born in Vienna in 1882, but read Freud for the first time only after moving to Budapest in 1910. Married at the age of twenty-one, from marriage until the age of twenty-eight she lived in small towns in Slovakia and Silesia following her husband. In Budapest she entered into analysis with Ferenczi and continued training with him for years. Klein began to discover a real vocation for psychoanalysis: she decided not to follow her husband who moved again for work (to Sweden) and read a first report on child development at the Psychoanalytic Society of Budapest, into which she was admitted. In 1920, having received strong encouragement from Karl Abraham at the Psychoanalytic Congress in The Hague, she decided to move to Berlin, and later to undergo analysis with him as well. Unfortunately, the analysis with Abraham, begun in 1924, ended after nine months following the death of the latter. After Abraham's death, the Berlin psychoanalytic milieu seemed to be much less receptive to Klein. A third member of Freud's committee then entered her life. Klein met Ernest Jones in 1925 and also found appreciation from him about her work: she would end up being his children's analyst (Grosskurth, 1986). She thus moved in 1926 to England, where she acquired an important following and remained for the rest of her life.

At her debut on the scene of the psychoanalytic movement, even Melanie Klein seemed convinced that the role of psychoanalysis in the developmental age should consist essentially in directing toward sex education: "We can spare the child unnecessary repression by freeing (. . .) the whole wide sphere of sexuality from the dense veils of secrecy, falsehood and danger spun by a hypocritical civilization upon an affective and uninformed foundation" Klein, 1921/1948a, p. 13).

The turning point in Melanie Klein's work occurred when she decided to focus her attention on play. Sporadically, Freud (1917/1995b), Abraham (1911/1937), and Ferenczi (1908/1994a) had all offered observations on the unconscious significance of infantile play. Hug-Hellmuth (1921) had also used play and drawing as means of entering into confidence with the child to be treated, but had not gone so far as to develop an actual technique. Beginning in 1923, however, Klein noticed that interpreting play (or inhibition of play) seemed to provide relief from anxiety to children. For example, Melanie Klein suggested to little Rita that her reluctance to play was determined by her fear of being alone with a stranger in a room, and that this fear constituted a concern already present in her life. Rita was relieved and began to play more spontaneously (Klein, 1955; see also Klein, 1932/1960). It seemed evident that: (a) the play reflected unconscious concerns; (b) interpretation was appropriate even with young children, since it alleviated the effect of such concerns; and (c) the content of the interpretation reflected negative transference thoughts (in other words, transference toward the therapist was present even at an early age). In summary: "Like resistance to free associations of adults, (. . .) inhibitions of free play can be resolved when the underlying anxiety is lessened by interpretation" (Segal, 1979, p. 33).

Klein expounded extensively on the ideas she was developing about the technique of play in *The Psychological Principles of Infant Analysis* (Klein, 1926/1948b), and then in the subsequent book *The Psycho-Analysis of Children* (Klein, 1932/1960), which built on the concepts set out in the previous article. The environment in which child analysis sessions took place assumed paramount importance. The space was furnished in such a way that children could move freely and, if necessary, express aggression without hurting themselves. There were materials suitable for games (especially "make-believe" games): a sofa with small cushions, a sink with running water, containers, rags for cleaning, small toys, including human figures, vehicles and animals arranged on a low table. Even highly inhibited children would have been led, according to Klein, to observe and touch the toys. Their way of behaving would therefore immediately offer elements to begin to understand their psychical life. Instead of verbalizing, the child tended to act, through play. Action, which was more primitive than thought and speech, constituted the predominant part of infantile behavior. The role of play in the analysis of children could be compared to the role of dreams in the analysis of adults: "Just as associations to dream elements lead to the uncovering of the latent content of the dream, so do the elements of children's play which correspond to those associations afford a view of its latent meaning" (Klein, 1932/1960, p. 43).

There is no doubt that the technique of play in psychotherapy with children is an instrument now definitively acquired and used by the most diverse schools.

The reason why, since the Berlin period, "wherever Melanie Klein went, feelings ran high" (Gay, 1988, p. 468) was her extremely direct way of interpreting, aimed at making the fundamental themes of the child's psychical life conscious. That is to say: to touch on themes such as parental sexuality, jealousy toward brothers and sisters, and the death wish toward relatives. A clinical vignette may clearly illustrate the Kleinian way of verbalizing interpretations:

> At the very beginning of his first hour Peter took the toy carriages and cars and put them first one behind the other and then side by side, and alternated this arrangement several times. He also took a horse and carriage and bumped it into another, so that the horses' feet knocked together, and said: "I've got a new little brother called Fritz." I asked him what the carriages were doing. He answered: "That's not nice," and stopped bumping them together at once, but started again quite soon. Then he knocked two toy horses together in the same way, upon which I said: "Look here, the horses are two people bumping together." At first he said: "No, that's not nice," but then, "Yes, that's two people bumping together," and added: "The horses have bumped together too, and now they're going to sleep." Then he covered them up with bricks and said: "Now they're quite dead; I've buried them."
>
> (Klein, 1932/1960, p. 41)

This direct and at times almost brutal approach remained a constant in Klein's work. From Klein's point of view, the disturbed child was prey to unconscious fantasies that gave rise to persecutory anxieties, the interpretation of which, precisely because it was explicit and direct, aroused immediate relief. The relief was visible in the child's attitude, which manifested itself in a more varied and less inhibited play activity, which opened up to further interpretations in a virtuous circle. For this reason, "the analyst should not be afraid of making a deep interpretation even at the start of the analysis, since the material belonging to the deep layers of the mind will come back again later and be worked through" (p. 50).

If anything, it can be argued, on the basis of one of her followers (Meltzer, 1978), that in her work with children in latency Klein even tried to arouse at the beginning of therapy those persecutory anxieties that they felt more easily from the beginning, not least because of the situation (the unnatural presence in a foreign environment with a stranger). When, for example, little Richard began a session talking about the possibility that British ships were trapped by the Germans, close to taking Gibraltar (in 1940), Klein replied that his real thoughts were different. In reality, he was concerned "about what might happen to Daddy when he put his genital into Mummy. Daddy might not be able to get out of Mummy's inside and would be caught there, like the ships in the Mediterranean" (Klein, 1961, p. 28). In fact, Klein pointed out that latency-aged children, compared to younger children, presented particular difficulties of analysis, linked to less imagination, less willingness to play, less openness to the possibility of being cared for, less tendency to talk about oneself (parallel to the struggle with oneself to avoid masturbation). Klein suggested that one could make up for this with greater willingness to draw and a spontaneous tendency to substitute playful activity with toys for acting out roles, which would naturally enact Oedipal fantasies. Even a greater capacity for association would have made up for the technical problems and an ego not yet fully developed. During puberty, "we once again meet with a greater dominance of the emotions and the unconscious and a much richer life of the imagination" (Klein, 1932/1960, p. 122). Even the age of puberty, however, presented its peculiar difficulties, related to the characteristic attitude of defiance (the result of overcompensation of anxiety) that often led the young patient to want to abandon therapy. Fantasy activity was also less recognizable and less easily interpreted, as it was linked to activities "more adapted to reality" and to the "stronger ego interests" of teenagers (p. 124) such as sport activities.

Developmental theory and object relations

A pupil of Ferenczi and Abraham and supported by Jones, it is not surprising that Melanie Klein could consider herself a faithful follower of Freud and claim to have only consistently developed Freudian ideas. This conviction was so deep-rooted that it caused in her a naive and genuine disappointment when Sigmund Freud took a position in favor of his daughter Anna in the heated theoretical dispute between the two. It is certainly true that Klein was the first analyst to accept and actively use the Freudian concept of death drive, making it one of the focal points of her own theoretical construction: aggression assumed a central motivational role in Klein's vision. Most of Freud's followers, on the contrary, were very reluctant to follow him "beyond the pleasure principle" and within this majority should be included Ernest Jones himself. One can therefore understand his embarrassment: "I yield to no one in my admiration of Freud's genius" (Jones, 1948, p. 10), he wrote, and "I find it a little odd that I should be criticizing her for a too faithful adherence to Freud's views" (p. 12).

Kleinian theory soon assumed, however, connotations of profound originality with respect to classical psychoanalysis, to the point of being considered, by some, one of the decisive turning points toward a genuine paradigm shift toward the so-called *relational/structure model* (Greenberg & Mitchell, 1983).

The developmental theory advocated by Melanie Klein was not an alternative to the Freudian model, presenting itself as a kind of integration. Its connotations, however, actually changed the basic ideas of psychoanalysis. The fantasies of very young children, in the Kleinian view, made it possible to argue that the Oedipus complex manifested itself at a very early age. The child's states of anxiety would have originated in the fear of aggression toward the parents and would have derived from the superego (whose debut on the developmental scene was also anticipated by Klein). The infant would have reacted in fantasy to his own aggressiveness and to the damage it might have caused as if he had suffered from an internal conflict concerning the superego. Then paranoid cycles would be observed, that is, recurrent states of aggression and anxiety: the child would stage terrible fantasies in which spirals of aggression would manifest themselves.

Melanie Klein (1935/1948d, 1946/1975) thus ended up theorizing that the very first months of life were already marked by two different ways of approaching reality. She called them *positions*, rather than phases or stages of development. In the Freudian view, a stage, once passed, did not return in the individual history, although conditions of exception (pathological) were possible. According to Klein, on the other hand, the *paranoid-schizoid position* was the initial condition of psychological life and was replaced by the *depressive position* around the age of six months in a way that was far from definitive. The whole of existence would be marked by the possibility of regressing to the most primitive position and returning to the most advanced position, without these movements necessarily signaling the onset of a neurotic condition. When coming into the world, the human being would have been marked by a turbulent psychological life, characterized by unconscious fantasies about his own needs and difficulties. The Kleinian child moved between moments of hunger and satiety, experienced respectively as the presence of a bad maternal breast and a good maternal breast, considered different and separate (hence the prefix schizo-). The bad breast would have been considered sadistic (hence the root -paranoid) and the child would have fantasized about attacking and destroying it with his own feces. At around the sixth month of life, the infant would finally understand that good and bad breasts were not separate partial objects but belonged to a single whole object, namely the mother. This new position was defined as depressive because the infant felt a sense of guilt for his destructive fantasies toward the bad breast: he/she feared having damaged the mother. The dynamic of affections was radically modified because "not until the object is loved as a whole can its loss be felt as a whole" (Klein, 1935/1948d, p. 284).

The certainty of being confronted with a whole object would not be definitively acquired, however, and the infants would move again and again between the depressive and the paranoid-schizoid positions, when they felt (in moments of suffering) prey to the attack of part-objects, until they thought of their mother as a unique being and felt new feelings of guilt for the attacks fantasized against her. It should be noted that both positions would have originated during the oral phase, and that there was no clear differentiation between oral and anal tendencies: the expulsion of the bad object or the attack against it could have been fantasized either through the mouth or through the urethral organs and the anus.

The problems of infantile positions would not have stopped at early childhood, because "[i]n normal mourning, as well as in abnormal mourning and in manic-depressive states, the infantile depressive position is reactivated" (Klein,

1940/1948e, p. 337). Moreover, the adult who employed the defense mechanism of splitting would unconsciously re-enact the schizo-paranoid position. Those who employed splitting, in fact, were unable to tolerate the fact that the same person could have positive and negative sides, could behave in a way that was not perfectly consistent. The result was to see the other (or oneself) as perfectly good or as completely bad, behaving accordingly. In the Kleinian vision, this meant enacting unconscious fantasies of relationships with partial objects, comparable to the perfectly satisfying good breast and the bad breast, bearer of pain and anxiety. Although certain Kleinian notions had been identified in children, they have also been fortunate as contexts to describe the adult mind. For example, Klein's elaborations on the good/bad object (splitting) were later reused to study phenomena of adulthood such as authoritarianism (see Lauriola et al., 2015).

Anyway, the relationship with the object acquired an importance in the life of the drive that Freudian theory did not have. In summarizing, Klein wrote:

> In tracing, in the analyses of adults and children, the development of impulses, phantasies, and anxieties back to their origin, i.e. to the feelings towards the mother's breast (even with children who have not been breastfed), I found that object relations start almost at birth and arise with the first feeding experience; furthermore, that all aspects of mental life are bound up with object relations.
>
> (Klein, 1955, p. 21)

Anna Freud: education, Montessori method, and psychoanalysis

Sigmund Freud's youngest daughter, Anna, was born a decade after Melanie Klein, but naturally had the opportunity to learn about psychoanalysis before her future colleague. Her father opposed the idea of his daughter studying medicine, so Anna turned to educational university studies. Anna Freud, however, was quick to make clear her intention to undertake, in addition to the career of teacher, that of psychoanalyst. Sigmund did not put further obstacles in her way and even decided to analyze his daughter himself, starting in 1918. Thus began a rather long process of training analysis for the time, in which Sigmund Freud was joined by Lou Andreas-Salomé (1861–1937), who, already known as a friend of Nietzsche and Rilke, had approached the psychoanalytic movement. The father-daughter relationship took on quite unique contours. Anna became a privileged collaborator, replacing Otto Rank in the Committee when he left.

Anna Freud was a key figure in the history of the psychoanalytic movement in the second half of the 20th century. In order to understand her ideas about the world of the child, it is necessary to introduce a personality who has been almost completely marginalized by the history of psychology and psychoanalysis: Maria Montessori (1870–1952).

Maria Montessori had been trained in experimental psychology and pedagogy in Rome, primarily with the support of Giuseppe Sergi (1862–1935) and Sante De Sanctis. However, she soon realized that, in general, positivists tended to view the child as a "perverse little being" who needed to be "readjusted" in his development (Guarnieri, 2006). Montessori moved away from experimental research and developed an educational system that respected the child's development and was based on two pillars: observation and child-friendly intervention. Montessori, therefore, created in Rome schools for children as young as three years old, in which every object was "scaled up" to the child (La casa dei bambini/The house of the children). The first Casa dei Bambini was founded in 1907 (on Maria Montessori and the foundation of Children's Houses see Foschi, 2008, 2012). Thus, Montessori's educational thinking presented itself as an absolute novelty, but one that emphasized cognitive rather than emotional development.

The Montessori educational model was well established in Europe at a time when Anna Freud was being trained and psychoanalysis was beginning to deal systematically with the developmental years (see Honegger Fresco, 2002–2003). Anna Freud herself speaks of her relationship with the Montessori method in the introduction to the second edition of the biography of Maria Montessori written by Rita Kramer (1976/2017). Anna acknowledges that at the time she was taking her first steps into the world of the child, the Montessori method represented the best that research could offer. The most revolutionary aspect was the autonomy that Montessori recognized in the child and her great faith in children's ability to regulate themselves (A. Freud, 1976/2017). It should be emphasized, therefore, that Montessori's teaching methods focused primarily on promoting cognitive development, and the major difference between psychoanalysis and the Montessori method was Maria's rejection of the importance of drives in child development. Montessori emphasized above all a physiological and cognitive unconscious that could determine the development of maladaptive behavior. Less important in her conception remained the infantile activities of affective symbolization (see, e.g., Montessori, 1948/1970).

Maria Montessori's attention to the possible educational applications of psychoanalysis, however, was not extemporaneous. Montessori was aware of the evolution of Freudian thought and was attentive to the activities of those who were seeking new ways to apply it, especially in England. For example, in 1922, she became interested in spreading the ideas about psychoanalysis of Hugh Crichton Miller (1877–1959), who founded the Tavistock Clinic in London in 1920 (Montessori, 1922). Crichton Miller was an effective synthesizer of psychiatry, psychology, psychoanalysis, and education. From his books emerged a thorough understanding of the Montessori method, placed on the same level of importance as Freudian and Jungian psychoanalysis (Crichton Miller, 1922).[3]

Valuable evidence of the relationship between Montessori's educational thinking and psychoanalysis can also be found in a letter written in 1917 by Sigmund Freud to Maria Montessori, in which the father of psychoanalysis responded favorably to her invitation to help establish a Children's House for preschool children in Vienna.[4] In this letter, Anna was defined by her father as an analytical pedagogue and her disciple. Freud wrote to Montessori:

> My dear Frau Montessori, [i]t gave me great pleasure to receive a letter from you. Since I have been preoccupied for years with the study of the child's psyche, I am in deep sympathy with your humanitarian and understanding endeavors, and my daughter, who is an analytic pedagogue, considers herself one of your disciples. I would be very pleased to sign my name beside yours on the appeal for the foundation of a little institute as planned by Frau Schaxel. The resistance my name may arouse among the public will have to be conquered by the brilliance that radiates from yours.
>
> (E. Freud, 1960, pp. 319–320)

In the beginning, Anna Freud dealt with typical early postwar educational issues, especially related to juvenile crime and the care of war children, meeting scholars who would deeply influence her (Bernfeld, Aichhorn). During her university training, Anna also studied the educational thinking of the American pragmatists (Dewey, Kilpatrick). Such thinking, steeped in functionalism, was, however, in conflict with Montessori's, which had developed out of European positivism and was based on a psychiatric and psychological matrix. It was not designed to educate the child as desired by society.

Moreover, Montessori's thought introduced themes at the beginning of the 20th century that would later become central to Ego psychology: the preparation of a physically and psychologically suitable environment to foster the child's psychophysical development, the idea that intrusions into infantile development could lead to a deviation from normality, the extreme attention paid to the developmental tasks of young children, the fundamental importance of the child's observation, and the importance given to the exercise of sensoriality as the foundation for the construction of psychic reality were all themes elaborated since the first 1909 version of the Montessori method (Foschi, 2012; Peller, 1978).

In the 1920s, together with Dorothy Burlingham (1891–1979) and Eva Rosenfeld (1892–1977), and with the collaboration of young Peter Blos (1904–1997) and Erik H. Erikson (1902–1994), Anna founded the first psychoanalytically oriented school in Vienna in Eva's house and organized by Dorothy. In the 1930s, the official founding of the Jackson Kindergarten (children up to two years of age) followed, named after the school's sponsor, a friend of Lili Roubiczek-Peller (1898–1966), a pupil of Maria Montessori. The influences of Montessori's educational thinking on psychoanalysis were thus linked above all to the creation of the Vienna Children's House in 1921–1922 by a circle of teachers who collaborated with Lili Roubiczek-Peller, a Montessori pedagogue turned psychoanalyst. The Viennese school was an important Bauhaus-style children's home at Rudolfsplatz in Vienna that served as a link between the Montessori and Annafreudian schools (Honegger Fresco, 2002–2003). Lili and Anna were mutually supportive, and an exchange of knowledge was created in which Anna trained the Montessorians and Lili trained the Freudians. Both the Children's House and the Jackson Kindergarten helped to educate the neediest children of the Viennese population. They were furnished in the Montessori style and provided special medical and nutritional care – something that had been a specific feature of Montessori institutes since their inception in Rome. Lili Roubiczek became more and more psychoanalytically oriented and emigrated to the United States with many of Anna's former collaborators in Vienna (Blos, Erikson, Redl, Hoffer, Waelder, Spitz, Hartmann, Kris, etc.). The furnishings of the Jackson Nursery were then reused in London in the Hampstead War Nursery, where the Annafreudian current took shape: here psychoanalysts began to deal primarily with the development of children and their relationship with their parents. Among Anna's London students, we should also mention James Robertson (1911–1988), who was a pioneer in attachment studies,[5] collaborated with Anna's educational institutions, and produced a whole series of works concerning the importance of children's bonds in wartime. Later, Robertson collaborated with John Bowlby (1907–1990) at the Tavistock Clinic and produced, with the help of his wife Joyce Robertson (1919–2013), a number of films documenting the importance of attachment to the mother in the lives of hospitalized children.[6]

Anna Freud's first writings on child analysis (deriving from a series of lectures in 1926) saw the light when Klein had already had the opportunity to expound her ideas and to arouse controversy. In fact, Freud's daughter did not fail to observe that the Viennese analysts had discussed Klein's theses and found themselves, for the most part, in total disagreement with them (A. Freud, 1926/1974). Essentially, then, Anna Freud immediately expounded her own ideas on the psychoanalysis of children in direct reference to Klein's positions, and in an equally direct polemic against her (for a biography of Anna Freud see Young-Bruehl, 2008). If, for Klein, analysis as such was possible and appropriate for all neurotic children (and indeed advisable for the development of every child), for Anna Freud this principle was unacceptable. Her position was that analysis, when it comes to children, requires certain modifications and adaptations, or at least must be employed with certain precautions. When there was no technical possibility of adhering to such precautions, it was advisable not to undertake analysis (A. Freud, 1926/1975, p. 5).

Anna Freud started from the fact that it was not the child who asked to undertake an analytic therapy. Sometimes even the adult could be pushed to take such a step at the request of his relatives, or in any case by circumstances not directly related to his will. It often happened that it was not even the child who was suffering from his own symptoms: it could be the parents who were worried about his difficulties and aggressive behaviors. Therefore, the child would have lacked the understanding of the disease, the willingness to be analyzed, and the desire to heal. The need therefore arose for a preparatory phase, which Anna Freud called "breaking the child in" for analysis (p. 7), during which children could develop some understanding of the maladaptive quality of their own conduct and accept the analyst as an interesting and useful ally in their conflicts with others and a collaborator on the road to change (pp. 15–18).

Compared to the analysis of adults, the analysis of children would have presented a fundamental difficulty in the anamnestic phase: one would have been generally forced to rely on the parents to reconstruct the history of the disease. There were, however, even some undoubted advantages: children dreamed as much as adults and were not afflicted by the prejudice that dreams had no meaning. They easily produced daydreams and fantasies. They also willingly resorted to drawing, which would offer important glimpses into their inner world. However, if the child refused to make associations and to make up for this impasse, Anna Freud recognized the great value of observation of the child, but she attributed to it some very serious limitations. The representations of the child would not have been dominated by the libidinal goal of adults: therefore they would not necessarily have been attributable to the same type of interpretation. The clash of two small cars could be the symbolic translation of the sexual act but also the reproduction of an event that the child had witnessed (even if, as Anna Freud was forced to acknowledge, the event could very well be remembered and recalled for its symbolic value).

Anna Freud believed that one had to be actively concerned about children to establish a positive transference, understood as an "affectionate attachment" (p. 40), fundamental to the purposes of those educational tasks that would be just as necessary as analytic tasks. A true transference neurosis would not have been possible because the parents were still strongly present in the patient's life. Since the old edition of the primary affects had not been exhausted, a re-edition of the same affects having the analyst as their object was to be excluded. The negative transference was understood by Klein as proof of the ambivalent attitude toward the mother. On the other hand, according to Anna Freud, the negative transference would have been formed if the relationship with the mother had been satisfactory: "The more tenderly a little child is attached to his own mother, the fewer friendly impulses he has toward strangers." Moreover, the interpretability of the negative transference on the part of the adult would also have been linked to the neutral attitude, like an "empty screen," that his analyst had to hold (pp. 45–46). The child, on the other hand, was in a position to know perfectly well what his analyst allowed or forbade, approved or disapproved.

For all these reasons, Anna Freud defined the setting for the analysis of the child in a way that was quite different from that of the adult, attributing a fundamental value to education, which acts on both internal and external factors, harmonizing the mind and the environment in which the processes of growth occur (pp. 50–69). A Montessori influence still emerges strongly in these final considerations.

From the theoretical debate to the splitting of the British psychoanalytic society

Klein (1927/1948c) retaliated against Annafreudian criticism: in her opinion, the very idea that there should be a difference between the analysis of adults and the analysis of children was nonsense. Analytic work was based on the interpretation of unconscious conflicts and, if there was a difference between adulthood and childhood, it had to do with a greater weakness of the ego on the part of the child. Therefore, to appeal more to the conscious part of the psyche could not be technically correct. In fact, Klein argued, what Anna Freud called "acknowledgement of illness and of naughtiness" was anything but the result of genuine understanding on the part of the child, but was a derivative "from the anxiety which she has mobilized in him for her own purposes: castration anxiety and the sense of guilt" (p. 157). Not that such feelings should be avoided per se, Klein argued: the problem was rather that Anna Freud did not analyze them and therefore did not resolve them. She used them "to attach the child to herself" while she herself enlisted them "from the outset (. . .) in the service of analytic work" (p. 159).

In practice, according to Klein, the educational intent not only did not favor the results of infantile analysis, but was, on the contrary, incompatible with the analytical procedure, just as was the artificial creation of a positive transference (as everyone would recognize in the case of adult analysis). On the contrary, it was necessary to enter immediately *in medias res* because the transference dynamic was generated immediately:

> As soon as the small patient has given me some sort of insight into his complexes (. . .) I consider that interpretation can and should begin. This does not run counter to the well-tried rule that the analyst should wait till the transference is there before he begins interpreting, because with children the transference takes place immediately, and the analyst will often be given evidence straight away of its positive nature. But should the child show shyness, anxiety or even a certain distrust, such behavior is to be read as a sign of negative transference, and this makes it still more imperative that interpretation should begin as soon as possible.
>
> (Klein, 1932/1960, pp. 46–47)

After all, the admission that partial results were obtained with children was, on the one hand, the result of the prejudice (which had no theoretical or practical basis) of the impossibility of an equally profound psychotherapy. On the other hand, it was, in fact, an admission of therapeutic inefficacy.

In this bitter confrontation, Sigmund Freud discreetly sided with his daughter. In his letters to Jones, he accused the latter "of arranging a campaign against his daughter's way of analyzing children, defended her criticisms of Melanie Klein's clinical strategies, and resented the charge that she had been insufficiently analyzed." Moreover, being himself the analyst of his daughter, "[h]e was beginning to wonder whether these attacks on his daughter were not really attacks on himself" (Gay, 1988, p. 469). In a note added to his autobiography in 1935, however, he merely observed even-handedly: "Child analysis in particular has gained a powerful momentum owing to the work of Mrs. Melanie Klein and of my daughter, Anna Freud" (Freud, 1925–1959, p. 70).

The contrast between Melanie Klein and Anna Freud precipitated when the Freuds and several Viennese analysts were forced to emigrate and London became for some years the center of the psychoanalytic movement. Klein had already acquired a large following in England: Joan Riviere (1883–1962), Susan Isaacs (1885–1948), and Paula Heimann (1899–1982) were three analysts destined for fame and quickly became her close collaborators. Donald Woods Winnicott (1896–1971) was one of her pupils. Edward Glover (1888–1972), one of the best-known British psychoanalysts of the time, also welcomed Kleinian ideas at first (Glover, 1933). His attitude changed completely, however: Glover could not accept that someone like Klein, not having studied medicine, would dare to argue about psychotic states (Segal, 1979). Anna Freud, on the other hand, could count on the prestige of the name and the support of the newly immigrated Austrian psychoanalysts. Two opposing groups thus formed in the British Psychoanalytic Society and it soon became clear that a clarifying theoretical debate was needed.

World War II made an immediate confrontation impossible: some members of the Psychoanalytic Society were called to the front; others, like Klein herself, left London, targeted by German bombing during the Battle of Britain. In Pitlochry, Scotland, where she resided for a year, Melanie Klein analyzed little Richard, who became her most famous clinical case. Although Richard's analysis lasted only four months, Klein had the almost unique opportunity in her hectic professional life to write down detailed notes after each session. The material formed the basis for two of her best-known writings (Klein, 1945/1948f, 1961). In 1943, when the risk of bombing had diminished and the psychoanalysts had almost all returned to London, Ernest Jones, president of the Psychoanalytic Society, decided to organize the theoretical confrontation that everyone had been waiting too long for. The result was the "Controversial Discussions," which engaged the Society until 1944: long and circulated only in cyclostyled form, they were finally collated into a volume many years later (King & Steiner, 1991).

At this point, what was at stake was no longer only child psychoanalysis, but psychoanalysis *tout court*, because both sides were contributing to modifying adult therapy as well. On the one hand, Anna Freud, according to an approach that would become dominant in the Ego psychology, tended to focus on the ego, instead of the id: her interpretations were aimed at the superficial layer of the unconscious rather than the deep one. On the other hand, Melanie Klein "developed Freud's conception of transference analysis into 'pure transference analysis,' a movement which, in particular, involved the discarding of all forms of reassurance, on the one hand, and educational pressure, on the other, with both children and adults" (Money-Kyrle, 1978, p. 409). Kleinians also promoted the extensibility of the psychoanalytic method to psychosis. As Hanna Segal summarizes:

> Both sides of the controversy quoted Freud repeatedly, but the quotations were different. One could say: Which Freud? Whose Freud? Riviere remarks that Klein's opponents tended to refer to Freud's early work, while she and her co-workers referred more often to his late work. This is particularly clear in the case of the dead instinct.
>
> (Segal, 1979, p. 95)

Neither faction was able to prevail. The discussion then moved on to negotiation, in order to prevent the British Psychoanalytic Society from splitting. Anna Freud and Melanie Klein, with the help of the mediator Sylvia Payne (1880–1976), reached a compromise, a sort of *cuius regio eius religio*. After the religious wars of the 17th century, in fact, the Peace of Augusta had sanctioned that every nation officially assume the religious beliefs of the sovereign. Similarly, within the Psychoanalytic Association, each leader would control its own "territory" by training analysts in the light of their theoretical beliefs. Around the two theoretical leaders were organized two groups, which would be assigned equally to the committees and the board of directors. After a few years, however, there also appeared a group of Independents or Middle Group, to which would belong the most creative minds of British psychoanalysis of the 20th century (Fairbairn, Winnicott, Bowlby, among others). The three groupings remained a central feature of the British Society but their boundaries have become less rigid and overlapping and fertile interchanges occur among them (Bateman & Holmes, 1995). The British one was destined to become a model for the International Psychoanalytic Association worldwide. The proliferation of theoretical approaches referring to Freud found the IPA always willing to establish situations of compromise and pluralist representation, except for the voluntary exit of theorists (as would happen with Ellis and Beck), or except for isolated cases, but no less clamorous, such as those of Karen Horney (1885–1952) and Jacques Lacan (1901–1981).

The impact of fascism on the history of psychotherapy: mass emigration of psychoanalysts and the foundation of the Göring Institute

The period between the 1930s and the 1950s was characterized by the ideological clash between totalitarianism and the free world. German psychiatrists, on the other hand, were initially engaged in eugenics programs that involved the sterilization of large masses of undesirable citizens (retarded, sick, schizophrenic, marginalized people). Later they also contributed to the physical elimination of adults and children on psychopathological, racial, and/or political grounds. The quest for racial purification resulted in the killing of several hundred thousand German citizens of various ethnicities and cultures. The regime had made compulsory a type of euthanasia prescribed to individuals considered unfit and propagandized by various means, including movies, to convince the population that the eugenics program was designed for their own good and for the greatness of Germany. The name of the Nazis' eugenics elimination program was "Aktion T4," from Tiergartenstraße 4, the street where the program's main offices were located. Aktion T4 involved doctors, nurses, and psychiatrists throughout Germany and all Nazi-occupied territory, leading to the killing by various practices of several hundred thousand people, including many children, considered undesirable by the Nazi regime (Lifton, 1986). While Nazi psychiatrists were engaged in eugenics programs, other psy-scientists who were not colluding with eugenics moved psychotherapy to the postwar period.

Thus, during World War II, psychology and psychotherapy also played a role in the countries of the Nazi-Fascist Pact. Italian and German psychologists met in Rome in 1941, isolating themselves from the research of the rest of the world (Gundlach, 2010). Among those who organized the meeting should be mentioned Father Agostino Gemelli (1878–1959), who also played a fundamental role in the history of Italian psychology and of psychotherapy in Catholic culture (Foschi et al., 2018), and Matthias Heinrich Göring (1879–1945), Hermann's cousin, founder of the Deutsches Institut für psychologische Forschung und Psychotherapie (German Institute for Psychological Research and Psychotherapy), also known as the "Göring Institute," which, by dissolving the German and Viennese psychoanalytic societies, promoted an Aryan conception of psychotherapy in which, however, were present, in disguise, even Freudian, Adlerian, and Jungian psychoanalytic notions (Cocks, 1985). While between 1932 and 1936 the number of psychologists in Germany declined by about one third, mainly due to the forced emigration of German academics of Jewish origin (Geuter, 2008, p. 41), it has been historiographically established that there was also an expansion of psychology and psychotherapy (Cocks, 1985). The modernization of the state as a function of the Reich's grandeur was a hallmark of Nazi Germany, and psychologists presented themselves as a useful category for this project, entrenching themselves as professionals. They laid the foundations of their training with the recognition of a university curriculum in psychology at the beginning of World War II. The German army (the Wehrmacht) was the context in which psychologists mainly worked. Psychological testing, in particular, was seen as a useful tool in the evaluation and selection of soldiers and officers. Psychology as practiced in the universities, on the other hand, dealt mainly with personality and diagnostic methods, again mainly for selective purposes. It was only when the ranks of the army dwindled drastically, due to casualties, that psychologists lost the social mandate given to them (Geuter, 2008).

The Institute chaired by Matthias Göring, in particular, while on the one hand replaced "Jewish" psychoanalysis with a hybrid psychotherapy, on the other hand kept alive and gave prestige to a discipline that would later be restarted by the organization wanted by Göring himself. Psychotherapy in the second half of the 20th century therefore also has dark roots, born from the reformulation in Nazi Germany of an Aryan psychotherapy. During the Third Reich, non-Jewish psychoanalysts who had survived the purges adapted to Nazism, continuing to work at the Göring Institute (which also reused the premises of the Psychoanalytic Institute of Berlin). In return, they received prestige and social recognition, just like the Nazi psychologists who were involved in academic and applied research. The Göring Institute promoted the organization of a lay psychotherapy in which non-doctors were also accepted. After the institution of the course in psychology, in 1941, the title of psychologist, obtained by those who had also carried out practical training, became a prerequisite for the possibility of specializing in psychotherapy. Therefore, psychotherapeutic training was also organized, with the establishment of seminars and the regulation of training analysis. In fact, psychoanalysis, individual psychology, and analytical psychology continued to be practiced in separate sections of the Institute. Alongside these, relaxation techniques (autogenic training), hypnosuggestion, massage, and music therapy were practiced. The lexicon of psychoanalysis was also aryanized: the term "depth psychology" (originally coined by Bleuler) was used to encompass all psychodynamic therapies; the "family complex" replaced the Oedipus complex; "developmental psychology" replaced psychoanalysis (Cocks, 1985).

The psychotherapists of the Third Reich dealt with any clinical phenomenon, developing short and focused psychotherapy techniques to be placed side by side with the longer and more expensive depth psychotherapy. The psy-scientists of the Göring Institute were employed in many fields of German society, from industry to war aviation, from pro-Nazi propaganda to child psychotherapy. Programs were organized against homosexuality and psychogenic impotence, phenomena not in line with the Nazis' idea of man (Cocks, 1985; see Schönpflug, 2017).

Nazi depth psychotherapy moved between (a) a Nazi medicine that was inspired by a holistic doctrine of nature and wanted to regenerate the nation by extolling the virtues of the Aryan race and (b) traditional German medicine, all oriented toward determinism and biology. Psychotherapy was seen as an opportunity to promote the anthropology of a new Nazi man, a loyal subject of the ethical and totalitarian state who put his ego at the service of the community. The techniques were modified and a *kleine Psychotherapie* (minor psychotherapy) was created, as opposed to a *große Psychotherapie* (major psychotherapy), both of which were functional to the idea of building an efficient citizen suited to the society conceived by the Nazis. As we will see, paradoxically in contemporary society, influenced by neoliberalism and ordoliberalism, a short, smart, globalized psychotherapy is spreading in search of demonstrable efficacy, characteristics that resemble those introduced by the aryanization of psychotherapy.

Nazi psychotherapy was thus professionally organized, but also completely at the service of totalitarianism. Jewish psychologists and psychotherapists who did not adapt to the new regime were purged and persecuted (Cocks, 1985).

In 1933, Jung had become president of the Allgemeine Ärztliche Gesellschaft für Psychotherapie (AÄGP, General Medical Society for Psychotherapy), which, founded in the second half of the 1920s, had gathered hundreds of young physicians who were critical of biological psychiatry and interested in psychotherapy. Important names in the history of psychoanalysis and psychology had joined the society (Alexander, Goldstein, Stekel, Rojo, Horney, Reich, Adler, Kretschmer, Lewin, etc.). With the advent of Nazism, the Society collaborated with the Göring Institute. During Jung's presidency, it became, first, a "supranational" society (Überstaatliche Allgemeine Ärztliche Gesellschaft für Psychotherapie), then an international one (Internationale Allgemeine Ärztliche Gesellschaft für Psychotherapie). The name changes marked a division of power: Jung was assigned to manage the International Society; Göring instead coordinated the German component of this society (Deutsche Allgemeine Ärztliche Gesellschaft für Psychotherapie), which was hegemonic, dictated the lines, and reduced the number of participants in the life of the International Society, which he tended to control from the outside. In any case, after a couple of international congresses in Copenhagen (1937) and Oxford (1938), Jung resigned from the presidency (1940), and his books ended up being banned by the Nazi regime like Freud's. In the war years the Society was dissolved, only to be revived at the end of World War II.

The psychologists of the Göring Institute appreciated some aspects of Jungian theory: for example, the idea of archetypes could be used as a basis for racism, and the importance given by Jung to creativity and freedom of the unconscious could be assimilated to the idea of the superman, dear to the regime. Some of the interviews given by Jung in 1933–1934 in which collusions emerged between his own theory and the anthropology propagated by the emerging Nazism became famous. Jung in this early period contrasted an Aryan psychotherapy with a Jewish one (McGuire & Hull, 1977).

Jung, like many others, seemed politically naive at the beginning of Nazism. In the 1930s he had already defended himself against accusations of cooperation with the regime, claiming that his intervention favored Jewish psychotherapists in maintaining their positions under the cover of the International Society of which he was president and, finally, recalling that without his work in 1933–1934 the Nazi government could have erased at the stroke of a pen the entire history of psychotherapy in German-speaking countries. Jung, in truth, with the publication of *Wotan* (1936/1964), had already written that, by affiliating themselves to Hitler (whom he considered a "possessed"), the Germans would be led to ruin, up to affirming in 1939 that the German "psychosis" had reached its climax (Cocks, 1985, pp. 176–181).

Jung was, however, only one of hundreds of psychotherapists who continued to work during Nazism, collaborating with German colleagues. The idea of neutrality in analysis had in fact led many to apolitical attitudes that did not grasp the danger of the exceptional laws implemented by Hitler after the seizure of power and that transformed Germany in a few days into a totalitarian regime (Germany was turned into a dictatorship within three months: 30 January–24 March 1933). Jung probably thought he could find in this context, heavily influenced and directed by political ends, the space for some reforms in psychotherapy, for example promoting technical changes in psychoanalytic practice and the entrance of more non-doctors into the International Society of Psychoanalysis. Jung's was a nonconformist program in a context that instead aimed to create a conventional anthropology that conformed to Nazi culture.

During the years of Nazism, German culture lost its objective hegemony in the history of psychotherapy, due to the diaspora of the great names of psychoanalysis, almost all of Jewish origin. London and New York became the capitals of psychotherapy, and, as we will see, the psychoanalysts who were forced to emigrate contributed to founding, after the end of World War II, various trends and schools of contemporary psychotherapy. With almost all analysts forced to flee because of Nazism, creativity in psychotherapy had emigrated abroad. What remained in Germany was the institutional component, which had surprisingly been able to survive Nazism and take root in German culture. The Göring Institute was successful in proposing an eclectic and secular psychotherapy, an alternative to organicist psychiatry, which offered brief and focused treatments, a technical and theoretical background that from its ashes (the Institute was destroyed by Allied bombing on the eve of the liberation of Berlin) gave way to the psychotherapy of Federal Germany to develop in the postwar period. The history of psychotherapy in the Third Reich is therefore a paradigmatic one within the more general history of psychotherapy and shows how it can adapt to opposing political regimes and how its transformations are never neutral but are determined by the cultures of which psychotherapy is an expression.

The outset of psychoanalysis in the United States

The history of the influence of psychoanalysis in the United States assumed peculiar connotations from the very beginning, that is, from the famous Clark Lectures to which Freud and Jung were invited in 1909, thus having the opportunity to expound their ideas directly before the Gotha of American academic psychology.[7] The reactions of American psychologists, although obviously not uniform, were generally aligned on two fundamental traits: a significant interest in Freudian ideas, combined with suspicion toward the method used by Freud to obtain his *data* and develop his theories. Emblematic, in this regard, is the attitude of one of the most important historical figures of American psychology, Edward Titchener (1867–1927), who highlighted, in a letter to psychiatrist Adolf Meyer (1866–1950) dated 19 September 1909, the "dogmatic fallacies" of Freud, without completely rejecting the proposals of the psychoanalytic movement, demonstrating, indeed, a positive disposition, for example, toward some of Jung's theorizations, such as the concept of complex (Leys & Evans, 1990, p. 125). It can probably be said that an underlying ambivalence was the most prevalent attitude. The reaction of another of the fathers of American psychology, William James, would seem in this sense typical: on the one hand, he expressed his satisfaction to Ernest Jones with the historical importance of the role of psychoanalysts, while on the other hand, he did not hide from others his impression of Freud as a man obsessed with fixed ideas (Shakow & Rapaport, 1964).

After Freud's journey, the influence of psychoanalytic ideas had a slow but significant rise in the United States, thanks in part to a favorable cultural atmosphere. In the first decades of the century, literary movements (such as realists and muckrakers), and social and cultural movements in general, modified an environment previously marked by Victorian and Puritan principles. Freudian ideas became an integral part of the Zeitgeist. Perhaps the cultural climate was, after the Clark Lectures, one of the main vehicles of influence of psychoanalysis on American academic psychology (Shakow & Rapaport, 1964). It was precisely the intrusive pressure of the general public's interest in Freudian ideas, however, that led to strong resistance to the reception of psychoanalysis by the American academic establishment. This tendency was certainly sustained by the long-standing unavailability of translations or at least reliable accounts of psychodynamic ideas. We can schematically state that the penetration of psychoanalysis in the United States followed two separate paths for psychologists and psychiatrists, corresponding to the very clear separation of roles between the two specializations for almost the entire 20th century (the figure of the psychotherapist with psychological training has been authorized in relatively recent times).

In American psychology, the behavioral paradigm was dominant: obviously it could only show skepticism toward a discipline that not only focused on the mind but even advocated the idea of an unconscious. Either for this reason or because of simple incomprehension, due also, as already mentioned, to the lack of availability of texts, psychoanalytic ideas penetrated with extreme difficulty. When they did break through, they were rather absorbed by other psychological theories, only to find themselves largely modified with respect to their context of origin. This was the case, for example, with the theoretical constructs on motivation proposed by Hull (1943), Dollard and Miller (1950), and Mowrer (1950), which only partly shared the Freudian concept of drive. There remained, however, very strong reservations about the reliability of clinical research methods, and attempts were made to use experimental, or at least quantitative, methods to seek possible confirmations or refutations of psychoanalysis. The results of these efforts, however, were mixed: for example, Sears

(1943) seemed to be less convinced than Hilgard (1952) about the reliability of experimental confirmations of Freudian theories (inaugurating an alternation of opinions that has continued, to this day, to characterize the debate among researchers).

According to Shakow and Rapaport, the attitude toward psychoanalysis on the part of American psychology scholars was also strongly conditioned by the particular historical situation of their discipline. They aspired to a solid scientific status, but also to methodological openings that would open up research areas that were impracticable using the pure experimental method. "There arose confusion in the use and meaning of the terms 'good' and 'bad' science – 'bad' science being taken to be which characterized psychoanalysis" (Shakow & Rapaport, 1964, p. 192). This evaluation, moreover, coming from two significant exponents of the American psychoanalytic movement, is nevertheless indicative of the attitude held by their own environment in the face of methodological criticism coming from outside. Academic psychology could consider the theoretical field of psychoanalysis as a set of more or less fruitful hypotheses on which to work, should they be empirically confirmed. Psychoanalysis for a long time did not consider necessary any dialogue with academic psychology, either on the theoretical level or on the methodological or epistemological one. As will be seen, the first to systematically attempt a dialogue with psychologists and philosophers of science would be the leader of Ego psychology, Heinz Hartmann (1894–1970).

Completely different was the attitude of the psychiatric milieu. The lectures of Freud and Jung in 1909 (followed by others given by Jung in 1912 and finally by Ferenczi in 1926) constituted the first act of an evolution that would slowly push the country to assume the theoretical leadership of psychotherapy, and not only psychoanalysis. In fact, Freud's influence made possible the emergence of very different forms of therapy, also as a direct reaction to psychoanalytic ideas: Albert Ellis (1913–2007) and Aaron Beck (1921–2021), for example, trained as psychoanalysts before becoming the two key figures in the birth of cognitive-behavioral psychotherapy.[8]

The process of development of psychoanalysis in the United States saw a stunted beginning and a subsequent explosion. In 1920, at the annual conference of American psychoanalysts in New York, only ten people were present. Abraham Brill even proposed the dissolution of the section. Just before World War II, 30% of the 560 members of the IPA were already in the United States. Forty years later, out of the 4000 members, more than 50% were of U.S. nationality (Fine, 1979).

Among American psychoanalysts we can observe from the beginning the birth of two currents, two profoundly different ways of using Freudian thought. There was, first, the birth of the American branch of the psychoanalytic movement, under the initial leadership of Brill, who were faithful to Freud's ideas except as regards the possibility of "laymen" (not doctors) becoming analysts: this group gave rise to the American Psychoanalytic Association. Secondly, thanks to the figure of Harry Stack Sullivan, a very different tradition of research developed, which, initially minority or even marginal, would later prove to be very fruitful: *interpersonal psychoanalysis*. However, it "does not constitute a unified, integral theory, as does classical Freudian drive theory. It is instead a set of different approaches to theory and clinical practice held together by shared underlying assumptions and premises" (Greenberg & Mitchell, 1983, p. 79). The so-called interpersonal or *culturalist* psychoanalysts, in fact, were convinced that Freud's theory of motivation, as his ideas about the nature of human experience and early developmental difficulties, was erroneous. Like the British object relations theorists, the culturalist psychoanalysts believed that

> drive theory provides an inadequate and essentially misleading foundation for psychoanalytic theorizing and clinical technique. They also shared a common belief that classical Freudian theory underemphasized the larger social and cultural context which must figure prominently in any theory attempting to account for the origins, development, and warpings of personality.
>
> (ibid.)

When a significant number of European analysts who were forced to emigrate during the 1930s chose the United States as their destination, the theoretical scene changed. The American Psychoanalytic Association, the U.S. section of the IPA, saw the emergence of Ego psychology; Sullivan's impulse merged into a broader and more multifaceted perspective, which would be generally defined as *neo-Freudian*.

Harry Stack Sullivan and the birth of interpersonal psychoanalysis

In the history of psychotherapy there is no lack of cases of outsiders who become characters of great historical importance, and Harry Stack Sullivan (1892–1949) may well be the most conspicuous example of this category. Born in Norwich, a town in Chenango County (200 miles from New York), in 1892, he completed his high school studies in the province, obtaining in 1908 a scholarship to study medicine at the prestigious Cornell University, where, however, he remained one year without taking exams. Between 1909 and 1911 he literally disappeared from circulation. According to the reconstruction proposed by his biographer and former collaborator Helen Perry (1983), he was hospitalized in a psychiatric hospital following a psychotic episode, or even a full-blown manifestation of schizophrenia. In 1911, he resumed his medical studies at the Chicago College of Medicine and Surgery, which had a much more modest scientific profile than Cornell, and was closed in the same year in which Sullivan graduated, in 1917 (Chapman, 1976). Such an unprestigious period of training was followed by four rather lean years of practice, apparently still marked by moments of crisis for reasons of mental health (Perry, 1983). In

1921, Sullivan went to St. Elizabeth's Hospital in Washington, directed by William Alanson White (1870–1937), a psychiatrist with an eclectic approach, who directed him toward psychiatry. Sullivan retained a lifelong veneration for him, as evidenced by the constant references in his writings that define White as one of the decisive figures in the development of modern psychiatry. If such an evaluation may seem exaggerated in retrospect, it is true that White transformed St. Elizabeth's into the "Burghölzli of the American continent" (D'Amore, 1976, p. 84), the first American institution where psychoanalytic theories were the foundation of psychiatric therapy. The following year Sullivan began his work as a psychiatrist at Sheppard Hospital, near Washington, where from 1929 he was able to run a small department organized entirely according to the ideas he had been developing in the meantime.

Initially, Sullivan dealt essentially with young male schizophrenics, as can be seen from his publications of the 1920s. Therefore, one can understand Marco Conci's statement that "the essential key to Sullivan's work with his patients was therefore represented by his personal vicissitudes, and the capacity for identification with patients and self-analysis that followed" (2000, p. 152). In fact, in his early writings Sullivan linked the onset of male schizophrenia to existential problems, which proved to be disastrous, faced during preadolescence and adolescence, and set the therapeutic course as an attempt to compensate for the failure to solve those problems:

> Out of his own experience, he assumed that the young male patients on his ward had missed out a relationship of reciprocal trust in the preadolescent period. Thus he tried to create such an experience, to begin with what he considered to be the basic experience of trust – the preadolescent friend.
>
> (Perry, 1983, p. 195)

Despite the extreme specialization at the beginning (which will always be matched by an attitude of caution toward generalizations), Sullivan's early writings were already characterized by basic ideas that would remain relatively constant in his theoretical-clinical thought. Indeed, the first public lecture (followed by the first publication in 1924) focused on a series of clearly oriented convictions and lines of research. Sullivan made it clear that the fundamental epistemological premise to which he adhered was that of a *critical realism* (i.e., ready, obviously, to adapt when faced with the discovery of perceptual and interpretative fallacies in the consideration of reality). The presuppositions that Sullivan considered necessary to accept his point of view were just as clearly stated: the postulate of the existence of the unconscious; a teleological conception of human existence (Sullivan explicitly referred to Jung's concept of libido); the ontogenetic hypothesis, based on the progressive organization of the mind according to a "vital sequence of experience" that is substantially similar for different human beings (Sullivan, 1924/1962a, p. 9). In order to understand pathology, and in particular schizophrenic pathology, as Sullivan suggested, it was necessary to reconstruct what the patient was trying to do through psychosis: "If the element of purpose and means is eliminated, there results sterile brain physiology" (p. 8). This meant opposing the entire psychiatric tradition that sought in heredity and brain lesions the etiology of schizophrenia, but also "the epilogue of the stimulus-response psychology" (ibid.).

In the same, very significant, debut lecture, Sullivan offered his own view of schizophrenia as "a series of major mental events always attended by material changes in personality, but in itself implying nothing of deterioration or dementia" (p. 12). In conclusion, "this illness is one of mental structure", it consists of a

> disorder of motivation, in turn reflected in the thought content and in the purposive activity – behavior. The mental structure is dissociated in such fashion that the disintegrated portions regress in function to earlier levels of mental ontology, without parallelism in individual depth of regression.
>
> (p. 13)

Based on his own early clinical experiences, Sullivan maintained that the prognosis of schizophrenia was not necessarily inauspicious (as both psychiatry and psychoanalysis had claimed up to then) and that a cure was possible, since early intervention could prevent the definitive regression of the personality. He also stressed that, just as the onset of the pathology was to some extent determined by the environment, so also the successful reintegration of the patient into the world must be considered closely linked to the context in which he would live the recovery phase. Sullivan therefore proposed as a research project the study of the patient and the pre-psychotic environment.

The influence of Freudian thought on Sullivan was immediately evident (no one ever doubted his identity as a psychoanalyst, albeit heterodox), as well as the diversity of orientation, which led Greenberg and Mitchell (1983), as we have seen, to build the image of a perfect counterpart of Freud. Rarely, however, has the strong influence exerted on him by Jung been perceived. Conci writes instead, very appropriately:

> It is possible for us to identify as many as three planes on which to set the discourse of Jung's influence on Sullivan. Firstly, the interpersonal orientation of his thought, secondly, his contestation of the Freudian concept of libido and the consequent reconceptualization of the concept of psychosis, in terms of the accessibility of patients affected by it to the psychotherapeutic relationship and, thirdly, in terms of the very possibility (. . .) of being able to develop an alternative psychoanalytic point of view to that of Freud. Not to mention (. . .) the intimate link that Jung thematized after his break with Freud, in a work like *Psychological Types*, between the theoretical system and personality of the individual author – in the field of dynamic psychology.
>
> (Conci, 2000, p. 276)

In his writings of the 1920s, Sullivan, also comforted by Jung's greater thera-peutic optimism than Freud's (Sullivan, 1925/1962b), developed an ontogenetic theory and treatment technique of schizophrenia that bent psychoanalytic ideas to a certainly new interpretation. While for Freud the decisive factors for health or illness were intrapsychic, for Sullivan they were *interpersonal* (first occurrence of the term in Sullivan, 1926/1962c). Sullivan continued to consider sexuality fundamental to individual development, not only as a possible source of neu-rosis but also as a protective factor: in his view, schizophrenic disorder "seems never to occur in those who have achieved if only for a short time a definitely satisfying adjustment to a sex object" (Sullivan, 1926/1962c, p. 104). Sullivan, however, considered Oedipus a "cultural artifact" (Sullivan, 1925/1962b, p. 94). The possible castrating effect of the family environment was better interpreted in a metaphorical sense than in the literal Freudian sense of castration anxiety. It was related to the parents' maladaptation to cultural conditioning related to sex-uality. Prolonging maternal care beyond the age at which it was needed could also have devastating effects (Sullivan, 1925/1962b). In short, Sullivan wrote: "We have not seen maladjustment which was without a foundation of erro-neous attitudes which parents or their equivalent had thrust upon the child" (1926/1962c, p. 104). In 1926, Sullivan had the opportunity to listen to the lectures given by Ferenczi, for the first time speaking on American soil, and felt a deep affinity with his ideas, to the point of pushing Clara Thompson (1893–1958) (met three years earlier) to become his pupil. Thompson joined Ferenczi in Europe and, upon her return, became one of Sullivan's main interlocutors. Also in 1926, Sullivan came into contact with the anthropologist Edward Sapir (1884–1939), who was destined to inspire the idea of thinking of psychiatry as one of the social sciences. In fact, Sullivan ended up considering himself a social scientist who specialized in psychiatry (Perry, 1983).

In 1928 and 1929, Sullivan participated (also on the organizational level) in two Colloquia on Personality Investigation that were held in New York and were attended by representatives of the various social sciences. Sullivan had become convinced that personality was largely a product of culture (1931/1962f, 1931/1962g). Psychopathology began to be explicitly conceived by him as a function of the events that had characterized a person's life, events experienced in real relationships with significant others and that had to some extent under-mined the individual's self-esteem (Sullivan, 1929/1962d, 1929/1962e). It was to New York that Sullivan moved between 1930 and 1939 and here he had the opportunity to start a dialogue with other fundamental figures in the history of psychotherapy and psychoanalysis: Erich Fromm, Frieda Fromm-Reichmann (1889–1957), and Karen Horney, who had all emigrated to the United States from Europe.[9] Together with them and Clara Thompson, Sullivan constituted a group that has been loosely termed the "neo-Freudian" movement. In com-mon with Sullivan, the Europeans showed (1) the conviction that classical psy-choanalysis needed to be reformed, because Freud was strongly conditioned by the historical and social situation in which he found himself working, without being aware of it; (2) openness to disciplines capable of expanding the pure clinical perspective, such as anthropology and sociology. They would also have had in common the fate of being marginalized from the mainstream of the psychoanalytic movement.

Sullivan's destiny of marginalization was already evident when he was able to present his ideas in front of his American colleagues of the IPA. Sullivan (1931/1962h) argued the importance, in working with psychotics, of a therapeutic procedure that preceded the actual application of psychoanalytic technique. This procedure included (1) putting the patient in "a situation in which he is encouraged to renew efforts at adjustment with others," namely hospitalization in a controlled environment; and (2) "providing an orienting experience" to the patient, that is, being treated "as a person among persons," something usually lacking in his or her past (p. 285). Only then could direct efforts begin "in reconstructing the actual chronology of the psychosis" (p. 287). Schizophrenic patients should be "treated firstly to the end of socialization, and thereafter by more fundamental reorganization of personality" (p. 290). According to Sullivan, from this perspective, the training of nonmedical personnel was fundamental, as was the principle that "therapeutic situations must be integrated between individuals of the same sex" (p. 289).

Among the discussants, Gregory Zilboorg (1890–1959) bluntly asserted that the social healing Sullivan sought was not real healing and that Sullivan's method consisted of "nothing more than a series of preliminary measures" (Zilboorg, 1931/1962, p. 292). Abraham Brill, for his part, as chairman of the conference session, coldly commented that Sullivan's optimism about the possibility of curing schizophrenics was to be welcomed (Brill, 1931/1962).

Sullivan's work would begin to be considered on the level of its true merits (those of a leading figure) in the psychoanalytic field only from the Eighties of the 20th century, thanks to the extraordinary influence of the aforementioned book *Object Relations in Psychoanalytic Theory* (Greenberg & Mitchell, 1983). This did not prevent his texts from exerting a profound, albeit subterranean, influence: Laing considered Sullivan's writings on schizophrenia the only truly valid texts on psychosis; Bateson was certainly influenced by the idea of the schizophrenogenic mother that arose in the interpersonal tradition (Fromm-Reichmann, 1948). Ellis referred explicitly to his works.[10] But in general, Sullivan was considered with some disregard, if, for example, Alexander and Selesnick wrote that his contribution "had no particular sociological sophistication" (1966, p. 365).

Sullivan's activity since the 1930s can be increasingly defined as an attempt at the "fusion of psychiatry and social science," a clever label created by Gordon Allport (1950) and taken up by Helen Perry as the title of a collection of Sullivan's essays (1964c) that she edited. The journal *Psychiatry*, which Sullivan contributed to founding in 1938, was probably the first interdisciplinary journal to deal with mental health (and for a long time it would remain almost the only one in the field). Sullivan's definition of psychiatry in an encyclopedia entry as early as 1934 reflected an extremely open conception of the discipline: "the scientific study of peculiarities of personality and of interpersonal relations" (p. 7). The last chapter of the unfinished and posthumously published book *The Interpersonal Theory of Psychiatry* (Sullivan, 1953) was visionarily entitled "Towards a Psychiatry of Peoples," expressing the hope that mental health professionals would not only be concerned with ex post care, but would contribute *ex ante* to the necessary prevention of mental distress, and engage in this endeavor on an international scale.

After moving to New York in 1932, Sullivan broadened the scope of his clinical experience to include less severe cases. The subject matter of his contributions also gradually expanded, albeit at a cautiously slow pace: the first contribution in which the word "schizophrenia" or an equivalent term did not appear was published five years after his transfer to New York (Sullivan, 1937/1964a).

Sullivan then developed theoretical insights for a theory of the "thinking and doing of persons, real or illusory" (Sullivan, 1938/1964b, p. 32) in its development, and for a theory of care, as an enterprise in which the therapist is also directly involved from a human perspective.

In Sullivan's view, human life was characterized by more or less adequate processes of adaptation to the world around us. Psychotic-type thoughts were rare but not absent from the experience of so-called "normal" people. Even they commonly alternated perfectly adequate personal relationships with distorted interactive modes, which Sullivan named with the neologism *parataxic*, wanting to avoid the terms *neurosis* and *neurotic*, which he considered "misleading and much abused" (p. 41, footnote). As with Freud, the evolutionary approach was the most correct one for understanding the origins of mental health problems: placing the processes of adaptation to the interpersonal world at the center of his conception, however, he produced radical changes with respect to the Freudian view.

Sullivan's theory of motivation was based on the idea that human acts fell into two basic categories, depending on the purpose for which they were intended. In a series of lectures in 1939, Sullivan stated:

> The most general basis on which interpersonal phenomena, interpersonal acts, may be classified is one which separates the sought end states into the group which we call satisfactions and those which we call security or the maintenance of security. Satisfactions in this specialized sense are all those end states which are rather closely connected with the bodily organization of man. Thus the desire for food and drink leads to certain performances which are in this category. The desire for sleep leads to such performances. The state of being, which is marked by the presence of lust, is also in this group. (. . .) On the other hand, the pursuit of security pertains rather more closely to man's cultural equipment than to his bodily organization. By cultural I mean what the anthropologist means – all that which is man-made.
> (Sullivan, 1946, pp. 20–21)

From the very beginning of individual existence, human beings have achieved security in their relationships with other human beings, those who are most significant. Long before the child was able to use language, in fact, he communicated with his mother through an empathic relationship. The empathic bond with the caregiver led to an awareness of the other's well-being and induced one's own well-being, or conversely, it caused the other's discomfort and one's own discomfort. As development proceeded, human beings constructed what Sullivan called the *self-system*, which was the repertoire of interpersonal acts that the environment helped to organize. The self-system was based on the positive or negative reactions one encountered in interacting with caregivers. Strongly negative reactions generated distress. All the security operations that *dynamisms* of the self perform are essentially aimed at avoiding dealing with anxiety. Note that Sullivan used the term "dynamism" to identify what classical psychoanalysis usually identified as "(defense) mechanism." "Mechanism has never suited me because it always suggests a diesel engine," Sullivan once wittily commented (1956, p. 5).

A more tolerant environment would have led to a wider repertoire of actions, while the more the individual's actions were strongly disapproved of, the fewer would be the initiatives that the individual would have implemented without feeling anxiety; and the more would be the components of one's personality of which the Self would have refused awareness (Sullivan, 1946), which would therefore have been dissociated from consciousness. The narrower the repertoire of actions permitted by consciousness, the more easily the human being would tend to develop a form of severe psychopathology. In the last formulation of his thought, Sullivan (1953) postulated an early tripartition of the self-system into *good me*, *bad me*, and *not me*. The first consisted of those behaviors that evoked appreciative responses from the mother; the second consisted of those behaviors that evoked anxiety in the mother, but could occasionally be used to achieve certain ends; the third grouped those behaviors that evoked such a negative response and generated such intense anxiety that they had to be avoided at all costs. Therefore, it can be summarized that, in Sullivan's view, "personal psychopathology can best be understood in relation to the family climate in which each patient grew up" (Conci, 2000, p. 189). Put more icastically, "[t]he outline of the child's personality is sharply etched by the acid of the parents' anxiety" (Mitchell & Black, 1995, p. 72).

The analyst's role, as Sullivan interpreted it, was to increase the patients' awareness of how they were participating in interactions (Sullivan, 1953). The patient would begin to notice significant characteristics that he had always avoided. He would come to understand the extent to which his successful attempts to control anxiety in the short term were precluding a more satisfying life in the long run. His relationship with the analyst was often an effective means of demonstrating the self-limiting features of security operations related to personality traits (Mitchell & Black, 1995).

Sullivan assumed a significant role in the selection of military personnel for his country during World War II. After the end of the conflict, he resumed his activity, aimed at promoting the preventive role of psychiatry, even outside the United States. He died prematurely in 1949, in Paris, during a tour of conferences addressed precisely to that end (Perry, 1983).

Erich Fromm: psychoanalysis and freedom

Fromm, born in Frankfurt in 1900 (he died in Locarno in 1980), approached psychoanalysis in 1924 through his future wife Frieda Reichmann. After undergoing training analysis, he began his clinical activity in 1927. Two years later, Erich and Frieda were among the founders of the Psychoanalytic Institute of Frankfurt (the second born in Germany, after that of Berlin), which was housed – through a chain of acquaintances – in the seat of the Institute for Social Research, headquarters of the Frankfurt School[11] Interested in the application of psychoanalysis to social phenomena and himself a reader of Marx, Fromm soon became a collaborator of the Institute directed by Horkheimer, of which he was director of the social psychology section from 1930. Psychoanalysis, Marxism, and Jewish origin were common to almost all the Frankfurt scholars, who were naturally also forced to emigrate with the advent of the Nazi regime. In 1934, Fromm moved to America, where, together with Sullivan and Horney, he became one of the greatest exponents of the neo-Freudian group.

Fromm's first step toward the progressive relativization of Freudian thought occurred with an essay written in 1935, entitled "The social determination of psychoanalytic therapy," written for the journal of the Frankfurt group but received very coldly by Horkheimer and Adorno (Funk, 1992). Fromm explicitly argued that many characteristics of humanity considered universal by Freud should instead be thought of as typical of contemporary bourgeois society. *Escape from Freedom* started from this idea to address in a very understandable language the burning and topical issue of the crisis of Western democracies in the face of authoritarian movements (Fromm, 1941). This book, which gave Fromm immediate international popularity, also introduced important theoretical innovations in the psychoanalytic field. The most important of these was the notion of *social character*, defined as "the specific form in which human energy is shaped by the dynamic adaptation of human needs to the particular mode of existence of a given society" (p. 278). Human personality was interpreted as the result of the interaction of biological components, interpersonal influences, and social factors. Moreover, it was no longer possible to conceive the idea of a normal personality in an absolute sense: the social character of a given historical and geographical context often differed from that of a different context. According to Fromm, moreover, the social character of an epoch could not correspond to the needs of the epoch itself: on some historical occasions, the majority of the components of a social category would have presented psychological characteristics that were not adaptive to the epoch. This would not have been an extreme case, but a typical situation in times when authoritarian changes were being prepared.

Given the relevance of the intersubjective and social context, neurosis could not be considered a purely personal phenomenon, since it was capable of affecting vast layers of society. Even the cultural aspects, which Freud believed to be the result of sublimation, could assume a profound importance in the analysis: "We believe that ideals like truth, justice, and freedom, although they are frequently mere phrases or rationalization, can be genuine strivings, and that any analysis which does not deal with these strivings as dynamic factors is fallacious" (p. 294).

Fromm later criticized other crucial elements of Freudian theory, in particular the Oedipus complex, the theory of narcissism, and the psychology of women. The Oedipal complex would not have originated from sexual impulses but from a conflict with parental authority. The idea of narcissism as the result of libidinal investment in oneself instead of the object was a misunderstanding, since experience showed that the ability to love the other was proportional to the ability to love oneself. The conception of women as inferior due to anatomical causes and the lack of the consequent castration complex were simply a rationalization of social prejudices against women. So far was the Freudian view from being universal that one could assume the possibility of an inverted social relationship and a consequent male complex, as Fromm observed:

> Quite in contrast to Freud's assumption that 'penis envy' is a natural phenomenon in the constitution of the woman's psyche, there are good reasons for assuming that before male supremacy was established there was a 'pregnancy envy' in the man, which even today can be found in numerous cases.
>
> (Fromm, 1951, p. 233)

In *The Forgotten Language* (1951), Fromm proposed a theory of dreams alternative to the Freudian one. The dream would not be the reflection of a desire, but would express "any kind of mental activity (. . .) both of the lowest and most irrational and of the highest and most valuable functions of our minds" (p. 47).

Fromm also had a view of the analytic relationship as much less neutral than that theorized by Freud. The analyst, according to Fromm, rather than resembling a mirror or a white screen, had to develop an authentic and non-judgmental contact with the patient. Interpretations were to be marked neither by kindness nor by unpleasantness. The patients had to feel understood in a participatory way. They had not to feel alone in their suffering (Fromm, 1994. Symptoms according to Fromm were compromises, through which the individual neurotically rebelled against conformism. The therapist had to promote the liberation of individuals, their autonomy, to the point of making them productive, preserving them from conflict and alienation (Maccoby, 1996; see also Burston, 1991; Durkin, 2014).

Fromm's interest in the social sciences, his relativization of Freudian thought, and his welcoming attitude toward the analysand naturally placed him close to Sullivan's mentality. In fact, the two animated a group of analysts that took the name of Zodiac Circle together with Frieda Fromm Reichmann, Clara Thompson, and Karen Horney.

Karen Horney: another great outsider

Karen Horney was born in Hamburg in 1885 from a Norwegian father and a Dutch mother. The family was perhaps not a loving one, judging by her auto-biographical memories. However, it supported her by encouraging her medical studies, which was rather unusual for a woman in the historical and social context to which Horney belonged. After an analysis with Karl Abraham, she was among the founders of the Psychoanalytic Institute of Berlin. In 1932, she crossed the Atlantic to move first to Chicago and then to New York, where in 1934 she assumed the role of professor in the local Psychoanalytic Institute. Her positions, though, soon proved to be very distant from classical psychoanalysis. An essay on female masochism (Horney, 1933/2013) was highly critical of Freud. Horney considered Freud's proposed description of the female psyche to be patently superficial and unfounded, despite the innumerable merits of his pioneering and fundamental work. Evidently, not even the genius of Freud had been able to transcend the cultural prejudices of his time, avoiding the trap of interpreting female psychology as a deposit of the desires and sorrows of men.

The collaboration with Erich Fromm made Horney more sensitive to considering the influence of the social context on human development, broadening the relativization of Freudian thought, initially limited to prejudices about women, as she herself acknowledged retrospectively (Horney, 1945). Moving to the United States, in itself, also contributed to her belief that neurosis was a phenomenon strongly conditioned by the human environment: the problems brought to analysis by the Americans differed from those faced by the Germans. The influence of cultural factors on neurosis constituted the nodal point of *The Neurotic Personality of Our Time* (Horney, 1937).

With *New Ways in Psychoanalysis*, Horney (1939) abandoned libido theory and theorized a much lesser importance of infantile sexuality to the neurotic condition than Freud's. Horney, in particular, abandoned the concepts of fixation and regression to a particular stage of psychosexual development (Paris, 1999). The very role of sexuality in human life was largely downsized, such that sexual difficulties, in her view, were rather the result than the cause of personality disorders (Smith, 2007). In fact, Horney ended up asserting that in neurosis "sexual activities become not only a release of sexual tensions but also of manifold nonsexual psychic tensions" (Horney, 1950, p. 301).

As recently reconstructed by Dagmar Herzog (2017), between the 1930s and 1940s, Horney had become a leader of psychoanalysis in the United States, who nonetheless developed nonconformist ideas regarding psychosexual development (Herzog, 2017). For this reason, her books had created so much perplexity in the establishment of the American Psychoanalytic Association that she was deprived of teaching at the Institute in New York in 1941. Her followers were already so numerous, however, that in the same year she founded the American Institute for Psychoanalysis, which she directed until her death in 1952.

Horney contested the Freudian idea that the conflict from which the neurosis originated opposed desires and fears (that is, in metapsychological language, ego and superego):

> A psychic situation such as Freud postulates would imply that a neurotic retains the capacity to strive for something wholeheartedly, that he merely is frustrated in his strivings by blocking action of fears. As I see it, the source of the conflicts revolves around the neurotic's loss of capacity to wish for anything wholeheartedly because his very wishes are divided, that is, go in opposite directions.
>
> (Horney, 1945, p. 38)

She also expressed misgivings about the idea that unconscious conflicts were ubiquitous: under normal conditions, a person may be unaware of their conflicts but become aware of them without the need for external help, whereas "the essential tendencies producing a neurotic conflict are deeply repressed and can be unearthed only against great resistance" (p. 32). The difference between normal and neurotic condition, only quantitative for Freud, became qualitative for Horney. The human being in a reasonably favorable environment could acquire self-confidence toward the world and develop his real self. In an unfavorable environment he would tend toward the condition of *basic anxiety*, that is, "feeling isolated and helpless toward a potentially hostile world" (Horney, 1950, p. 301). This would have driven the human being to forced relational behaviors, that is, to feel they had to do something without this duty being real (Albert Ellis would have been very influenced by this idea).[12]

Horney's view of the possible outcomes of analytic therapy diverged from Freud's in an almost paradoxical way. On the one hand, Horney claimed her ability to recognize the considerable obstacles that the neurotic encountered in the attempt to resolve conflicts, obstacles that in her opinion Freud had not adequately recognized: Freudian psychoanalysis would have claimed to be able to heal by absurdly simple means (Horney, 1945). On the other hand, in Horney's eyes it was far easier than in Freud's for a patient to gain substantial and lasting benefits from analysis. Freudian therapeutic pessimism would have been linked to a radical as well as unjustified distrust of humanity. Horney also believed that the human ability to overcome difficulties and contradictions persisted throughout life and that therefore there were no contraindications to the analysis of mature people (who would indeed accept more easily than young people the principle that their problems did not come from outside and could therefore question themselves as the source of his own problems [Horney, 1945]). Horney also did not share the attitude of cold neutrality of classical analysts and ego psychologists: in her opinion the analyst had to be wholehearted. In this she anticipated the group of intersubjectivists (Smith, 2007).[13] Given these premises, the American Institute for Psychoanalysis became the association that brought together the American psychoanalysts most open to novelty and at the same time critical of the dogmatism of traditional psychoanalytic societies.[14]

Notes

1 See infra, Vol. 2, Ch. 7, pp. 79–80.
2 By a curious historical circumstance, among those who worked hardest to unmask the forgery could be counted Sir Cyril Burt (1883–1971), a British psychologist who rose to fame for studies that later turned out to be falsified.
3 On the importance of the Tavistock Clinic for the history of psychotherapy, see infra, Vol. 2, Ch. 7.
4 Freud's letter to Montessori seems to have the inscription "1917" in the header, as also reported by Ernst L. Freud (1960), however Freud's archives have currently classified it as 1927. The content of the letter, however, leads us to believe that the date of 1917 is correct, as the foundation of the Children's House in Vienna, to which the letter refers, would only take place in the two-year period 1921–1922.
5 On Attachment Theory, see infra, Vol. 2, Ch. 8, pp. 133–137.
6 See infra, Vol. 2, Ch. 8, p. 135.
7 See supra, Ch. 3, p. 96.
8 See infra, Vol. 2, Ch. 7, pp. 74–77 and Ch. 8, pp. 149–154.
9 Sullivan, during a trip to Berlin during the Christmas vacations of 1928, had already had the opportunity to meet some members of the local psychoanalytic community, including Horney herself and Franz Alexander (1891–1964) (Perry, 1964).
10 See infra, Vol. 2, Ch. 7, pp. 74–77.
11 See supra, Ch. 4, pp. 164–166.
12 See infra, Vol. 2, Ch. 7, pp. 74–77.
13 See infra, Vol. 2, Ch. 8, pp. 144–147.
14 In 2016, the American Institute for Psychoanalysis was finally recognized as a member of the International Psychoanalytic Association.

References

Abraham, K. (1937). Giovanni Segantini a psychoanalytic essay. *The Psychoanalytic Quarterly*, *6*(4), 453–512. (Original work published 1911)

Adler, A. (2015). *The education of children*. Routledge. (Original work published 1930)

Alexander, F. G., & Selesnick, S. T. (1966). *The history of psychiatry: An evaluation of psychiatric thought and practice from prehistoric times to the present*. Harper & Row.

Allport, G. W. (1950). *The individual and his religion: A psychological interpretation*. Macmillan.

Appignanesi, L., & Forrester, J. (1992). *Freud's women*. Basic Books.

Ash, M. G. (1998). *Gestalt psychology in German culture, 1890–1967: Holism and the quest for objectivity*. Cambridge University Press.

Back, K. W. (1987). *Beyond words: The story of sensitivity training and the encounter movement* (2nd ed.). Transaction Books.

Badolato, G., & Di Iullo, M. G. (1979). *Gruppi terapeutici e gruppi di formazione* [Therapeutic and training groups]. Bulzoni.

Bateman, A., & Holmes, J. (1995). *Introduction to psychoanalysis: Contemporary theory and practice*. Routledge.

Binswanger, L. (1909).Versuch einer Histerieanalyse [Attempt of analysis of an hysteria]. *Jahrbuch für Psychoanalytische und Psychopathologische Forschungen, 1*(1), 174–318; *1*(2), 319–356.

Binswanger, L. (1911). Analyse einer hysterischen Phobie [Analysis of an hysteric phobia]. *Jahrbuch für Psychoanalytische und Psychopathologische Forschungen, 3*(1), 228–308.

Binswanger, L. (1920). Psychoanalyse und klinische Psychiatrie. *Internationale Zeitschrift für ärtzliche Psychoanalyse, 7*(2), 137–165.

Binswanger, L. (1922). *Einführung in die Probleme der allgemeinen Psychologie* [Introduction to the problems of general psychology]. Springer.

Binswanger, L. (1936). *Erinnerungen an Sigmund Freud* [Memories of Sigmund Freud]. Francke.

Binswanger, L. (1957). *Der Mensch in der Psychiatrie* [The man in psychiatry]. Neske.

Binswanger, L. (1963a). Dream and existence. In *Being-in-the-world* (pp. 222–248). Basic Books. (Original work published 1930)

Binswanger, L. (1963b). Freud's conception of man in the light of anthropology. In *Being-in-the-world* (pp. 149–181). Basic Books. (Original work published 1936)

Binswanger, L. (1963c). Freud and the magna charta of clinical psychiatry. In *Being-in-the-world* (pp. 182–205). Basic Books. (Original work published 1930)

Blatner, A. (1995). Psychodrama. In R. J. Corsini & D. Wedding (Eds.), *Current psychotherapies* (5th ed., pp. 399–408). Peacock.

Borgna, E. (2006). Introduzione. In L. Binswanger (Ed.), *Melanconia e mania. Studi fenomenologici* [Melancholy and mania. Phenomenological studies]. Bollati Boringhieri. (Original work published 1960)

Brill, A. (1962). Discussion of H.S. Sullivan, 'The modified psychoanalytic treatment of schizophrenia'. In H. S. Sullivan (Ed.), *Schizophrenia as a human process* (pp. 292–293). W. W. Norton. (Original work published 1931)

Burrow, T. (1927). The group method of analysis. *The Psychoanalytic Review, 14*, 268–280.

Burston, D. (1991). *The legacy of Erich Fromm.* Harvard University Press.

Chapman, A. H. (1976). *Harry Stack Sullivan: His life and his work.* Putnam.

Cicciola, E. (2019). *La scoperta dell'intelligenza. Alfred Binet e la storia del primo test* [The discovery of intelligence. Alfred Binet and the history of the first test]. Fefè.

Cocks, G. (1985). *Psychotherapy in the Third Reich: The Göring Institute.* Oxford University Press.

Conci, M. (2000). *Sullivan rivisitato* [Sullivan revisited]. Massari.

Crichton Miller, H. (1922). *The new psychology and the teacher.* Seltzer.

D'Amore, A. R. T. (1976). William Alanson White, pioneer psychoanalyst. In A. R. T. D'Amore (Ed.), *William Alanson White: The Washington years 1903–1937* (pp. 69–94). U.S. Government Printing Office.

Danziger, K. (1990). *Constructing the subject: Historical origins of psychological research.* Cambridge University Press.

Dollard, J., & Miller, N. E. (1950). *Personality and psychotherapy.* McGraw-Hill.

Dreikurs, R. (1956). The contribution of group psychotherapy to psychiatry. *Group Psychotherapy, 9*, 115–125.

Durkin, K. (2014). *The radical humanism of Erich Fromm.* Palgrave Macmillan.

Ferenczi, S. (1913). Ein kleiner Hahnemann (A little cock-man). *Internationale Zeitschrift für Psychoanalyse, 1*, 240–246.

Ferenczi, S. (1994a). Psycho-analysis and education. In *Final contributions to the theory and technique of psycho-analysis* (pp. 280–290). Karnac. (Original work published 1908)

Fichtner, G. E., & Pomerans, A. J. (Eds.). (2003). *The Sigmund Freud-Ludwig Binswanger correspondence 1908–1938.* Other Press.

Fine, R. (1979). *A history of psychoanalysis.* Columbia University Press.

Foschi, R. (2008). Science and culture around the Montessori's first "Children's Houses" in Rome (1907–1915). *Journal of the History of the Behavioral Sciences, 44*(3), 238–257.

Foschi, R. (2012). *Maria Montessori.* Ediesse.

Foschi, R., & Cicciola, E. (2006). Politics and naturalism in the 20th century psychology of Alfred Binet. *History of Psychology, 9*(4), 267–289.

Foschi, R., Innamorati, M., & Taradel, R. (2018). 'A disease of our time': The Catholic Church's condemnation and absolution of psychoanalysis (1924–1975). *Journal of the History of the Behavioral Sciences, 54*, 85–100.

Freud, A. (1974). Four lectures on child analysis. In *The writings of Anna Freud* (Vol. 1, pp. 3–69). International Universities Press. (Original work published 1926)

Freud, A. (2017). Foreword. In R. Kramer (Ed.), *Maria Montessori. A biography* (p. 5). Diversion Books. (Original work published 1976)

Freud, E. L. (Ed.). (1960). *The letters of Sigmund Freud.* Basic Books.

Freud, S. (1955a). Analysis of a phobia in a five-year-old bou. In *The standard edition of the complete psychological works of Sigmund Freud* (Vol. 10, pp. 5–149). Hogarth. (Original work published 1909)

Freud, S. (1955b). A child recollection from "Dichtung und Wharheit". In *The standard edition of the complete psychological works of Sigmund Freud* (Vol. 17, pp. 145–156). Hogarth. (Original work published 1917)

Freud, S. (1955c). Group psychology and the analysis of the ego. In *The standard edition of the complete psychological works of Sigmund Freud* (Vol. 18, pp. 69–143). Hogarth. (Original work published 1921)

Freud, S. (1957a). Leonardo da Vinci and a memory of his childhood. In *The standard edition of the complete psychological works of Sigmund Freud* (Vol. 11, pp. 63–137). Hogarth. (Original work published 1910)

Freud, S. (1957b). On the history of the psycho-analytic movement. In *The standard edition of the complete psychological works of Sigmund Freud* (Vol. 14, pp. 7–66). Hogarth. (Original work published 1914)

Freud, S. (1959). An autobiographical study. In *The standard edition of the complete psychological works of Sigmund Freud* (Vol. 20, pp. 3–74). Hogarth. (Original work published 1925)

Fromm, E. (1941). *Escape from freedom.* Rinehart.

Fromm, E. (1951). *The forgotten language. An introduction to the understanding of dreams, fairy tales, and myths.* Rinehart.

Fromm, E. (1994). *The art of listening.* Constable & Robinson.

Fromm-Reichmann, F. (1948). Notes on the development of treatment of schizophrenics by psychoanalytic psychotherapy. *Psychiatry, 11*, 263–273.

Funk, R. (1992). Vorwort (Foreword). In E. Fromm (Ed.), *Schriften aus dem Nachlass* (Posthumous works). Beltz, Weinheim.

Gay, P. (1988). *Freud: A life for our time.* W. W. Norton.

Geuter, U. (2008). *The professionalisation of psychology in Nazi Germany.* Cambridge University Press.

Glover, E. (1933). "The psycho-analysis of children" by Melanie Klein. Authorized translation by Alix Strachey. *International Journal of Psychoanalysis, 14*, 119–129.

Greenberg, J. R., & Mitchell, S. A. (1983). *Object relations in psychoanalytic theory.* Harvard University Press.

Griesinger, W. (1845). *Pathologie und Therapie der psychischen Krankheiten, für Ärzte und Studierende* [Pathology and therapy of mental diseases, for physicians and students]. Krabbe.

Grosskurth, P. (1986). *Melanie Klein: Her world and her work.* Knopf.

Guarnieri, P. (2006). Un piccolo essere perverso. Il bambino nella cultura scientifica italiana tra Otto e Novecento [A perverse little being. The child in the Italian scientific culture between the nineteenth and twentieth centuries]. *Contemporanea, 9*(2), 253–284.

Gundlach, H. (2010). Psychology and its professionalization in times of war. The convention of German and Italian psychologists in Rome in 1941. *Physis, 47,* 319–337.

Heidegger, M. (2010). *Being and time.* Suny Press. (Original work published 1927)

Herzog, D. (2017). *Cold War Freud. Psychoanalysis in an age of catastrophes.* Cambridge University Press.

Hilgard, E. R. (1952). Psychoanalysis as science. *Engineering and Science, 16,* 11–17.

Honegger Fresco, G. (2002–2003). Anna Freud e l'esperienza Montessori [Anna Freud and the Montessori Experience]. *Il Quaderno Montessori, 20*(76), 47–64.

Horney, K. (1937). *The neurotic personality of our time.* W. W. Norton.

Horney, K. (1939). *New ways in psychoanalysis.* W. W. Norton.

Horney, K. (1945). *Our inner conflicts.* W. W. Norton.

Horney, K. (1950). *Neurosis and human growth.* W. W. Norton.

Horney, K. (2013). The problem of feminine masochism. *The Psychoanalytic Review, 100*(5), 675–694. (Original work published 1933)

Hug-Hellmuth, H. (1921). On the technique of child analysis. *International Journal of Psycho-Analysis, 2,* 281–305.

Hug-Hellmuth, H. (1924). *New paths to the understanding of youth.* Franz Deuticke.

Hug-Hellmuth, H. (1971). *A young girl's diary.* Milford. (Original work published 1919)

Hull, C. L. (1943). *Principles of behavior.* Appleton.

Husserl, E. (2012). *Ideas: General introduction to pure phenomenology.* Routledge. (Original work published 1913)

Innamorati, M. (1993). *Il concetto di Io in Kierkegaard* [The concept of ego in Kierkegaard]. Ateneo.

Jones, E. (1948). Introduction. In M. Klein (Ed.), *Contributions to psycho-analysis 1921–1945* (pp. 9–12). Hogarth.

Jung, C. G. (1964). Wotan. In *The collected works of C. G. Jung* (Vol. 10, pp. 179–193). Routledge & Kegan Paul. (Original work published 1936)

King, P., & Steiner, R. (1991). *The Freud-Klein controversies 1943–1945.* Routledge.

Klein, M. (1948a). The development of a child. In *Contributions to psycho-analysis 1921–1945* (pp. 13–67). Hogarth. (Original work published 1921)

Klein, M. (1948b). The psychological principles of infant analysis. In *Contributions to psycho-analysis 1921–1945* (pp. 140–151). Hogarth. (Original work published 1926)

Klein, M. (1948c). Symposium on child analysis. In *Contributions to psycho-analysis 1921–1945* (pp. 152–184). Hogarth. (Original work published 1927)

Klein, M. (1948d). A contribution to the psychogenesis of manic-depressive states. In *Contributions to psycho-analysis 1921–1945* (pp. 282–310). Hogarth. (Original work published 1935)

Klein, M. (1948e). Mourning and its relation to manic-depressive states. In *Contributions to psycho-analysis 1921–1945* (pp. 311–338). Hogarth. (Original work published 1940)

Klein, M. (1948f). The Oedipus complex in the light of early anxieties. In *Contributions to psycho-analysis 1921–1945* (pp. 282–310). Hogarth. (Original work published 1945)

Klein, M. (1955). The psycho-analytic play-technique: Its history and significance. In M. Klein, P. Heimann, & R. Money-Kyrle (Eds.), *New directions in psychoanalysis* (pp. 3–22). Maresfield Library.

Klein, M. (1960). *The psychoanalysis of children.* Grove. (Original work published 1932)

Klein, M. (1961). *Narrative of a child analysis.* Hogarth.

Klein, M. (1975). Notes on some schizoid mechanisms. In *Envy and gratitude and other works 1946–1963* (pp. 1–24). Hogarth. (Original work published 1946)

Kramer R. (2017). *Maria Montessori. A biography.* Diversion Books. (Original work published 1976)

Lauriola, M., Foschi, R., & Marchegiani, L. (2015). Integrating values and cognitive style in a model of right-wing radicalism. *Personality and Individual Differences, 75*, 147–153.

Lazell, E. W. (1921). The group treatment of dementia praecox. *Psychoanalytical Review, 8*, 168–179.

Lewin, K. (1931). The conflict between Aristotelian and Galilean modes of thought in contemporary psychology. *Journal of Genetic Psychology, 5*, 141–177.

Lewin, K. (1935). *A dynamic theory of personality.* McGraw-Hill.

Lewin, K. (1936). *Principles of topological psychology.* McGraw-Hill.

Lewin, K. (1942). Field theory of learning. *Yearbook of the National Society of the Study of Education, 41*, 215–242.

Lewin, K. (1945). The research center for group dynamics at Massachusetts Institute of Technology. *Sociometry, 8*(2), 126–136.

Lewin, K., & Korsch, K. (1939). Mathematical constructs in psychology and sociology. *The Journal of Unified Science, 8*(1), 397–403.

Leys, R. E., & Evans, R. B. (Eds.). (1990). *Defining American psychology: The correspondence Between Adolf Meyer and Edward Bradford Titchener.* Johns Hopkins University Press.

Lifton, R. J. (1986). *The Nazi doctors: Medical killing and the psychology of genocide.* Basic Books.

Maccoby, M. (1996). *The two voices of Erich Fromm: The prophetic and the analytic.* In M. Cortina & M. Maccoby (Eds.), *A prophetic analyst: Erich Fromm's contributions to psychoanalysis* (pp. 61–93). Jason Aronson.

Marsh, L. C. (1931). Group treatment of the psychoses by the psychological equivalent of the revival. *Mental Hygiene, 15*, 328–349.

Marx, K. (1998). Theses on Feuerbach. In *The German ideology, including Theses on Feuerbach.* Prometheus. (Original work published 1845)

McGuire, W., & Hull, R. F. C. (Eds.). (1977). *CG Jung speaking: Interviews and encounters.* Princeton University Press.

Mead, M. (1934). The use of primitive material in the study of personality. *Journal of Personality, 3*, 3–16.

Mecacci, L. (1992). *Storia della psicologia del Novecento* [History of psychology of the twentieth century]. Laterza.

Meltzer, D. (1978). *The Kleinian development: Part II, Richard week-by-week.* Clunie.

Merton, R. K. (1957). The role-set: Problems in sociological theory. *The British Journal of Sociology, 8*, 106–120.

Mitchell, S. A., & Black, M. J. (1995). *Freud and beyond: A history of modern psychoanalytic thought.* Basic Books.

Molaro, A. (2016). *Psicoanalisi e fenomenologia* [Psychoanalysis and phenomenology]. Raffaello Cortina.

Money-Kyrle, R. (1978). British schools of psycho-analysis: Melanie Klein and her contributions to psycho-analysis. In *The collected papers* (pp. 408–415). Clunie Press.

Montessori, M. (1922). Lettera a Giulio Cesare Ferrari del 27 febbraio [Letter to Giulio Cesare Ferrari of February 27]. In *Aspi – Archivio storico della psicologia.* Retrieved January 16, 2021, from www.aspi.unimib.it/collections/object/detail/4663/

Montessori, M. (1970). *La mente del bambino. Mente assorbente* [The mind of the child. Absorbing mind]. Mondadori. (Original work published 1948)

Moreno, J. L. (1923). *Der Königsroman* [The king's novel]. Verlag der Vaters.

Moreno, J. L. (1946). *Psychodrama: First volume*. Beacon House.

Moreno, J. L. (1953). How Kurt Lewin's 'research center for group dynamics' started. *Sociometry*, *16*(1), 101–104.

Moreno, J. L. (1964). Preface to the third edition. In *Psychodrama: First volume*. Beacon House.

Moreno, J. L. (1987a). Sociometry. In J. Fox (Ed.), *The essential Moreno: Writings on psychodrama, group method, and spontaneity* (pp. 20–31). Springer. (Original work published 1937)

Moreno, J. L. (1987b). *Spontaneity and catharsis*. In J. Fox (Ed.), *The essential Moreno: Writings on psychodrama, group method, and spontaneity* (pp. 39–59). Springer. (Original work published 1940)

Moreno, J. L. (1987c). The role concept, a bridge between psychiatry and sociology. In J. Fox (Ed.), *The essential Moreno: Writings on psychodrama, group method, and spontaneity* (pp. 60–65). Springer. (Original work published 1961)

Mowrer, O. (1950). *Learning theory and personality dynamics*. Ronald Press.

Needlemann, J. (1963). Introduction. In L. Binswanger (Ed.), *Being-in-the-world* (pp. 1–6). Basic Books.

Paris, B. J. (1999). Karen Horney's vision of the self. *American Journal of Psychoanalysis*, *59*, 157–166.

Peller, E. L. (1978). The children's house. *The NAMTA Quarterly*, *3*, 47–55.

Perry, H. S. (1964). Introduction. In H. S. Sullivan (Ed.), *The fusion of psychiatry and social science* (pp. 8–32). W. W. Norton.

Perry, H. S. (1983). *Psychiatrist in America: The life of H. S. Sullivan*. Belknap Press.

Pertegato, E. G., & Pertegato, G. O. (Eds.). (2013). *From psychoanalysis to group analysis. The pioneering work of Trigant Burrow*. Karnac.

Pratt, J. H. (1907). The organization of tuberculosis classes. *The Boston Medical and Surgical Journal*, *157*, 285–291.

Rogers, C. R. (1970). *Encounter groups*. Harper & Row.

Rossi, P. (1898). *L'animo della folla* [The soul of the crowd]. Riccio.

Schilder, P. (1939). Results and problems of group psychotherapy in severe neurosis. *Mental Hygiene*, *23*, 87–98.

Schönpflug, W. (2017). Professional psychology in Germany, national socialism, and the second world war. *History of Psychology*, *20*(4), 387–407.

Sears, R. R. (1943). *Survey of objective studies of psychoanalytic concepts*. Social Science Research Council.

Segal, H. (1979). *Melanie Klein*. Fontana.

Shakow, D., & Rapaport, D. (1964). *The influence of Freud on American psychology*. International Universities Press.

Slavson, S. R. (1943). *An introduction to group therapy*. Commonwealth Fund.

Smith, W. (2007). Karen Horney and psychotherapy in the 21st century. *Clinical Social Work Journal*, *35*, 57–66.

Sullivan, H. S. (1946). *Conceptions of modern psychiatry*. W. W. Norton.

Sullivan, H. S. (1953). *The interpersonal theory of psychiatry*. W. W. Norton.

Sullivan, H. S. (1962a). Schizophrenia: Its conservative and malignant features. In H. S. Sullivan (Ed.), *Schizophrenia as a human process* (pp. 7–22). W. W. Norton. (Original work published 1924)

Sullivan, H. S. (1962b). Peculiarity of thought in schizophrenia. In H. S. Sullivan (Ed.), *Schizophrenia as a human process* (pp. 26–99). W. W. Norton. (Original work published 1925)

Sullivan, H. S. (1962c). The onset of schizophrenia. In H. S. Sullivan (Ed.), *Schizophrenia as a human process* (pp. 104–136). W. W. Norton. (Original work published 1926)

Sullivan, H. S. (1962d). Research in schizphrenia. In H. S. Sullivan (Ed.), *Schizophrenia as a human process* (pp. 186–202). W. W. Norton. (Original work published 1929)

Sullivan, H. S. (1962e). Achaic sexual culture and schizophrenia. In H. S. Sullivan (Ed.), *Schizophrenia as a human process* (pp. 206–215). W. W. Norton. (Original work published 1929)

Sullivan, H. S. (1962f). Schizophrenic individuals as a source for data for comparative investigation of personality. In H. S. Sullivan (Ed.), *Schizophrenia as a human process* (pp. 218–232). W. W. Norton. (Original work published 1931)

Sullivan, H. S. (1962g). Environmental factors and course under treatment of schizophrenia. In H. S. Sullivan (Ed.), *Schizophrenia as a human process* (pp. 246–255). W. W. Norton. (Original work published 1931)

Sullivan, H. S. (1962h). The modified psychoanalytic treatment of schizophrenia. In H. S. Sullivan (Ed.), *Schizophrenia as a human process* (pp. 272–290). W. W. Norton. (Original work published 1931)

Sullivan, H. S. (1964a). A note on the implications of psychiatry, the study of interpersonal relations, for investigations in the social sciences. In *The fusion of psychiatry and social science* (pp. 15–29). W. W. Norton. (Original work published 1937)

Sullivan, H. S. (1964b). The data of psychiatry. In *The fusion of psychiatry and social science* (pp. 32–55). W. W. Norton. (Original work published 1938)

Sullivan, H. S. (1964c). *The fusion of psychiatry and social science* (pp. 32–55). W. W. Norton.

Van Ginneken, J. (1992). *Crowds, psychology and politics, 1871–1899*. Cambridge University Press.

Wender, L. (1936). The dynamic of group psychotherapy and its application. *Journal of Nervous and Mental Diseases, 84*, 54–60.

Young-Bruehl, E. (2008). *Anna Freud: A biography*. Yale University Press.

Zilboorg, G. (1962). Discussion of H.S. Sullivan, 'The modified psychoanalytic treatment of schizophrenia'. In H. S. Sullivan (Ed.), *Schizophrenia as a human process* (pp. 291–292). W. W. Norton. (Original work published 1931)

Index

For Product Safety Concerns and Information please contact our EU
representative GPSR@taylorandfrancis.com
Taylor & Francis Verlag GmbH, Kaufingerstraße 24, 80331 München, Germany